W9-BKP-144

PRAISE FOR
What Helped Get Me Through

• • •

"*So much wisdom, strength, and courage can be gained from listening to others who have been there.* This book provides much-needed inspiration for people with cancer, or any illness for that matter, and all those who love and care for them."

—Ann H. Partridge, MD, MPH,
Assistant Professor of Medicine,
Harvard Medical School

"*I wish I had had a book like this when I was diagnosed!*"

—Steve Mazan, Comedian, Cancer survivor

"*For all patient health collections.*"

—*Library Journal*

"Dr. Silver provides insight into the cancer experience that instills hope and will inspire people newly diagnosed with cancer in her latest book *What Helped Get Me Through*. **This practical guide includes information shared by the experts themselves—people with cancer— that conveys an understanding of what is important to healing and recovery during and after treatment.** Reclaiming aspects of one's life after a cancer diagnosis and heightening an appreciation for life after cancer are important issues related to cancer survivorship.

—Elyse Caplan, Education Director,
Living Beyond Breast Cancer,
Cancer survivor

"When one is truly inspired and wants to be a survivor, information derived from the experience of others is vital. The natives know how to help one another because of their experience. *Read and learn from the wisdom of others, and save yourself from having to learn the hard way.*"

—Bernie Siegel, MD,
Author of *Love, Medicine & Miracles*
and *Help Me to Heal*

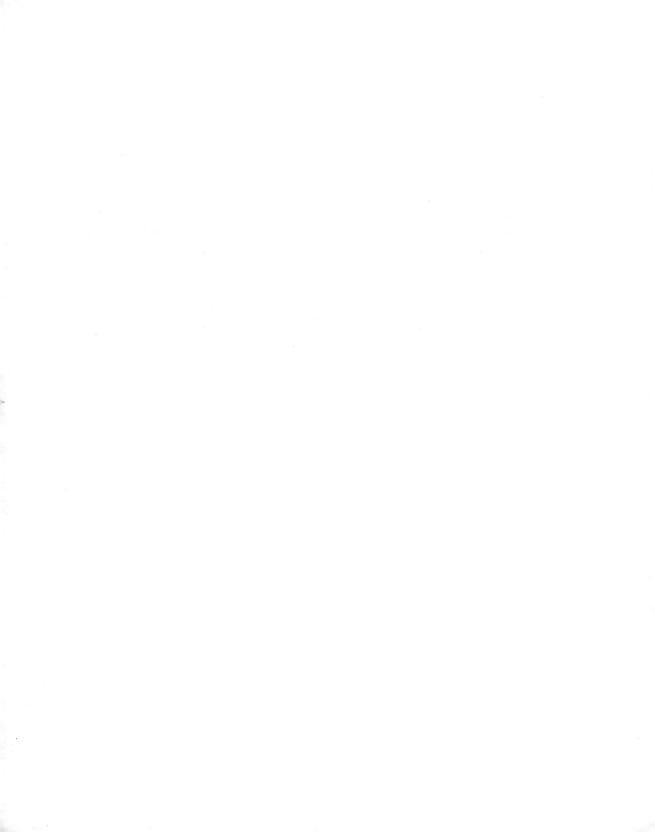

What Helped
Get Me Through

What Helped Get Me Through

Cancer Survivors Share Wisdom and Hope

Edited by Julie K. Silver, MD

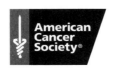

Published by the
American Cancer Society
Health Promotions
250 Williams Street NW
Atlanta, GA 30303-1002

Copyright ©2009 American Cancer Society

All rights reserved. Without limiting the rights under copyright reserved above, no part of this publication may be reproduced, stored in or introduced into a retrieval system, or transmitted in any form or by any means (electronic, mechanical, photocopying, recording, or otherwise) without the prior written permission of the publisher.

Printed in the United States of America

Edited by Julie K. Silver, MD
Cover design and composition by Rikki Campbell Ogden/pixiedesign, llc

5 4 3 2 1   09 10 11 12 13

Library of Congress Cataloging-in-Publication Data

What helped get me through: cancer survivors share wisdom and hope/edited by Julie K. Silver.
   p. cm.
 Includes index.
 ISBN-13: 978-1-60443-004-2 (pbk.: alk. paper)
 ISBN-10: 1-60443-004-4 (pbk.: alk. paper)
 1. Cancer—Patients—Biography. I. Silver, J. K. (Julie K.), 1965-

RC265.5.W53 2009
362.196'994—dc22

           2008030285

AMERICAN CANCER SOCIETY

Strategic Director, Content: Chuck Westbrook
Director, Cancer Information: Terri Ades, MS, FNP-BC, AOCN
Director, Book Publishing: Len Boswell
Book Marketing/Rights Manager: Candace Magee
Managing Editor, Books: Rebecca Teaff, MA
Books Editor: Jill Russell
Book Publishing Coordinator: Vanika Jordan, MS Pub
Editorial Assistant, Books: Amy Rovere

For more information about cancer, contact your American Cancer Society at **800-ACS-2345** or **http://www.cancer.org**.

Quantity discounts on bulk purchases of this book are available. Book excerpts can also be created to fit specific needs. For information, please contact the American Cancer Society, Health Promotions Publishing, 250 Williams Street NW, Atlanta, GA 30303-1002, or send an e-mail to **trade.sales@cancer.org**.

NOTE TO THE READER

• • •

Hundreds of cancer survivors participated in a survey that formed the basis for this book. The information presented here represents their viewpoints and experiences and does not imply endorsement by the American Cancer Society. The information presented is not intended as medical advice and should not be relied upon as a substitute for talking with your doctor. This information may not address all possible actions, treatments, medications, precautions, side effects, or interactions. All matters regarding your health require the supervision of a medical doctor or appropriate health care professional who is familiar with your medical needs. For more information, contact your American Cancer Society at 800-ACS-2345 or http://www.cancer.org.

To my wonderful husband and children and my devoted friends and supportive colleagues who have taken this difficult cancer journey with me. You have helped me more than I am able to describe.

Contents

Preface xiii

Acknowledgments xvii

1 How I Nurtured Myself 1

2 How My Family Helped 23

3 How Friends Made a Difference 39

4 Care and Support from the Health Care Team 65

5 What Helped My Children Cope 93

6 Balancing Work and Family 115

7 How I Changed My Diet 131

8 How I Changed My Exercise Routine 145

9 What I Did to Relieve Stress 159

10 How Being Spiritual Helped 177

11 What I Wish I Had Known at Diagnosis 203

12 What Would Have Helped but Was Too Hard to Ask For . . 227

13 How My Body and Intimacy Were Affected 243

14 What Helped Me Heal 269

15 How Cancer Changed My Life 291

16 What It Means to Be a Survivor 313

Resources 335

Contributors Index 345

Index 351

PREFACE

• • •

The breast surgeon came into the exam room with tears in her eyes. I wanted her to say what other doctors had told me in the past, "Go home, you're fine." I was praying that I was a hypochondriac—a young doctor who had seen too much and now mistakenly thought she was seriously ill, maybe even dying. Instead, she softly said, "You are right; you have breast cancer."

I was thirty-eight years old, and I had been going to doctors for the previous two years to check out something I felt on my breast. I didn't have a family history of breast cancer or any other type. Statistically, I wasn't supposed to get cancer. The doctors considered my lack of a family history of cancer and couldn't feel what I believed was there, but they were thorough and sent me for mammograms and an ultrasound. It took two years for the tests to show what I suspected shortly after I'd had my youngest child—I had cancer.

Grief makes it difficult to process and store events in our brains in the way that we normally do. I remember my husband was devastated but extremely loving and supportive. When I told each of my three children who were three, seven, and eleven years old, they didn't seem to understand what I was telling them. Over time and with repeated explanations from me and my husband, they began to understand more about what our family was going through and why.

I remember a surreal phone call I had with my mother when I told her about my diagnosis. Since we live on opposite coasts—she in California and I in Massachusetts—I had asked my brother and sister to be with her when I called. As I was talking to my mom, she was looking at my brother who cradled his head in his hands. Before I could tell her that I had cancer, she said, "Julie, I have to hang up now. Something is really wrong with your brother, and he needs me."

Waiting for my test results was agonizing. After a two-year delay in my diagnosis, I knew I didn't have a best-case scenario. What I didn't know was whether I had a worst-case one. Every time I looked at my children, I wondered how many weeks, months, or years, I'd be able to see their sweet little faces. Their laughter continued to ring through our house. I had never imagined that hearing my children play would torment me, but all I could think of was when would I stop hearing those sounds?

Now, when I give speeches to cancer survivors, I encourage them to understand that though we all long for a best-case scenario cancer diagnosis (if we have to have one at all), this is very often not the situation in which we find ourselves. Nevertheless, the odds are that there are treatments that can help.

If you are reading this book, chances are that either you or someone you love has been diagnosed with cancer. Perhaps you are in shock, wondering what to do next. What will help? This is something I thought about constantly—considering things from every imaginable angle and worrying about how best to get myself and my family through this crisis.

When television news reporter Kelley Tuthill was diagnosed with breast cancer, her sister, Melissa, sent me an e-mail, telling me that her family was in crisis mode and wanted to do whatever they could to help Kelley through this difficult experience. I wrote back a long e-mail, with a number of suggestions about how family members and friends can make a difference. When I read what I had written, I realized that I wanted to ask other cancer survivors for their thoughts on this subject. What would five-, ten- and twenty-year survivors say about what really helped them? I knew what had helped me through a breast cancer diagnosis in my thirties, but I wanted to hear from others, too. More than that, I wanted to create the guide I wished I had been able to read when I was first diagnosed—a book that offered hope and inspiration from survivors who had been there and could reach back and help pull me through.

I started by talking with the director of Book Publishing at the American Cancer Society, Len Boswell. Len and I had had previous conversations about the importance of publishing books that are survivorship oriented. I thought that a guide called *What Helped Get Me Through* would be a worthwhile book for the American Cancer Society to publish. Len and his wonderful editorial team, including Rebecca Teaff, enthusiastically agreed.

Thus, with the help of one of my assistants, Anna Rubin, I set up a Web site where survivors could fill out an online survey. Anna sent announcements to various support groups, newsletters, advocacy organizations, and cancer Web sites, asking for volunteers who would be willing to fill out the survey and share with others what really helped them get through their cancer diagnosis.

Hundreds of people participated in this project, and it came as no surprise to me that every single person who completed a survey had something important to say. Therefore, I included at least one quote from everyone who participated. There were a few surveys that people did not completely fill out or didn't provide enough information to be useful, so I discarded those. Of note is that I lightly edited the quotes for spelling, punctuation, grammar, and appropriateness.

As you read the words of the survivors, you'll see that only their first names are listed. I wanted them to be able to find their quotes in the book but to remain anonymous to others. All of the names and other identifying information such as their occupation and specific cancer diagnosis are real. I left out the last names so that the survey participants could freely express their thoughts and feelings and have no reservations about being very candid. If you read Chapter 13 entitled "How My Body and Intimacy Were Affected," you'll see why it was important to many survey participants to withhold their last names.

In addition to the cancer survivors who filled out surveys, I contacted many medical experts, cancer advocates, and celebrities. Some were hard to reach, and I wasn't able to get through. However, I made an extensive effort to reach a wide cross-section of important people in the field of oncology. Although the American Cancer Society is the publisher of this book, I wanted its range to be as broad as possible, that is, to include the insights of some amazing people who are affiliated with other organizations that support cancer research and treatment.

I am truly honored to say that Lance Armstrong (Lance Armstrong Foundation); Nancy Brinker, Hala Moddelmog, and Eric Winer (Susan G. Komen Foundation); Terry Music and Carolyn Runowicz (American Cancer Society); Elyse Caplan (Living Beyond Breast Cancer); Ellen Stovall (National Coalition for Cancer Survivorship); Diane Blum (CancerCare); and many others contributed quotes. You'll read their thoughts throughout this book on what really helps people get through the cancer experience.

I sought to be as inclusive as possible so that readers could hear from the leaders in the field of oncology—particularly those who are dedicated to survivorship issues. I also asked my colleagues who work in the field of oncology for their assistance. They have so much great advice, and you'll read their quotes in the boxes throughout the chapters.

It is my desire that this book will provide hope and reassurance to those who are struggling with the cancer experience. I like to think of this guide as a way of having those who've survived cancer reaching out and pulling up those who are going through it now. As a doctor who is also a survivor, I think of this book as an infusion of wisdom and hope that will help you and your family navigate the cancer experience with as much resilience and optimism as possible.

Julie K. Silver, MD

ACKNOWLEDGMENTS

• • •

In addition to the people whom I have acknowledged in the Preface, I'd like to thank Rebecca Teaff for her excellent editorial guidance throughout this project and Amy Rovere for her editorial support. I am also grateful to Chuck Westbrook who oversees the books program at the American Cancer Society, Vanika Jordan who has handled many production tasks, Jill Russell who provided editorial assistance, and to Candace Magee and Leslie Wolfe Arista whose excellent efforts in public relations have made it possible for many survivors and their friends and families to learn about this book.

Ross Zafonte, DO, chair of the department of Physical Medicine and Rehabilitation at Harvard Medical School, has been consistently supportive of my academic work. My academic assistant, Mary Alice Hanford, helped keep track of the participants' surveys and other information. It is an honor to work with my colleagues at Dana-Farber Cancer Institute, and I am particularly grateful to those who offered assistance with this guide in the form of expert advice for readers.

Selma Schimmel from Vital Options® International was enormously helpful in providing me with suggestions and contact information for the many experts who have contributed to this book.

Of course, this guide would not be possible without the generosity of so many cancer survivors who were willing to fill out surveys and share with readers what really helped get them through this difficult experience. I am grateful to all of them and want them to know how powerful their words will be in providing hope and inspiration for thousands of people.

Finally, I am in debt to my family, friends, and colleagues for their amazing support and help when I was diagnosed with breast cancer in 2003.

CHAPTER 1

· · ·

How I Nurtured Myself

People facing cancer not only need love and nurturing from others, they need it from *themselves*. Some people may link self-nurture to narcissism, fearing that it's unhealthy or immoral to spend much time thinking about what they need. However, psychologist Frances Cohen Praver has a more modern view of the nurture versus narcissism controversy. She writes, "A shift in attitudes finds that contemporary analytic thinkers value narcissism as a healthy aspect of mature behavior. We now refer to narcissism as high self-esteem, which inspires expression of the self…Healthy narcissism facilitates aspirations and goals" (Praver 2004, 96).

I recall doing an interview with Ellen Michaud, former editor-at-large of *Prevention Magazine*, when she was writing the book *Sleep to be Sexy, Smart, and Slim*. I explained to Ellen how important sleep is during cancer treatment and thereafter because it helps boost the immune system, as well as improve fatigue, a common and debilitating symptom in cancer survivors. After hearing my comments, Ellen decided to devote an entire chapter in her book to the importance of sleep in fighting cancer. I also told her that while getting a good night's rest is an important way for people to nurture themselves, it can be hard to accomplish because of worry, pain, hot flashes, and a host of other issues.

I thought back to when I was going through treatment and my children were quite young. When they awoke from a nightmare in the middle of the night, I could hardly say to them that I couldn't help because I needed uninterrupted sleep. It was a traumatic time for them. They had a mother who was fighting a life-threatening disease. My children's need for comfort interfered with my own ability to sleep and nurture myself.

Certainly, there is a difference between "healthy selfishness" and a narcissistic "I come first" attitude. Even so, sometimes the lines seem blurry, making it difficult to decide when it's okay to nurture yourself. The fact is most people tend to be better at caring for others than they are at paying attention to their own needs and desires. If you are erring in one direction or another, it's likely that you are not giving yourself enough attention.

One way to make peace with the idea of taking time to nurture yourself is to know that the stronger and healthier you are, the better able you will be to nurture others in the future. If you are currently undergoing treatment or have undergone treatment in the past, it is important that you add things to your schedule that are strictly designed to make you feel good.

Cancer survivors who participated in this book described the many ways they nurtured themselves. Basically, it really breaks down to this: what makes one person happy doesn't necessarily make everyone happy. We all have individual personalities, and the things that provide comfort and bring us joy vary widely.

As you read this chapter, consider the things you can do for yourself that will help you feel loved, secure, and happy. The objective is not to pretend to be lighthearted during a very difficult time, but rather to nurture yourself in any manner that will help lighten your load.

Not Enough Nurture

Not everyone took the time to nurture themselves. Lindy explains her situation: "I was thirty-five years old and had stage III breast cancer. Twenty-three years ago, that was uncommon. I'm afraid I didn't do much of anything to nurture myself because I tried to give the appearance that I was okay." Though Lindy is describing how she felt more than two decades ago, many people share this sentiment even today.

In my medical practice, people often tell me that they don't have the time to spend on healing. They've been sick and are so far behind in all the things they need to do, including work and family responsibilities. Yet taking the time to heal is incredibly important. Saying yes to all your old commitments may mean saying no to healing as well as possible. Thus, nurturing yourself can translate into taking the time out of your day that you need to focus on your own health needs—both physical and emotional. Some people are better at doing this than others, but it's worth giving yourself permission to spend the time you need to feel better. Think of focusing on your health as a gift you give not only yourself but also your loved ones. Remember that the stronger and healthier you are—no matter what kind of cancer you have or what stage it is—the more you can nurture others.

This chapter is one of my favorites because I thoroughly enjoyed reading the many ways that the survey participants nurtured themselves. Often it was something really simple, like making a necklace of beads to represent positive milestones, as Cathy describes in the next section. Keep reading, and let Cathy and many others inspire you to love and nurture a really wonderful person—*you*.

• • •

WHEN PEOPLE FOUND OUT I had cancer, most assumed it was breast cancer. Not many people, including myself, had heard of pancreatic cancer. When they had, they assumed men were the only ones to get it. I started a beaded necklace. This necklace has a bead for every positive event I have made it to: birthdays, holidays, anniversaries. I even celebrated the one-year anniversary of my surgery as another birthday.

Cathy, retail district manager
Diagnosis of pancreatic cancer at age 45 in 2005 in Columbus, Ohio

• • •

I'M NOT ONE of those quiet people who keep stress to themselves. I talk to anyone who will listen to me. Most think that isn't wise, but that's how I deal with it. I told everyone. I would have told the mailman if I could have caught him.

Kathie, nurse and social worker
Diagnosis of kidney cancer at age 53 in 2005 in Kingston, New York

• • •

I TOOK ONE DAY at a time.

James, retired police officer
Diagnosis of lymphoma at age 66 in 2007 in Sheridan, Wyoming

PRIOR TO MY DIAGNOSIS, we had planned a special vacation to Hawaii with our children and grandchildren to celebrate my wife's retirement. We went for two weeks. I call it "Maui in the shade." I let the beauty of Hawaii minister to my soul, and then had several surgical procedures immediately upon our return.

Robert, fire chaplain
Diagnosis of melanoma (skin cancer) at age 57 in 2003 in La Habra, California

• • •

I SURROUNDED MYSELF with positive, caring people. My husband would not let anyone with a negative attitude come around. We were honest, knew the prognosis was extremely poor (six months to live), but kept a positive attitude.

Beth, health educator
Diagnosis of liver cancer at age 32 in 1990 in Fort Hood, Texas

• • •

I NURTURED MYSELF BY being friendly and outgoing with all the family and friends who asked to help and were there just to talk to. I believed that going bald was no big deal in relation to what was happening in my body.

David, journeyman sheet metal worker
Diagnosis of breast cancer at age 63 in 2005 in Missoula, Montana

• • •

MY WHOLE LIFE IS different as a result of this experience. I actually needed something to happen to make me realize that I didn't know how to care for myself in many ways. Now, I appreciate everything and everyone. I also let go of anger and resentment, which was a normal part of my life. I have set boundaries with people who drain me and cut people who are toxic out of my life. I am now a vegetarian and eat healthy foods rather than the junk I used to eat. I don't care what people think of me anymore. I have a new hobby—photography—that I always wanted to try but never did, and I have peace of mind.

Jennifer, psychotherapist
Diagnosis of breast cancer at age 39 in 2004 in Pennington, New Jersey

I WENT ON VACATION for a twelve-day cruise of the North Sea.

Mark, retired nuclear pharmacist
Diagnosis of chronic lymphocytic leukemia at age 59 in 2001 in Bay Shore, New York

• • •

I WENT OUT for walks between the once-a-month chemo sessions and focused on building up my strength before the next dose. I tried to rest when I felt I needed to, and I used breast cancer Web forums to give me the information and support I wanted and needed. I was not keen on sitting in a circle talking to others who'd had breast cancer. I wanted to do it all my way. After all, it was MY cancer.

Pearl, nurse
Diagnosis of breast cancer at age 32 in 2004 in Glasgow (Scotland)

• • •

I WAS DIAGNOSED with colon cancer, which had metastasized heavily throughout the liver. I would have died within three or four months had we not discovered it and done something about it. At the beginning, I did nothing at all to help or nurture myself except to rest, to try to eat as best I could, and to go for my chemotherapy once each week. I was too consumed with fatigue and melancholy to even think about self-help. But over time, as the chemotherapy began to destroy my cancer and improve my overall health, I began to engage myself to a greater degree in my treatment, to ask questions to better understand it all. I even wrote a weekly health report that I sent out by e-mail to my kids, family, and close friends. I sent this report to my doctor and medical team as well for their critique and/or corrections, to be sure I understood everything correctly. My weekly health reports were the single most interesting, enjoyable, and helpful activity I could imagine. In writing it all down, I began to see the questions I needed to ask to "round out" my understanding of my situation. It also brought me, my family, my support group, and my caregivers much closer together. My doctor helped and encouraged me in it.

Mike, retired real estate developer and cattle rancher
Diagnosis of colon cancer at age 66 in 2006 in Red Lodge, Montana

I WAS AN INFORMATION seeker. I wanted as much information as possible, and my doctor provided me what I asked for. If he did not know the answer, he would point me in the direction to receive it. I formulated goals—both short-term and long-term—and I got involved in the cancer community almost immediately by volunteering for the Leukemia & Lymphoma Society (LLS) and the National Marrow Donor Program (NMDP). Focusing my energies on using my experience to help others deal with theirs was very rewarding.

Todd, oncology social worker
Diagnosis of chronic myelogenous leukemia at age 25 in 1997 and kidney cancer at age 33 in 2005 in Warwick, Rhode Island

• • •

> "Focusing my energies on using my experience to help others deal with theirs was very rewarding."

I TREATED MYSELF LIKE a very precious and tender person. I really put all of my energy into taking care of myself and making sure my needs came first (not my usual style). I did not do this in an especially selfish way although I was, in fact, very self-absorbed and very okay with that. I wrote in a journal. I cut out inspirational quotes and pasted them on the walls of my dressing room. I read books by other survivors. I burned songs onto a CD to listen to during chemo—songs that meant something to me and inspired me. I called a designer who was having a studio sale to ask if I could come at a time when no one else was there, so that I wouldn't have to be exposed to lots of people in a crowded dressing room. She was very kind and accommodating, and I had my own private sale! I took long walks with my dog in the park near my home every day. I really became aware of how precious I am and how precious my life is. That has never left me—what a blessing.

Cathi, clinical social worker
Diagnosis of breast cancer at age 52 in 2003 in Waban, Massachusetts

> Don't be afraid; embrace your treatment, and never give up.
>
> **SHARON OSBOURNE** is the wife of musician Ozzy Osbourne and is best known for her role in the reality MTV series *The Osbournes*. A self-described "housewife superstar," she received a diagnosis of colon cancer at age 49 in 2002.

ONE NEW ACTIVITY I did was scrapbooking. My aunt who is also a survivor handed me a kit when my cancer was diagnosed and told me to keep myself busy. By scrapbooking, I was able to see pictures of my husband and children, and that kept me motivated to fight the fight.

Shelly, program coordinator for adults with disabilities
Diagnosis of breast cancer at age 32 in 2004 in Concord, New Hampshire

• • •

THE MAIN THING I did solely for myself was to get on the bike and ride, long and hard. When I was on the bike, I found that I could focus on the riding, then the scenery and wildlife, and stop thinking about having cancer. As I would be returning home and making the final turn before arriving at the farm, thoughts of the cancer would resurface. It seemed that I could go no more than a few minutes at a time without thoughts of the cancer coming to mind. When I was on the bike, after about fifteen minutes or so, I could stop thinking about the cancer and focus on the ride itself.

Bill, administrator
Diagnosis of prostate cancer at age 62 in 2007 in Jefferson, Wisconsin

• • •

MY FIRST (and only) child was only three months old when I was diagnosed, so she truly was the silver lining in a time that seemed to have lots of dark clouds in it. From the minute I found out I had breast cancer, I vowed that my daughter wouldn't suffer from [my being ill] at all and that I would make the most of the time I had with her, even if I was bald and nauseated! Through nurturing her, I nurtured myself and made it through a difficult treatment and recovery period.

Sarah, paralegal
Diagnosis of breast cancer at age 28 in 2000 in Miami, Florida

I LOOKED AT THIS time as ME time. I decided to focus on healing...this was my time to rest, get stronger, and not worry about anything else. I thought, well, if I have to stay in bed because I'm sick from the treatment, I will look at it as time to read all those books I never get around to, to watch all the movies I don't have time to...and I did just that. By telling myself it was my vacation from work and other responsibilities, it almost became a vacation.

Linda, retired
Diagnosis of breast cancer at age 54 in 2003 in Placentia, California

After twenty years of working with people during radiation, I've learned that the most crucial thing they can do to enhance their well-being is to get enough sleep. In my experience, survivors who make sleep a priority end up having fewer physical difficulties and enhanced coping skills; overall, they tolerate all cancer treatment much more easily. For some people this means a "power nap" at midday or right after their radiation treatment; for others, it might mean the short-term use of sleeping pills to ensure they get the sleep they need. But for most survivors, it just means shutting off the endless "to do" list an hour earlier every night and carving out the ultimate "me first" time. Shakespeare described a sleep that "knits up the raveled sleeve of care" (*Macbeth*, 2.2.46–51). In this case, sleep "knits up the raveled sleeve of radiation!"

ROBIN SCHOENTHALER, MD, is a radiation oncologist with Massachusetts General Hospital at the Emerson-Hospital-MGH Radiation Oncology Center in Concord, Massachusetts, and an instructor at Harvard Medical School.

I GOT A DOG. The dog made me smile even when I was feeling really bad.

Kirsten, distribution assistant
Diagnosis of colon cancer at age 49 in 2006 and endometrial (uterine) cancer at age 50 in 2007 in Buford, Georgia

• • •

I SHOPPED. A lot!

Evelyn, executive assistant
Diagnosis of colon cancer at age 33 in 2004 in Boston, Massachusetts

• • •

I WAS FIFTEEN YEARS old and diagnosed with Ewing's sarcoma in my femur with mets [metastases] to my lungs and skull. I had three recurrences of tumors to my lungs in 1996, 2000, and 2006. I always made sure to have something fun to look forward to on my calendar. It was very difficult to maintain a schedule because I'd get neutropenic and need to be hospitalized unexpectedly, but I'd always try to focus on the next "fun" thing to get me through the times when I was feeling awful. It might have been camp in August, or Thanksgiving in November, or *The Nutcracker* in December, or my Make-A-Wish trip in June. I was always trying to keep my head looking forward to brighter times in the future.

Andrea, hospital administrator
Diagnosis of Ewing's sarcoma (a form of bone cancer) at age 15 in 1992 in Norfolk, Massachusetts

• • •

I JOINED A SUPPORT group that really helped me understand a lot of those feelings I didn't even know I had. I marked each milestone with a purchase that I probably would not have made otherwise. I let the house go to pieces and worried only about me.

Pat, office manager
Diagnosis of breast cancer at age 53 in 2001 in Canton, Michigan

I NURTURED MYSELF by staying in a positive frame of mind. I would go out to dinner with friends, as this was a wonderful way for me to share my concerns for the road ahead.

Laura, housecleaner
Diagnosis of esophageal cancer at age 45 in 2002 in Schenectady, New York

• • •

THE MOST IMPORTANT SELF-HELP thing I did was to educate myself. I read books, pamphlets, and [information from] reputable Web sites. I made lists of questions and asked my doctors everything until I understood what I needed to know. I focused on one thing at a time; I shared everything with my husband and most things with everyone else. I couldn't keep secrets; I needed that energy for what I was facing, and I needed the support from others that they could only give if they knew what was going on. I developed an attitude of realistic optimism or optimistic realism, I still don't know which—it means understanding and accepting the reality of the cancer and all that entails and still moving forward in a positive, "can do" way. The smartest thing I did was to talk with other breast cancer survivors through the American Cancer Society's Reach to Recovery® program and at the support group at the cancer center where I was receiving my care.

Kathi, retired special education teacher
Diagnosis of breast cancer at age 49 in 2003 in Wrightstown, Wisconsin

• • •

"I always made sure to have something fun to look forward to..."

JUST A LOT of rest and warm baths.

Nicki, homemaker
Diagnosis of thyroid cancer at age 20 in 2005 in Union, Missouri

• • •

WHAT HELPED ME the most was the accurate information I found on the Internet.

Rochelle, manicurist
Diagnosis of melanoma (skin cancer) at age 34 in 2007 in Las Vegas, Nevada

I TRIED TO GET through every day as normally as possible. During the summer and the first radiation treatments, I remember sleeping a lot (I also had two major surgical procedures in two weeks). During the second series of radiation treatments, I was in my senior year in high school. I went to radiation before school, then went to school and got sick and vomited during the first class, and finished the day. Thirty-four years later during breast cancer surgeries/reconstruction, I did a lot more things to conscientiously help myself like trying to get enough sleep, exercise when I was able (I went to the gym), and I ate fairly healthy.

Charose, nurse
Diagnosis of Hodgkin disease at age 17 in 1972 and breast cancer at age 51 in 2006 in Omaha, Nebraska

• • •

I MADE GOALS. I wanted to attend my cousin's wedding. I wanted to go to the beach for the weekend. I wanted to visit my family in Philadelphia. I wanted a friend to visit for the weekend.

> "I made goals. I wanted to attend my cousin's wedding."

Sheri, actress
Diagnosis of Hodgkin disease at age 29 in 1993 in Columbia, Maryland

• • •

I AM A PERSON who usually does everything herself, but I knew I would need help with this [diagnosis]. I wrote a letter to all my friends and told them what I needed from them to get through it. I asked for phone calls, visits, cards, anything that they thought would help me. I had two close friends who went with me for all my six rounds of chemo treatments (even one that didn't end until 4:00 AM). Also, a few days after each chemo treatment, I would treat myself to a gift or whatever would please me. One time it was a new book; another time it was a nice dinner out. After all treatments were over, my big treat was to go to San Francisco with my family. Planning that trip kept me going day by day.

Joyce, educational assistant at an elementary school
Diagnosis of breast cancer at age 41 in 1995 in Knoxville, Tennessee

When I was hospitalized for a month in 1997 for a bone marrow transplant, I took my manuscripts, my journal of spiritual affirmations, a Bible, a dictionary and thesaurus, beautiful new nightgowns in bright silks and flowered satin, scarves to wrap around my bald head, and CDs and tapes of classical music, hymns, and Gregorian chants. From Jessye Norman's *Spirituals in Concert*, I listened to "In That Great Getting Up Morning" to help me rouse myself each day and the moving "There is a Balm in Gilead," to help me sleep peacefully each night. I took my ballet shoes so that holding onto a hospital handrail as a barre, I could execute with grace, slowly, a few *grandes battements* and *rondes de jambe a terre* and *developpés*. And, of course, art books. These things composed my armor of enrichment as I went to do battle with Goliath. I took no novels that might be depressing. No cruelty. No death. Something of that too-sensitive child still existed.

SUSAN VREELAND is a lymphoma survivor and a *New York Times* bestselling novelist whose most recent book is *Luncheon of the Boating Party*. She received her cancer diagnosis at age 50 in 1996.

THORNE BAY, ALASKA, is located on an island approximately fifty nautical miles northwest of Ketchikan. There were no movies, malls, or any of the other amenities found in most areas. Therefore, there wasn't a lot of "special" to do for myself. Friends and family visited, though, and that was enough.

Ruthanne, bookkeeper
Diagnosis of breast cancer at age 51 in 1995 in Thorne Bay, Alaska

I DID STAND-UP COMEDY prior to being diagnosed. It made my situation somewhat easier when I saw it as comedic.

Laurie, medical assistant
Diagnosis of breast cancer at age 43 in 2006 in Sacramento, California

• • •

I BOUGHT A WIG and named it Fi-Fi, and nobody knew I had cancer. I wanted normalcy to remain constant in my life. I bought myself a new bed, because I figured if I was going to be sick, I was going to be very comfortable.

Jerri, state employee
Diagnosis of breast cancer at age 48 in 2006 and endometrial (uterine) cancer at age 50 in Standish, Michigan

• • •

I SEARCHED THE INTERNET for breast cancer support groups. I spent lots of time in prayer and also in connection with the Internet support group.

Jan, retired hospice chaplain
Diagnosis of breast cancer at age 55 in 2006 in Wichita, Kansas

• • •

I TREATED MYSELF WELL during the good times. My last two chemo treatments were delayed because I needed transfusions. So after the chemo treatments, I bought myself presents—you know, things you might want but would find a better use for the money. I got an MP3 player and a flat-screen monitor—these were my rewards for getting through chemo.

Carmela, technical writer
Diagnosis of endometrial (uterine), bladder, and ovarian cancer at age 48 in 2005 in Clinton Township, Michigan

> "I bought myself a new bed because I figured if I was going to be sick, I was going to be very comfortable."

> ## "I nurtured myself by responding to what my body was telling me it needed to heal... rest, sleep, and (eating and drinking) protein to keep physically nourished."

MY HUSBAND TALKED ME into getting a hot tub, so I would "take time to smell the roses," and I did spend more time in it than I expected to—that was a special and unexpected thing.

Teri, retired kindergarten teacher
Diagnosis of chronic lymphocytic leukemia at age 51 in 1999 in Fort Langley, British Columbia (Canada)

• • •

I NURTURED MYSELF by responding to what my body was telling me it needed to heal....rest, sleep, and (eating and drinking) protein to keep physically nourished. After having lost significant weight throughout the treatment, I went out and treated myself to a new wardrobe!

Bryna, management development consultant
Diagnosis of tongue cancer at age 35 in 1985 in Brockton, Massachusetts

• • •

I DID A LOT of praying and meditating.

Dorothy, receptionist
Diagnosis of breast cancer at age 44 in 2005 in Chesapeake, Virginia

• • •

I SPENT A LOT of time in prayer and reading the scriptures. I also began to define my deepest convictions in the form of poetry. Always an avid reader, I searched for books and other publications written by people who had been down the path I was now on.

Barbara, homemaker
Diagnosis of breast cancer at age 38 in 1986 in Conway, Arkansas

I GOT INVOLVED WITH a local support group.

April, disabled
Diagnosis of breast cancer at age 34 in 1999 in Wichita, Kansas

I wrote a song about fear, followed by hope and spiritual togetherness with all the women who have ever gone through this wrenching experience. The song is called "Scar," and I recorded it on an album called *The Bedroom Tapes*. It was a homage to all those men and women who are dealing with fear and [a poor] self-image, then finally coming to terms with and making a change in self-image and having a new kind of belief in humanity.

CARLY SIMON is a Grammy award–winning singer. She was age 52 when her breast cancer was diagnosed in 1997. Her song "You're So Vain" was a number-one single on the pop charts in 1973.

WHEN I WAS FINALLY feeling well enough to go back to work as a contractor, one of the first things I did was something I absolutely could not afford. I purchased a pool table—a lifelong dream—for my basement, and it became kind of a rallying point for my entire family as being in the "anger free zone." This was the best money I ever spent.

Jerry, computer software instructor
Diagnosis of acute myelogenous leukemia at age 43 in 2003 in Anoka, Minnesota

• • •

I NURTURED MYSELF (and still do) by relaxing in a nice warm bubble bath every night.

Marie, retired
Diagnosis of ovarian cancer at age 59 in 2004 in Lebanon, Ohio

I WAS NOT WORKING (on disability), and so I looked more into support opportunities. I joined Gilda's Club. I went to Look Good...Feel Better® by the American Cancer Society and really started paying attention to makeup and dress.

Judy, chaplain
Diagnosis of colorectal cancer at age 48 in 2003 in Cudahy, Wisconsin

• • •

I TOOK A BREAK between my diagnosis and surgery and my radiation treatments to go to China to tour and participate in a dragon boat race. Then, I took a girl-trip to Alaska right after finishing radiation. Even though I was a bit depleted, it was a wonderful celebration of "graduation."

Robin, college professor
Diagnosis of breast cancer at age 50 in 2006 in Costa Mesa, California

What helped get me through was my innate and very deep love for life mostly, my belief that life is worth fighting for, as well as my knowledge that even cancer is treatable and beatable. And I think, too, my ability and willingness to think outside the box and do my own research, to ask questions and discover on my own how to really survive and thrive.

JAMIE RENO is a *Newsweek* correspondent, author, and singer-songwriter. He received a diagnosis of stage IV, low-grade, follicular non-Hodgkin lymphoma at age 35 in 1996.

I HAVE ALWAYS DONE things for others, so it was really hard for me to allow others to do things for me. I really did nothing special for myself. I was determined to get back to normal as quickly as possible.

Fran, postmaster
Diagnosis of breast cancer at age 42 in 1999 in LaVergne, Tennessee

FOR FUN, I LIVED on my computer in the breast cancer chat rooms.

Kathleen, retail manager
Diagnosis of breast cancer at age 48 in 2007 in Washington Township, New Jersey

• • •

I WROTE IN MY journal daily. This was a way for me to express my inner feelings.

Jocelyn, social worker
Diagnosis of breast cancer at age 43 in 2006 in Macedon, New York

• • •

I TRIED TO DO absolutely nothing the first week after chemo.

Jennifer, housekeeper
Diagnosis of breast cancer at age 40 in 2004 and skin cancer at age 41 in 2005 in Craig, Colorado

• • •

WHENEVER I'M DOWN, I engage in shopping therapy. I bought myself anything I wanted...within reason, of course.

Laura, unemployed psychiatric social worker
Diagnosis of breast cancer at age 43 in 2006 in Avon, Connecticut

• • •

I SURROUNDED MYSELF with my animals. They made me laugh.

Yvonne, paralegal
Diagnosis of colon cancer at age 48 in 2004 in San Antonio, Texas

> "I have always done things for others, so it was really hard for me to allow others to do things for me. I really did nothing special for myself."

> "Cancer is a wake-up call to slow down, assign tasks to others, reach out and ask for support."

I THINK IT IS very important to carve out time for myself. We have a tendency to care for others first. Cancer is a wake-up call to slow down, assign tasks to others, reach out and ask for support.

Iris, artist
Diagnosis of liver cancer at age 50 in 2007 in Sante Fe, New Mexico

• • •

I WATCHED TV SHOWS that kept my spirits up. I watched a lot of comedies and animal shows.

Brenda, government clerk
Diagnosis of breast cancer at age 58 in 2006 in Madison, Tennessee

• • •

I TRIED TO PLAN new things for my husband and me after treatment. We bought a new bed (I did not want that old one any more), and we moved to a new home.

Karen, real estate broker
Diagnosis of breast cancer at age 38 in 2001 in Loganville, Georgia

• • •

I ATTENDED SPORTING EVENTS, which I love.

Karen, medical assistant
Diagnosis of breast cancer at age 43 in 2001 in Cincinnati, Ohio

• • •

MY ADVICE IS TO remember that only you can fight your cancer. Other people can do the laundry, make meals, and even wipe away tears. You must—even if it's the first time in your life—think of yourself first. No one can fight this battle as well as you can.

Deborah, physician
Diagnosis of breast cancer at age 47 in 2007 in Overland Park, Kansas

NO MATTER HOW MANY people I had around me during the day to make sure I was okay, going to sleep was the hardest part. I was left alone with my thoughts, and my fear seemed to spiral out of control. I always watched Seinfeld DVDs before I went to sleep so I could go to sleep laughing, with good thoughts in my head. It helped tremendously to keep my spirits up.

Jennifer, publicity coordinator
Diagnosis of melanoma (skin cancer) at age 21 in 2004 in San Diego, California

Take a deep breath! Don't panic. In most cases, a cancer diagnosis is not an emergency. It's important to take the time you need to find the treatment team you trust and a plan you feel good about. You will get a lot of advice from friends, relatives, and family— they mean well but don't always understand your medical situation. Thank them for their input, but rely on your team of doctors for the advice you need.

SUSAN PORIES, MD, FACS, is an assistant professor at Harvard Medical School and a breast surgical oncologist at Mount Auburn Hospital in Cambridge, Massachusetts, and the Beth Israel Deaconess Medical Center in Boston, Massachusetts.

I ATTENDED AMERICAN CANCER SOCIETY programs such as Look Good...Feel Better® and hospital workshops and support groups.

Jo Ann, retired
Diagnosis of breast cancer at age 60 in 2006 in Lanoka Harbor, New Jersey

• • •

I NURTURED MYSELF by going to Myrtle Beach with my friend.

Jo Anne, nurse's aide
Diagnosis of breast cancer at age 51 in 2003 in Brownstown, Michigan

I READ INSPIRATIONAL BOOKS to teach me self-motivation and faith in myself. The books helped me to pull from my inner core all the strength I felt I could muster and show everyone that I could hold my smile and not cry.

Alejandra, clerical worker
Diagnosis of uterine cancer at age 36 in 2005 in Torrance, California

• • •

I LEARNED TO SAY NO during my diagnosis and treatment. I did not take on another project but became my own project. For the first time in years, I had to focus on *me* and, being a wife and mother, that was initially not easy. Every day I would have a good breakfast and a nutritional dinner that would nurture my body and be good to my taste buds. I drank tea and wrote in my journal. I read funny books and looked at meaningful movies. Took good naps and enjoyed time. I enjoyed the fact that I didn't have "bad hair days." Being bald brought on freedom for me, and I was able to enjoy the sunshine and wind on my scalp.

Tracey, radiation oncology information analyst
Diagnosis of breast cancer at age 37 in 2002 in Villa Park, Illinois

It is important to try to maintain your daily routines during cancer treatment, provided you feel well enough. Preserving your normal schedule, if that is important to you, can help you take control of your life when you may feel out of control upon hearing your cancer diagnosis. Taking time out for the parts of your life that have the most meaning for you can aid in your recovery.

ELYSE CAPLAN oversees educational programming for breast cancer information and awareness for Living Beyond Breast Cancer (LBBC). Elyse was 34 years old when her breast cancer was diagnosed in 1991. At the time, her sons were 2, 5, and 8 years old.

I BOUGHT A $4,000 bed, because the chemo caused neuropathy in my feet, and I wanted to be comfortable.

Sheila, legal secretary
Diagnosis of breast cancer at age 65 in 2006 in Walnut Creek, California

• • •

I CRIED A LOT. I was extremely exhausted and could barely get out of bed most days for the first six weeks of treatment. Holding my baby girl did more emotional good for me than anything else. We could not afford many extras during that time, but every now and then, I would get an ice cream shake or Frosty.

Carlyn, administrative assistant
Diagnosis of Hodgkin disease at age 30 in 2004 in Willow Spring, North Carolina

It would have been easy for me to feel sorry for myself and expect others to feel sorry for me...but I soon realized that it was much healthier simply to be nice to myself and to my circle of caregivers. After realizing that I needed to go through chemo, radiation, and surgery, I made a decision to keep my life as close to "normal" as possible outside of the "invasions." I continued to work, but with the complete support of my workplace; I paced myself to my capacity to perform. I stayed home and in bed when I needed to, I worked half days when full days were too hard, and I talked about my experience when people asked. These things helped me make it through.

TERRY MUSIC was 46 years old when her breast cancer was diagnosed. She is the chief mission delivery officer of the American Cancer Society.

> **"For the first time in years, I had to focus on *me*..."**

I SLEPT A LOT! I bought the softest and warmest lounge clothes and throw I could find. I also bought the coolest and most silky gowns and robes for those "hot flash" moments that sometimes seemed to last an entire day.

Pam, retired dental hygienist
Diagnosis of breast cancer at age 57 in 2005 in Lakeland, Florida

Reference

Praver, F. C. 2004. *Crossroads at midlife.* Westport, CT: Praeger Publishers.

CHAPTER 2

• • •

How My Family Helped

As I mentioned in the Preface, the idea for this book came to me when Kelley Tuthill's sister, Melissa, asked me what would help Kelley when she received her breast cancer diagnosis. Kelley, a Boston-based reporter who chronicled her journey on television and through her blog, has been an inspiration to many cancer survivors. I e-mailed Melissa a list of ideas about what helped me. Then I thought, maybe others would have some great advice for her. Which is how this book was born.

In this chapter, survivors tell us what their family members did that really helped them through their diagnosis and treatment. There were a lot of stories about wonderful spouses. Dorinda, an ovarian cancer survivor, wrote about how her husband was there for her through "every test, procedure, and treatment." He even left the treatment center one day in the middle of a snowstorm just to get her a chocolate malted.

Many people wrote about how some loved ones were more helpful than others. Kathie, a kidney cancer survivor, realized that her mother and stepfather were in denial through most of her ordeal. They traveled more than three hundred miles to be with her after her surgery, but basically "just stared" at her. In retrospect, she realized they had done the best they could. Her boyfriend was very kind to her family, uncritical of them, and was really there for her throughout her treatment.

Though serious illness may tear families apart, it can just as easily bring them together. Pearl, a young Scottish breast cancer survivor wrote, "My brother was the first person I telephoned about my diagnosis, and we have become so close ever since." Social worker Todd, a two-time cancer survivor (chronic myelogenous leukemia and kidney cancer), wrote that he was twenty-five years old at the time of his diagnosis and still lived with his mother. "She did everything for me," he said. "She was a mom…my advocate, my strength, my rock!"

Some people admitted that it was hard to accept help from their families. Sherri, who had a diagnosis of endometrial cancer at age forty-two, recalled that there were daily chores she didn't always enjoy before her illness—tasks like carpooling, cleaning, and nagging her daughter to do her homework. Yet, when she had to rely on others to do those things, she came to appreciate what a privilege it was to be able to do them herself.

Many survivors felt obligated to demonstrate courage and resilience for their families. Federico received a diagnosis of testicular cancer when he was thirty-two years old. He shared how he tried to continue to do special things for his wife, even as she helped him through his illness. His caveat to cancer patients is to keep in mind that "the cancer not only affects the sick, but also the caregivers around them."

In this chapter you'll hear more from cancer survivors like Matt who wrote that all of his siblings were tested for bone marrow donor matching, and his youngest brother ended up being the donor. It was "pretty darn special," said Matt.

Families *are* special and if someone you love has cancer, the stories in this chapter can help you to figure out the best way to support him or her through this difficult time.

• • •

KNOWING MY HUSBAND and family were there for me to lean on and cry with helped me the most when I was first diagnosed. My husband was always there for me and never faltered. He helped care for our baby and was a constant source of love and comfort when I needed it the most. When my hair fell out and I became bald from the chemotherapy, he shaved his head so that I wouldn't have to be the only bald one in the house. He is an amazing man, and I couldn't ask for a better partner in life.

Sarah, paralegal
Diagnosis of breast cancer at age 28 in 2000 in Miami, Florida

MY HUSBAND SHOWED ME just what true love means. He was with me for every doctor's appointment and every chemotherapy treatment. He became my sole motivation for each day. I lived to see his smiling face and to hear his gentle kind words of encouragement after long nights of nausea and pain. He never left me alone. When my hair began to fall out, he went with me to have my head shaved, and so did he. When all my hair fell out, he shaved his head every other day so he would be just like me. He held my hand while the chemo drugs were being administered. He would sit and talk with everyone around us so that we had distractions from what the nurses were doing to get us through the treatment. He cooked meals for a whole year so I didn't have to deal with the smells and the feelings of nausea. His greatest help to me was his daily hug in the morning with this statement: "Hello, Beautiful. Thank you for fighting so hard so that we can all be together again today!"

> ## "My husband made sure in every way that I knew I was loved..."

Dorothy, receptionist
Diagnosis of breast cancer at age 44 in 2005 in Chesapeake, Virginia

• • •

I RECEIVED MY BREAST cancer diagnosis at the age of twenty-seven. I was a single mother of a ten-year old, and I had recently broken up with Michael, my long-time boyfriend. Michael, my ex, immediately stepped up to the plate. He lived down the street, so he was with me as often as he could be. When I started daily radiation treatments, he would either come or call me as soon as he knew I was out. When I started weekly chemo treatments, he was there every day. When I needed surgery, his was the face I saw when I got out. We were married April 1, 2007! Michael and, of course, my son support me to this very day. We are closer and more in love then ever before. I honestly believe that Michael and I would never have gotten married if I hadn't gotten sick. He had already moved out and decided that he was never going to marry me. He has said that he never knew the extent of his love for me until he thought he was going to lose me.

Megan, procurement manager with a fortune 500 company
Diagnosis of breast cancer at age 27 in 2005 in Milford, Connecticut

MY WIFE'S FAMILY and our friends were wonderful support. During my first surgery, they made a schedule of who would watch our children and who would deliver meals when I returned home. They gave so much and asked for nothing in return except that I fight this through.

Mike, management professional
Diagnosis of rectal cancer at age 38 in 2006 in Rochester, New York

• • •

MY HUSBAND MADE SURE in every way that I knew I was loved and that he would be by my side no matter what.

Kelly, financial services executive
Diagnosis of chronic lymphocytic leukemia at age 50 in 2003 and basal cell carcinoma (skin cancer) at age 53 in 2007 in Arlington, Virginia

• • •

I HAD MY UNBELIEVABLY supportive husband. He was there for every test, procedure, treatment, and doctor visit. He handled the insurance issues and, best of all, he fed me the absolute best meals. One day, my husband left the treatment center in the middle of a snowstorm to walk to an ice cream shop. He returned with a large chocolate malted for me. That was a real treat.

Dorinda, retired teacher
Diagnosis of ovarian cancer at age 50 in 2005 in Edison, New Jersey

• • •

MY MOM WAS MY ROCK (and still is). She quit her job, stayed home to care for me, grieved with me, didn't leave me alone in the hospital for a single night, advocated for me, catered my menu to the limited food I would eat, helped me shop for hats, rubbed my bald head when I needed consoling, listened to me whine and whimper, gave me hope in the future, and helped me come to terms and contentment with whatever life threw my way.

Andrea, hospital administrator
Diagnosis of Ewing's sarcoma (a form of bone cancer) at age 15 in 1992 in Norfolk, Massachusetts

MY HUSBAND. He was my nurse, my Pollyanna. He was great, especially for a guy who hates hospitals, blood and guts!

Peggy, pathologist's assistant
Diagnosis of breast cancer at age 47 in 2003 in St. Augustine, Florida

• • •

MY MOTHER MADE ME do my little laps around the house to get exercise; she slept with me and pulled me out of bed when I was too weak to lift myself up. She made me half sandwiches when that was all I could eat. She bathed me and combed my hair! She did everything!

Evelyn, executive assistant
Diagnosis of colon cancer at age 33 in 2004 in Boston, Massachusetts

• • •

MY TWIN SISTER WAS also diagnosed at the same time with invasive breast cancer. You certainly don't want your sister to get breast cancer, but if you have to go through it, it's nice to have someone you love going through the same thing with you for support back and forth. My eighty-five-year-old mom gave all her time [to us] dividing herself between two cities, and we had our surgeries and recovered.

Deb, nurse practitioner
Diagnosis of melanoma (skin cancer) at age 21 in 1974 and breast cancer at age 52 in 2006 in Evansville, Indiana

• • •

KNOWING THAT MY SEVENTY-NINE-YEAR-OLD husband, who is physically disabled, needs me so much. I also have Crohn's disease and had to stop the chemo for that to start chemo for cancer. I was fecally incontinent, had to live on hospital-prescribed fruit juice for four months, and could eat no solid foods. My husband prepared and cooked all his own food and never made me feel guilty that I was ill. He always made me feel I would conquer this disease and inspired me with his love and caring.

Elizabeth, retired administrator
Diagnosis of breast cancer at age 58 in 2003 in Plymouth, Devon (England)

IT WAS MY SISTER who started doing research on the Internet and helping me sort through the mounds of information we found. She traveled over one and one-half hours to stay four days with me after the surgery so my husband could continue to work. And she coaxed me to join a breast cancer support group in which I still participate a year after treatments. I absolutely cannot forget to mention my husband, "my rock," who was with me every step of the way, came to every appointment I had, and did all the housework and cooking for me so I could concentrate on myself.

Kelley, massage therapist
Diagnosis of breast cancer at age 36 in 2006 in Rochdale, Massachusetts

• • •

MY HUSBAND. He was there for me, no matter how difficult it was for him. He is a very quiet person who doesn't express his emotions, but he was always there for me—to let me cry, to hold me.

Eileen, technology specialist
Diagnosis of breast cancer at age 34 in 1984 and acute myelogenous leukemia at age 49 in 1999 and basal cell carcinoma (skin cancer) at age 55 in 2005 in Framingham, Massachusetts

What helped me most in going through cancer treatment each time was having a supportive network of family and friends, access to excellent medical care, and a great desire to be well again. My family helped me by being present, listening well, and keeping my sense of humor piqued at all times. Oh yes, and keeping the M&Ms dish full!

ELLEN STOVALL, president and CEO of the National Coalition for Cancer Survivorship, had three separate cancer diagnoses: Hodgkin disease at age 24 in 1971, recurrent Hodgkin disease at age 36 in 1983, and breast cancer at age 61 in 2007. Ellen has been married for more than forty years and has one son who was 4 weeks old at the time of her first cancer diagnosis.

WHILE I WAS IN the hospital one Christmas break, my father and brother built me a clubhouse where I could play with my friends.

Randy, respiratory therapist
Diagnosis of Hodgkin disease at age 6 in 1965 in Ewa Beach, Hawaii

• • •

MY SISTER-IN-LAW HELPED with bathing my baby, putting her to bed, and making dinner. My sister-in-law just assumed all the roles I normally have without question. My mom came in from out of town and made sure I had everything I needed to make me as comfortable as possible. She had even nagged me to get the mole removed, which is how I found out about the cancer in the first place. Neither of them let me overdo things, which is what I normally do.

Rochelle, manicurist
Diagnosis of melanoma (skin cancer) at age 34 in 2007 in Las Vegas, Nevada

• • •

MY MOTHER was a stay-at-home mom and went with me to my treatments. She is such a calm, quiet soul. She would cook anything that I thought would be good to eat when I was having treatments and such trouble eating. Even as an adult, with my breast cancer, she was such a support. But I think for the breast cancer diagnosis, my husband was most helpful to me, and I was so grateful for that. He even got me a gold medallion, engraved with "two-time winner" (two-time cancer survivor). He gave me his opinion when asked about treatment options, but he wanted me to make the decisions that I was most comfortable with.

Charose, nurse
Diagnosis of Hodgkin disease at age 17 in 1972 and breast cancer at age 51 in 2006 in Omaha, Nebraska

• • •

MY PARENTS WERE THERE every step of the way: taking me to chemo, going to the doctors, and researching my disease (even though my mom had two open heart surgeries within a week of each other during my treatment).

Sheri, actress
Diagnosis of Hodgkin disease at age 29 in 1993 in Columbia, Maryland

> ## "He was the one to tell me I looked beautiful when I couldn't face looking at myself; he was the one to love me..."

MY MOM WAS SO worried, so she and I would go sit by the lake and talk.

> **LaDonne, retired**
> *Diagnosis of kidney cancer at age 40 in 1978 in Mundelein, Illinois*

• • •

I DON'T THINK MY brother knew what to do to help, although he was very supportive and loved to tell people that I had survived cancer.

> **Kathleen, teacher**
> *Diagnosis of Hodgkin disease at age 40 in 1997 in Lisbon, Connecticut*

• • •

MY HUSBAND AND SISTER. They listened to me and went to every doctor's appointment, test, and treatment—that is huge.

> **Eileen, teacher**
> *Diagnosis of breast cancer at age 43 in 2006 in Hilton, New York*

• • •

GOD GAVE ME the most peace throughout my cancer treatment, but my husband was incredibly supportive through it all. He was the soft place to fall; he was the strength and comfort when I just couldn't do anymore; he was the one who allowed me to laugh at myself and at life when times were tough; he was the one to tell me I looked beautiful when I couldn't face looking at myself; he was the one to love me no matter what. What an amazing man he is. Thank you, God, for blessing me with him.

> **Julie, real estate agent**
> *Diagnosis of thyroid cancer at age 34 in 1996 and breast cancer at age 43 in 2005 in Torrance, California*

MY HUSBAND WAS UNABLE to be with me during the surgical procedures because he had to stay in Germany and take care of our three young children. But he was with me through my treatment and stuck by me even when I tried to push him away. I felt it would be easier for everyone if I just pushed everyone away. My husband brought me a kitten (Sammy) as I was just starting treatment. I still have her, and she is always by my side. I had a difficult time in the beginning. I didn't want to accept the diagnosis, and I was so unsure of the future. Doctors gave me a 61 percent chance of surviving five years. I wrote some in a journal and wrote poetry. At first, I went to a survivors group, but found that too depressing. I became extremely close with my mom during that time, and it has made our relationship stronger.

Danielle, financial service specialist
Diagnosis of melanoma (skin cancer) at age 30 in 2000 in Ramstein (Germany)

• • •

BOTH MY MOTHER-IN-LAW and my aunt had previously had breast cancer. They and several other women also diagnosed with breast cancer from my community were helpful in answering my questions, and I also got answers from the American Cancer Society's Web site.

Marla, executive assistant
Diagnosis of breast cancer at age 35 in 1994 in Jasper, Indiana

• • •

MY BROTHER HELPED ME the most. He was with me when we initially met with the oncologist, and he went with me for a second opinion. He was so positive and strong.

Julie, account executive in advertising/marketing
Diagnosis of laryngeal cancer at age 46 in 2002 in New York City, New York

• • •

MY WIFE GAVE ME purpose (her) to get well. I had a full life and am not afraid to die, but I realized she really needs me around!

James, retired police officer
Diagnosis of lymphoma at age 66 in 2007 in Sheridan, Wyoming

MY COUSIN'S GENEROUS OFFER to use her condo in Hawaii for a week! What a great family vacation we had! We could not have afforded it otherwise.

Kathryn, homemaker
Diagnosis of multiple myeloma at age 39 in 2001 and basal cell carcinoma (skin cancer) at age 45 in 2007 in St. Charles, Missouri

• • •

I ASKED ALL of my family and friends to please keep me motivated, to give me encouragement, and to push me to get up and get on with my life. Not a day goes by when someone doesn't call or come over.

Audrey, disabled
Diagnosis of lung cancer at age 51 in 2007 in Baltimore, Maryland

• • •

I WAS IN COLLEGE when I received the diagnosis of Hodgkin disease. My parents insisted that I remain enrolled in school while going through treatment. They wanted me to have as "normal" a life as possible, so that cancer wouldn't be my sole focus. After learning about my illness in the summer, I returned to Brown University that fall as a senior and took a light course load, lived off campus, attended parties, etc. Every couple of weeks, I boarded a train to New York to receive my chemotherapy treatments, rested a day at home, then headed back to Providence. My radiation regimen took place at the end of the first semester, and then we took a family vacation. Looking back, I really appreciate my parents' approach. It enabled me to be a college kid with cancer, rather than a cancer patient in college.

Debbie, journalist
Diagnosis of Hodgkin disease at age 20 in 1979 in New York City, New York

• • •

MY HUSBAND HELPED the most by being there for me. We negotiated and discussed everything. He was able to understand that I needed him but still had to make all my own decisions regarding my care.

Barbara, nurse
Diagnosis of breast cancer at age 58 in 1995 in Stoneham, Massachusetts

I WAS DIVORCED WHEN I went through my cancer the first time. When I was rediagnosed with metastatic cancer, my ex-husband and I became closer. We are now best friends! We decided that since we really don't know how long I have left on this wonderful earth that we should at least be under the same roof for the sake of the kids. Our youngest is only ten years old, and it has made a big difference in our family to be back together.

April, disabled
Diagnosis of breast cancer at age 34 in 1999 in Wichita, Kansas

When I received my cancer diagnosis, my family meant (and means) everything to me. They were hugely supportive then and now. Hope is everything when you're sick. Hope is not simply an unrealistic expectation. Hope is what you feel when you know your doctors and other care partners are doing everything that is possible and reasonable to help you get well. Hope stems from that support you get from your family and friends.

DAVID JOHNSON, MD, director of the Division of Hematology & Oncology at Vanderbilt-Ingram Cancer Center in Nashville, Tennessee, had a diagnosis of non-Hodgkin lymphoma at age 41 in 1989.

SHORTLY AFTER MY DIAGNOSIS, I found myself in the ICU (intensive care unit), clinging to life. I don't pretend to remember a lot of it, but when I awoke I was met by my parents and five of my six brothers and sisters, most of whom came from out of state. That was when I knew I was in serious trouble. I could not let them all down. I had to hang in there.

Jerry, computer software instructor
Diagnosis of acute myelogenous leukemia at age 43 in 2003 in Anoka, Minnesota

MY PARENTS WOULD BUY us groceries and donate funds to pay the bills. Without them, we could not have survived.

Yvonne, paralegal
Diagnosis of colon cancer at age 48 in 2004 in San Antonio, Texas

Faith, hope and love. Our relationships and connections are the key. They give our lives meaning.

BERNIE SIEGEL, MD, is the author of many books, including the bestseller *Love, Medicine and Miracles*.

MY MARRIAGE BECAME MUCH stronger. We were married right out of high school and argued a lot.

Fran, postmaster
Diagnosis of breast cancer at age 42 in 1999 in LaVergne, Tennessee

• • •

"My sister is amazing. ...she always calmed me down and left me reassured."

MY SISTER IS AMAZING. I can't remember how many times I called her crying hysterically, and she always calmed me down and left me reassured. I often feel bad because I don't do this with many people—she gets the brunt of my "bad days." I only hope she knows I would do the same for her.

Laura, unemployed psychiatric social worker
Diagnosis of breast cancer at age 43 in 2006 in Avon, Connecticut

• • •

MY HUSBAND LET ME cry and feel sorry for myself.

Jo Ann, retired
Diagnosis of breast cancer at age 60 in 2006 in Lanoka Harbor, New Jersey

MY HUSBAND HAD FAITH that I would pull through. I worried that it was denial on his part and so, I put all my affairs in order, including setting up a family trust and writing in a notebook, page after page of detailed instructions on operating the washing machine, DVD player, satellite TV remote, and unsticking the icemaker...well, you get the idea. The very act of doing all this mundane work was the best thing I could do to keep from dwelling on all the "what if's" that were fighting for possession of my mind.

Judy, retired accounting clerk
Diagnosis of lung cancer at age 64 in 2004 in Norwalk, California

• • •

MY HUSBAND
(1) fixed meals without complaint when I was tired;
(2) took me to work and waited when I was called out at night as a hospice chaplain;
(3) changed his work schedule to be available for me;
(4) pushed me all around in the wheelchair when I was too weak to walk;
(5) held me when I cried. And much, much more.

Judy, chaplain
Diagnosis of colorectal cancer at age 48 in 2003 in Cudahy, Wisconsin

• • •

MY GRANDMA CAME IN during the surgery to talk to me since I was awake. She helped keep my mind off of what was going on around me.

Mary Anne, word processor
Diagnosis of melanoma (skin cancer) at age 26 in 2007 in Dixon, California

• • •

MY OLDER SON WAS the most help for me. He turned out to be my angel and was there for me when my husband had a hard time dealing with my cancer. I was in great hands with God and my son.

Luann, stay-at-home mom
Diagnosis of colon cancer at age 50 in 2003 in Charleston, West Virginia

> ## "My marriage was tested a lot, and my husband came through. We are stronger and value the time we have together."

I AM FORTUNATE/UNFORTUNATE to have an older sister who is an eighteen-year survivor. My cancer was diagnosed on March 28th, and I was getting married on October 13th. I was too busy to let cancer get in the way! My fiancé and I put a "healing garden" in my back yard after my first chemo. It was my place to rest while I watched the flowers bloom.

Linda, purchasing agent
Diagnosis of breast cancer at age 47 in 2007 in Antioch, California

• • •

ALTHOUGH I COME FROM a very modest background, my family believes in the incredible power of being there in times of need. We have a saying in Family Medicine: "You can pretend to know and you can pretend to care, but you can't pretend to be there."

Deborah, physician
Diagnosis of breast cancer at age 47 in 2007 in Overland Park, Kansas

• • •

WHEN I LEARNED of my diagnosis, I was getting married in three weeks! I was so caught up in the wedding and seeing family that I couldn't feel too sorry for myself. I had my first lumpectomy the week following my wedding, followed by chemo and radiation therapy. I was recently diagnosed with a lump in my other breast and, while they found some cells that were abnormal, they will not know if it is cancer until they do another lumpectomy. I feel immensely stronger. My husband's sense of humor was great. He made me laugh, even though I was going through treatment. My marriage was tested a lot, and my husband came through. We are stronger and value the time we have together.

Sheila, legal secretary
Diagnosis of breast cancer at age 65 in 2006 in Walnut Creek, California

I helped myself, first, followed very closely by my amazingly loving and supportive wife Gabriela, who has been with me for every single doctor's appointment, every moment of laughter, every tear, every crisis, every bit of good news and bad, every round of chemo, every moment of fear, and every moment of joy. I'm a pretty strong person, but I do not think I'd be here if not for my beautiful wife, who is truly an angel.

JAMIE RENO is one of the nation's most successful and honored journalists. A longtime San Diego correspondent for *Newsweek*, Jamie has covered the 9/11 investigation, the war in Iraq, the last four presidential campaigns, and many other major stories. Jamie received a diagnosis of stage IV, low-grade, follicular non-Hodgkin lymphoma at age 35 in 1996.

MY EIGHTY-NINE-YEAR-OLD GRANDMOTHER came and stayed at my home to take care of me for two weeks after my husband had to go back to work.

Lisa, administrative assistant
Diagnosis of breast cancer at age 38 in 2000 in Owings Mills, Maryland

• • •

MY HUSBAND LET ME express my fear in the middle of the night. He was fully present as I cried. My husband's sister was at our home one night when I was really having emotional problems—crying, screaming at my husband. She was a support for him when I wasn't really being rational.

Judi, nurse
Diagnosis of breast cancer at age 40 in 2000 in Pen Argyl, Pennsylvania

"My wife gave me purpose (her) to get well."

> ## "Fit your cancer treatment into your life in all its fullness—not your life into your cancer treatment."

MY HUSBAND HAS BEEN to every doctor's appointment since I was referred to the oncologist. He has been to every radiation treatment since. I do not have cancer alone; he has borne the burden as well.

Jennifer, federal officer with U.S. Customs and Border Patrol
Diagnosis of cervical cancer at age 36 in 2007 in Montreal, Quebec (Canada)

• • •

FAMILY MAKES ALL the difference. For with them, you have care and respect for you and not the condition that you happen to have. They are there for the long haul, no matter what. So what am I saying? Fit your cancer treatment into your life in all its fullness— not your life into your cancer treatment.

Kyle, pastor
Diagnosis of kidney cancer at age 60 in 2004 in Johnstown, Pennsylvania

My husband was absolutely wonderful and, surprisingly, not afraid—he tends to be a worrier.

HALA MODDELMOG is a breast cancer survivor and president and CEO of Susan G. Komen for the Cure®.

CHAPTER 3

· · ·

How Friends Made a Difference

Joni Rodgers, who wrote the book *Bald in the Land of Big Hair* about her struggle with lymphoma, summed up being a friend to someone going through cancer in this way: "Hi, I'm Joni, and I'm a sucking black hole of emotional need right now. My hobbies are taking drugs, napping, and calling people I hardly know for emergency child-care. Wanna be my friend?" (Rodgers 2001, 61).

There is no doubt that it can be a demanding calling to be a good friend to someone who is going through a serious illness such as cancer. However, it was heartening to know that everyone who filled out a survey for this book had a story about how their friends came through for them. Elena, who had a diagnosis of inflammatory breast cancer at age forty-four, wrote about how a dear friend accompanied her and her husband to appointments with three oncologists. The friend had lived through a breast cancer diagnosis and treatment three years earlier. She was able to take detailed notes, so that Elena and her husband could just listen. "It is so hard to absorb information when you are in shock," said Elena. "We were able to review what each doctor said by reading [my friend's] thorough notes that explained everything." Elena's comments represent a common theme among the survey participants: it was very meaningful to many of them to have friends accompany them to various health care appointments—either to be supportive, take notes, or simply stave off boredom.

Some friends eased the trauma of losing hair and other difficult things that cancer treatment can bring about. Sandra, also a breast cancer survivor, shared a story about how her friend helped her find the perfect wig. A friend offered to shop with her for wigs, but Sandra was indecisive about whether to seek help or do it alone. In the end, her friend accompanied her. Together they learned that synthetic wigs are often scratchy and uncomfortable and cannot be colored to match one's actual hair color. They also learned that human hair wigs are very expensive and, in Sandra's case, not covered by insurance. So her friend made a little box, decorated it and wrote "for Sandra's wig" on it, and passed it around their church community. Very soon, there was $1,200 in there—all anonymously given so Sandra did not have the burden of writing thank you notes. "My beautiful wig was so like my natural hair that no one could tell," she said. "Even my oncology nurse was confused and asked me what cycle I was on when I came in with hair when she expected to see me without. It was a huge help to my frail, bruised ego."

Most people going through cancer treatment will miss out on important events. My middle child still remembers that I missed her second grade play the night after I had surgery. No one could take my place, but friends and family members did what they could. They came over to my house the night of the play and helped my daughter get dressed and fixed her hair. They took pictures and recorded the play for me to watch with her later.

Others shared their stories of how friends made it easier to miss important events. Cathy, the pancreatic cancer survivor who made the beaded necklace to mark her milestones, gave this example, "I had tickets to a Beach Boys concert but was not able to go because my blood counts were low. I gave the tickets to family friends. They told the security people for The Beach Boys about me, and Mike Love signed a T-shirt and the drummer ended up giving them the sticks he used at that concert. Both are now in a shadow box hanging in my hallway."

As Joni Rodgers implied in her book, it is not always easy to ask friends for the help you need. Ann learned this lesson when she received a diagnosis of breast cancer. Ann noted, "I was a stay-at-home mom when my cancer was diagnosed. My husband worked sixty-hour weeks. So, I did everything else. I needed help with a million things, especially cleaning and yard work. Acquaintances would constantly call me to drill me on my condition and details of my treatment. The conversations were particularly long and hard to deal with when talking to one individual. But each time I would hear the same statement [no matter who called]: 'Let me know if there is anything I can do.' I would always answer the question with something specific that I needed, like 'The grass is really long' or 'It would be nice if you would invite my son over to play with your son at *your* house'. Rarely, did anyone ever get it. I realized that 'Let me know what I can do' is really a hollow offer."

One of my colleagues, psychiatrist Paula Rauch, co-authored the book, *Raising an Emotionally Healthy Child When a Parent Is Sick*. In her book, Dr. Rauch advises parents who are ill to appoint someone to be the "Minister of Information." That person would be in charge of passing along any information that you want others to know about your condition and would also have a list of specific things that would be helpful to you. So, when friends ask what they can do to help, the Minister of Information is able to suggest something specific (Rauch 2006, 58). However, it's important to note that not all friends will follow through.

Ann has this advice for well-intentioned friends: "I think if people know of someone going through treatment for cancer (or another chronic illness) they should not make that empty offer, but actually *do* something. If you notice the weeds in the yard are beginning to look like the Little Shop of Horrors, pitch in and do some weeding. Stop calling to satisfy your curiosity, and think about what is going on in the life of the cancer patient. A vague offer of help is hard to respond to. You really need to make a step to show your sincerity."

Beth, a breast cancer survivor, agrees that people need to be given specific tasks, but she also concurs that not everyone will be able to follow through. Beth advised, "If people offer to help in a generic way, then tell them you can use help with meals, cleaning, laundry, yard work, grocery shopping, running kids to wherever, getting to doctor's appointments, keeping track of prescriptions. Whatever it is that needs to be done or you just want to have done, but don't feel up to managing. It might take a few requests before you hit on the right person for the right thing, but you won't know until you ask, and you'll quickly weed out the talkers from the doers. Try to remember that the talkers don't wish you well any less than the doers, but they may not have the stamina it takes to truly help or may be challenged by their own issues that get in the way."

People also shared how friends helped them long distance. Cathy wrote how cards and letters from friends helped. She said, "It is amazing how getting the mail and seeing a card in the midst of all the bills can make your day." Kenneth, who had kidney cancer many years ago, explained that most of his friends thought he had little time left, so they sent cards. Kenneth proved them wrong, but still appreciated the notes and other gifts his friends sent.

Many survivors reported finding new friends. Linda wrote about how she enlisted the support of other breast cancer survivors. She noted, "Online survivors helped me the most. You could rely on these ladies to tell it to you straight, even at 2:00 AM in your pajamas." Many other people wrote about how they received tremendous support from friends who had survived the same kind of cancer that they had. Dorinda commented, "Finding a networking group of other ovarian cancer survivors was incredibly helpful."

I often tell people that the absolute best thing you can do for a parent with children still at home is to do something kind for their kids. Dr. Rauch suggests not only appointing a Minister of Information, but also a "Captain of Kindness," one who is in charge of being kind to the children and encouraging other friends to ease their burden of having a parent with cancer. Parents wrote in about how meaningful it was to them when people were kind to their children and distracted them.

Jennifer explained how difficult it is to go through cancer treatment while trying to raise young children. She had a diagnosis of breast cancer in her thirties. For her, having young kids and caring for them was the worst part of the diagnosis: "I believe that if I hadn't had to care for them, I could have handled the chemotherapy and the breast cancer diagnosis much easier. I had to use all my energy on them because they needed me to be Mom, and I really tried. So when my friends took them, then I could just relax into oblivion."

Listening also proved to be one of the more meaningful things that a friend could do. Ric has been fighting cancer for many years. His friends continue to ask about his health and listen to him. Ric wrote, "Many of my friends have been willing to ask questions about my cancer and treatment. Their brave and loving gift means there is never an uncomfortable moment when they want to understand what is happening but are hesitant to ask. After twelve years of continuous treatment, I'm bored talking about my cancer. It would be easy to become silent about what is happening. Fortunately, my friends ask."

As you read this chapter, you will see that there are many meaningful ways that friends can help. If you have a friend who is going through cancer treatment and recovery, find out what will truly help her. Even if you live far away, reach out over the phone, Internet, or by mail. The survivors made it abundantly clear that the support and help their friends offered were invaluable.

• • •

OUR FRIENDS AND FAMILY did not ask what they could do to help us. They simply did things, knowing full well we would not ask for anything. They brought meals, picked up our children for events and outings, and many other small actions. It's a good thing they were thinking for us; we sure weren't. We were too focused on the prize of recovery.

Mike, management professional
Diagnosis of rectal cancer at age 38 in 2006 in Rochester, New York

• • •

THE MOST IMPORTANT THING I did was to give myself the ability to be strong. When I had melanoma, I was only twenty-one years old, a blond, blue-eyed sun worshipper. At the time, I fell apart about my cancer diagnosis. I cried and pouted. Later I looked back on the person I was and declared, "If I ever get cancer again, I will be stronger." Of course, maturity and age helped me be a stronger person the second time. For me, that meant I didn't fall apart when I was diagnosed. It was "Let's make a plan and get going." Waiting for the diagnosis was the worst part. But I did something special by saying to myself, "You can still be a strong woman and say yes to help and support." I've never been very good at saying I needed help; I was always the one who held everyone together. But I realized that I could be a strong woman and fight, and I could do it with the help of others. I let people bring food, clean my house, and take care of my family.

Deb, nurse practitioner
Diagnosis of melanoma (skin cancer) at age 21 in 1974 and breast cancer at age 52 in 2006 in Evansville, Indiana

• • •

ONE FRIEND PUT a big container with a lid on my back porch. Several people would pick up treats for me or the kids when they went to the store and then anonymously drop them off on their way home. It was always a treat for the kids to come home from school and find a favorite snack or drink.

Sherri, elementary school teacher
Diagnosis of endometrial (uterine) cancer at age 42 in 2004 in Bruceville, Indiana

> ## "It is amazing how getting the mail and seeing a card ...can make your day."

CARDS AND LETTERS from friends helped. It is amazing how getting the mail and seeing a card in the midst of all the bills can make your day.

Cathy, retail district manager
Diagnosis of pancreatic cancer at age 45 in 2005 in Columbus, Ohio

• • •

AT MY WIFE'S REQUEST, friends in our little hometown loaned us furniture and came over to set up a special bedroom for me when I came home from surgery in a greatly weakened condition.

Mike, retired real estate developer and cattle rancher
Diagnosis of colon cancer at age 66 in 2006 in Red Lodge, Montana

• • •

IT WAS LIKE the movie *It's a Wonderful Life.* People came out of the woodwork to help me—bringing by meals, loading up my freezer so I would eat, fighting over who was going to take me to chemo. Some would sit there crying because they couldn't stand seeing me hooked up to an IV. In my usual fashion, I would make everyone laugh. That's my style. I received hundreds of cards and gifts, especially from my friends at work. Angels, prayers, bears, gift certificates. It was unbelievable.

Myra, service representative, internal technical support
Diagnosis of breast cancer at age 52 in 2003 in Sharon, Massachusetts

• • •

MY FRIEND CAME OVER to my house one day and brought me a blanket. I had been going through cold spells, where my hands and feet were cold all the time. That blanket became my lifesaver. Every time I picked it up, I thought of my friend who was there for me. It was my comfort zone.

Rosi, student accounts office assistant
Diagnosis of colon cancer at age 52 in 2007 in Austin, Texas

WHEN MY ANNUAL LEAVE, sick leave, and help from the Family Medical Leave Act were exhausted, my coworkers donated some of their annual leave so I would not lose my health insurance. I initially resisted offers but agreed after I was told that I would do the same for them, and I realized the other side. I was stunned to learn that 540 hours were donated. I have had to use less than 150.

Linda, genealogy associate at a historical library
Diagnosis of breast cancer at age 59 in 2006 in Sulphur, Louisiana

• • •

PEOPLE WHO BROUGHT ME hope in one way or another. Telling me they were praying for me, giving me books about survivors, treating me as if I would live a long time! People who believed I would beat it and encouraged me to go on fighting even when I wanted to give up. I hated to let my cheerleaders (that's what I called them) down! So I would get up each day and try again and again and again.

Dee, retired
Diagnosis of colon and kidney cancer at age 53 in 2000 in Wood Dale, Illinois

• • •

I LIVE ABOUT 130 miles from Anchorage, Alaska, which is where the major hospitals are located. For surgery, chemotherapy, and follow-up, I had to drive to Anchorage from Seward once per week. My friend Jeff became my "Tuesday man," driving me and my boyfriend to the treatments each week for six months. I didn't have enough leave time at my job, and my coworkers donated hours to my account so that I could keep my job and have the time off.

Mollie, retired state employment office manager
Diagnosis of breast cancer at age 47 in 2004 in Seward, Alaska

• • •

I SENT THE WORD out with my Christmas card to virtually everyone I had known over the years. I heard back in some form or another from almost all of them. That was very uplifting.

Linda, administrative assistant
Diagnosis of breast cancer at age 55 in 2006 in Superior, Colorado

My friend, Trish Tobin, whom I hadn't even met at the time, called me every day and told me what to expect; how I would feel during and after a chemo treatment; how I would feel initially about the stark, bare chest on my left side; and what to do about breast reconstruction. Most important was that warm, intelligent voice on the telephone every day becoming my hard rock and my comforting cushion. I did eventually meet her, and we are now best of friends.

CARLY SIMON is a Grammy award–winning singer and breast cancer survivor. Her cancer was diagnosed in 1997. Perhaps best known for her number one hit song in 1973, "You're So Vain," she's never revealed who the song is about.

YOUR REAL FRIENDS WILL feel frustrated because they can't help fix your cancer. Realize that. Let them do something to help; they want to. It will help you and make them feel good because they are doing something.

Greg, disabled
Diagnosis of mantle cell lymphoma at age 57 in 2005 and acute myelogenous leukemia at age 60 in 2008 in Orland Park, Illinois

• • •

CHEERLEADER CALLS from my friend helped. He is sicker than me with amyloidosis.

James, retired police officer
Diagnosis of lymphoma at age 66 in 2007 in Sheridan, Wyoming

• • •

NOAH, MY OLD ENGLISH Sheep dog, offered me warmth when the chills were so bad. He checks up on me at every opportunity of the day and takes me for walks.

Kyle, pastor
Diagnosis of kidney cancer at age 60 in 2004 in Johnstown, Pennsylvania

FINDING A NETWORKING GROUP of other ovarian cancer survivors was incredibly helpful. I also had two female friends, Sharon and Nancy, who were especially helpful. They called, visited, invited me to dinner, and loaned me books to read. Every Sunday during treatment, Sharon brought me communion and prayed with me. It helped me feel connected with my faith community. Nancy's husband would also call my husband and see how he was doing and ask him to lunch.

Dorinda, retired teacher
Diagnosis of ovarian cancer at age 50 in 2005 in Edison, New Jersey

• • •

PEOPLE I HADN'T HEARD from for awhile sent me presents—huge, girlie treats at that! Pampering products and books to help me through the five months of treatment.

Pearl, nurse
Diagnosis of breast cancer at age 32 in 2004 in Glasgow (Scotland)

• • •

I LOVED IT WHEN friends took walks with me. I was not very disabled by my treatment, so I did not need much in the way of doing. Mostly, I needed (and got) the "being with me."

Cathi, clinical social worker
Diagnosis of breast cancer at age 52 in 2003 in Waban, Massachusetts

• • •

THE TEACHERS AT MY children's school pooled their money together and gave my family gift cards for food. When I had surgery, they gave me a gift card so that I could buy button-front shirts. The teachers took my children under their wing and made them feel loved; they had special lunches with them and allowed them the opportunity to cry and express their emotions. My son's Cub Scout troop picked days where someone was responsible for making my family a meal and dropping it off.

Shelly, program coordinator for adults with disabilities
Diagnosis of breast cancer at age 32 in 2004 in Concord, New Hampshire

I AM A BACHELOR and live with a whacked-out border collie, Skip. I have a wide group of friends whom I have gotten to know through running and cycling. Via e-mail and phone, I maintained contact with these friends who live literally coast-to-coast. A number of them are either cancer survivors or spouses of cancer survivors or victims. The support I received from these friends was vital in maintaining an "even keel." Without their support, the emotional and psychological burden of living with cancer would have been much greater. Several of them are very strong Christians, and the sharing of their faith was also a source of comfort and strength.

Bill, administrator
Diagnosis of prostate cancer at age 62 in 2007 in Jefferson, Wisconsin

• • •

UNFORTUNATELY, I NOW KNOW that there are so many young women, especially young mothers, who have been through what I went through. I was only twenty-eight years old when I was diagnosed, and I had no family history or risk factors. It was difficult for me to find women my age who had gone through what I was facing, so I felt very alone in that aspect. A coworker sent me a card each week without fail just to let me know that she was thinking about me and praying for my recovery. Opening the mailbox and seeing her card every week always brightened my day.

Sarah, paralegal
Diagnosis of breast cancer at age 28 in 2000 in Miami, Florida

• • •

PEOPLE VISITING ME at the hospital and at home surprised and pleased me.

Bill, retired
Diagnosis of colon and lung cancer at age 63 in 2004 in Niceville, Florida

• • •

ONE POSITIVE THING that came out of this whole cancer [experience] is that I now know for sure who my real friends are—who I can't count on and who is flaky.

Evelyn, executive assistant
Diagnosis of colon cancer at age 33 in 2004 in Boston, Massachusetts

A LOT OF PEOPLE brought meals when I was first diagnosed. But that almost became more than my family could handle because my poor dad, who was trying to manage my three brothers while my mom was staying with me for weeks at a time in the hospital, had to keep track of who brought dishes and how to return the pans afterwards. My brothers were picky anyway and didn't like others' home-cooked food. Lots of other people sent me stuffed animals and other items. To this day I still feel bad that I was not able to adequately thank people for thinking of me. I got so much stuff but was so sick that I really couldn't use any of it, and I wasn't able to write or send thank you notes. What I remember being most special, though, was when people took the time to come visit. Most people seemed to be scared of the hospital and of me and of perhaps saying the wrong thing, but there were a handful of people who took the time to visit me there, and I still clearly remember those visits.

Andrea, hospital administrator
Diagnosis of Ewing's sarcoma (a form of bone cancer) at age 15 in 1992 in Norfolk, Massachusetts

• • •

AT THIS TIME, I found out who my friends were and who were not my friends. I lost three important people in my life because of the cancer. Not one of them was there to support me emotionally, so I realized I was better off without them. I am not sure why they did what they did, but I cannot let it bother me. There were many others who stayed by my side.

> **"I now know for sure who my real friends are..."**

Debra, administrative assistant
Diagnosis of ovarian cancer at age 51 in 2007 in Chicago, Illinois

• • •

THE STUDENTS in the running club at the school where I taught decided to run in my honor in a fundraising event for the American Cancer Society. Later, they invited me to speak to their group about my experience.

Kathi, retired special education teacher
Diagnosis of breast cancer at age 49 in 2003 in Wrightstown, Wisconsin

IT WAS HARD DEALING with others' attitudes about my cancer. I found out who were friends. I noted that some people didn't contact me as often or did not return calls. That was hurtful, but I guess they were afraid. It is difficult because there are not many liver cancer survivors. I would love to talk with some and I have been looking, but it's a really small group.

Iris, artist
Diagnosis of liver cancer at age 50 in 2007 in Sante Fe, New Mexico

• • •

ONE FRIEND ORGANIZED a blood drive on my behalf. Others gave blood or platelets at the hospital. They made sure to keep in touch with my husband without driving him crazy with phone calls.

Eileen, technology specialist
Diagnosis of breast cancer at age 34 in 1984, acute myelogenous leukemia at age 49 in 1999, and basal cell carcinoma (skin cancer) at age 55 in 2005 in Framingham, Massachusetts

• • •

"One friend organized a blood drive on my behalf. Others gave blood or platelets at the hospital."

PRAYERS FROM CONCERNED FRIENDS are always so special and comforting.

Charose, nurse
Diagnosis of Hodgkin disease at age 17 in 1972 and breast cancer at age 51 in 2006 in Omaha, Nebraska

• • •

WHEN LEAVING THE COUNTRY for a vacation that was already scheduled, I was surrounded by some family and friends who helped me celebrate life before the ten months of "hell" began.

Sheri, actress
Diagnosis of Hodgkin disease at age 29 in 1993 in Columbia, Maryland

MY BOYFRIEND WAS THERE throughout the whole ordeal and always reminded me to think positively—to know that he loved me always, and to be tough. One day, I was very, very sad and sick, crying, and having a bad time. He stood me in front of the mirror and told me to raise my arms and make fists. I was tough...be a tuffy! Afterwards, I felt better, and it made me laugh. He always tried to find ways to make me laugh.

Mollie, retired state employment office manager
Diagnosis of breast cancer at age 47 in 2004 in Seward, Alaska

• • •

I HAD A NETWORK of close friends who immediately came to my aid and were always there for me during the treatment process. My immediate family (parents and siblings) were not any help, nor was my husband. My two close friends went to every chemo treatment with me, including one at 4:00 AM. It was almost an all-day ordeal. One would take the morning shift, and the other would take the evening shift. We really had a great time, talking and doing jigsaw puzzles, anything to distract me. They would check up on me during the days after the treatment. One would send me a card every week. Other friends would call or send cards. I received over one hundred cards. One of the close friends had a round robin dinner list in which dinners were brought to my family weekly while I was having chemotherapy (which lasted from May–September). Anything I needed my friends provided. They were a godsend. After all chemo was completed, we had a party to celebrate and invited all my friends. It was really neat!

Joyce, educational assistant at an elementary school
Diagnosis of breast cancer at 41 in 1995 in Knoxville, Tennessee

Don't be afraid to ask for the help you need, whether it is an errand or a hand to hold—your friends and family really do want to help in any way they can.

SUSAN PORIES, MD, FACS, is a breast surgical oncologist and assistant professor at Harvard Medical School. She is the co-editor of the book *The Soul of a Doctor*, a collection of stories about young Harvard doctors-in-training.

MY TWO BEST FRIENDS helped me the most. They were there to listen to my concerns. Even if I drove them crazy with all my whining, they still accepted me for who I am and what I was going through. God love them.

Vera, personal assistant
Diagnosis of thyroid cancer at age 51 in 2002 in Milwaukee, Wisconsin

• • •

I HAD TWO FRIENDS, and we all kept our sense of humor, which was invaluable. Both assured me that if one in three* women would be touched by breast cancer, they were thankful I was the one.

Ruthanne, bookkeeper
Diagnosis of breast cancer at age 51 in 1995 in Thorne Bay, Alaska
*Actual estimate is now one in eight.

• • •

MY SYNAGOGUE ARRANGED for people to bring dinner to our house three times a week for many weeks following my surgical procedures. Members of our synagogue community, as well as other friends and neighbors, contacted a central person so that we did not have to personally be bothered with making the arrangements. It allowed me to see lots of people as they dropped off meals. Our family ate home-cooked, wonderful meals, and my husband and I did not have to think about shopping, cooking, or planning meals.

Janet, elementary school teacher
Diagnosis of colon cancer at age 42 in 1993 in Philadelphia, Pennsylvania

• • •

I HAD A DEAR FRIEND come and visit me at the hospital after my first mastectomy, and he brought me a gift. The gift was a "Hooters" T-shirt and job application. I know it sounds terrible, but it was the best moment because it allowed me to laugh in the face of such seriousness. And when all of my surgical procedures (five +) were completed, we celebrated at "Hooters" in Hollywood. It was perfect.

Julie, real estate agent
Diagnosis of thyroid cancer at age 34 in 1996 and breast cancer at age 43 in 2005 in Torrance, California

FRIENDS THAT I HADN'T seen in years seemed to appear in the unlikeliest places to offer their support or share their own experiences with their cancer and offer hope. I consider this a blessing from God.

Nancy, administrative assistant
Diagnosis of breast cancer at age 54 in 2006 in Fowlerville, Michigan

From the moment my cancer was diagnosed, I was touched by the outpouring of support from survivors. Women close to me and others who were friends of friends reached out to offer advice. I spent countless hours on the phone with various women talking about what I could expect in my own cancer journey. Truthfully, I don't know how I would have gotten through treatment without their expert tips. For example, a survivor warned me that one of my cancer drugs would be bright red and would be delivered via a syringe instead of a drip bag. Having that information ahead of time made that experience less frightening. The generosity and kindness of those survivors prompted me to go public with my experience, both on television and through the Internet. Information is power and, at a time of utter powerlessness, we all need someone to show us the way.

KELLEY TUTHILL, a reporter for WCVB TV in Boston, received a diagnosis of breast cancer at age 36 in 2006.

MY DEAR FRIEND BROUGHT me a "laughing stick." It was silly, but really helped me keep my sense of humor.

Cynthia, administrative assistant
Diagnosis of breast cancer at age 55 in 2003 in Highland Lakes, New Jersey

ONE OF MY CLOSEST friends encouraged me to think positively and to say a mantra during radiation treatment to will my cancer out of my body. I did this religiously!

Bryna, management development consultant
Diagnosis of tongue cancer at age 35 in 1985 in Brockton, Massachusetts

• • •

"My dear friend brought me a 'laughing stick.' It was silly, but really helped me keep my sense of humor."

VISITING ME in the hospital—it showed they cared.

Andrew, self-employed
Diagnosis of non-Hodgkin lymphoma at age 45 in 2005 in Greater Manchester, Cheshire (United Kingdom)

• • •

I REALLY APPRECIATED PEOPLE who called and treated me like normal. It may sound odd, but those who could joke and laugh with me about the cancer made it better. One friend called and said, "I was having a silly pity-party for myself and thought, 'Who can I call who has a worse life than I do right now?' And, immediately, I thought of you." I roared and laughed so hard it hurt. We are good friends, and just the way she said it confirmed that I was still very much alive.

Carmela, technical writer
Diagnosis of endometrial (uterine), bladder, and ovarian cancer at age 48 in 2005 in Clinton Township, Michigan

• • •

THE MEMBERS of my Sunday School class prepared a basket of small gifts, each one containing a familiar and encouraging scripture verse.

Barbara, homemaker
Diagnosis of breast cancer at age 38 in 1986 in Conway, Arkansas

MY CHURCH FAMILY MEMBERS were all there for me. For nine days following my surgery, a different family provided my meal, and each family brought enough for more than one meal. They also prayed for me before and after my surgery and following chemotherapy. I wouldn't have made it through without their concern and support.

Glenda, disabled
Diagnosis of ovarian cancer at age 60 in 2004 in Chanute, Kansas

• • •

I THINK THAT ALL the words of encouragement that were offered, not only to me but to my husband, were the most precious to our family. Sure, I had to deal with cancer, but my husband had to deal with me *and* the cancer. I truly am thankful for all the kindnesses he received.

Dorothy, receptionist
Diagnosis of breast cancer at age 44 in 2005 in Chesapeake, Virginia

I think a person with cancer needs to seek out support from friends and family. I had a group of people there to listen to me, cheer me on, and remind me I wasn't alone. I always felt that other people were invested in my survival. You can't overestimate the benefit of that kind of support and friendship.

LANCE ARMSTRONG received a diagnosis of advanced testicular cancer at age 25 in 1996. Just over three years later, he went on to win the Tour de France.

SOME FRIENDS GAVE ME a $300 gift certificate to a place where you can choose from several restaurants to call, and each delivers the food to you.

April, disabled
Diagnosis of breast cancer at age 34 in 1999 in Wichita, Kansas

PEOPLE FROM MY OFFICE went to Costco and stocked my home with at least six months of needed staples (bathroom tissue, paper towels, etc).

Maureen, manager
Diagnosis of breast cancer at age 40 in 2004 in Camarillo, California

• • •

A COUPLE OF SPECIAL family friends went to outrageous lengths to organize an unbelievable fundraiser for me that consisted of a "casino night" with donated prizes from dozens of area merchants. My wife's karate school held a well-publicized blood drive in their parking lot, which drew impressive numbers of donors and just plain well-wishers who all signed a big get-well banner for me. They also cooked meals for my family, so my wife could spend more time at the hospital. My wife's colleagues, recognizing there was no way she would be able to concentrate at work, donated their own paid time off so she would not have to work. I was coaching city rec-league basketball at the time of my illness, and my team signed a basketball and presented it to me. I still display it proudly. In the initial six weeks I spent in the hospital, I received over one hundred cards. I treasure them all. Well wishes are always appreciated, but I am especially grateful for those who backed them up with deeds that helped my family cope with the difficulty of having their husband/dad in cancer treatment—to all those who offered diversions for my kids, who spent time with my wife, and cooked for my family. Situations such as mine make it easy to recognize your true friends.

Jerry, computer software instructor
Diagnosis of acute myelogenous leukemia at age 43 in 2003 in Anoka, Minnesota

• • •

A GROUP OF GIRLFRIENDS and I went to see *Menopause the Musical*. We got up on stage when the audience was invited to join the cast doing high kicks at the end of the show. It was so relaxing to laugh and share a normal experience with my friends.

Barbara, nurse
Diagnosis of breast cancer at age 58 in 1995 in Stoneham, Massachusetts

IN ADDITION TO MY extraordinary spouse, I chose to share my cancer diagnosis only with four very special women: two had gone through cancer; the third was my best and most pragmatic, realistic friend; and the fourth was my boss who provided me with the most amazing support so I could continue to work.

Robin, college professor
Diagnosis of breast cancer at age 50 in 2006 in Costa Mesa, California

• • •

MY HAIRDRESSER and the company she works for gave me one of the nicest gifts. I went in for a haircut with my daughter, and they presented me with a bouquet of flowers and gave both of us a free haircut and manicure.

Cindy, staffing specialist
Diagnosis of cervical cancer at age 32 in 1989 and colorectal cancer at age 48 in 2005 in Maryville, North Dakota

• • •

MY GIRLFRIEND CAME to the hospital and shaved my legs and gave me a pedicure! Only a woman can appreciate how much better that made me feel.

Judy, retired accounting clerk
Diagnosis of lung cancer at age 64 in 2004 in Norwalk, California

• • •

MY BEST FRIEND HAD been diagnosed at exactly the same age, and she became a great support system for me.

Cheryl, homemaker
Diagnosis of breast cancer at age 49 in 2006 in Garland, Texas

"My girlfriend came to the hospital and shaved my legs and gave me a pedicure! Only a woman can appreciate how much better that made me feel."

MY BUSINESS FRIENDS through my Rotary Club were great.

Karen, real estate broker
Diagnosis of breast cancer at age 38 in 2001 in Loganville, Georgia

My spirit and my will to survive helped me the most. I was so determined to beat this disease, and I was definitely not ready to leave my family. Also, the incredible outpouring of support from friends and people I didn't even know helped me so much. I received many get well cards and letters, and I kept every one of them. They're so special to me.

SHARON OSBOURNE met rock star Ozzy Osbourne when she was 17 years old. She received a diagnosis of colon cancer at age 49 in 2002.

INITIALLY, THERE ARE a lot of people around. Lots of food, friends, flowers, noise. Once people think you're okay, it stops. That was very difficult.

Laura, unemployed psychiatric social worker
Diagnosis of breast cancer at age 43 in 2006 in Avon, Connecticut

• • •

A GOOD FRIEND COMMITTED one day a month to whatever I needed.

Judy, chaplain
Diagnosis of colorectal cancer at age 48 in 2003 in Cudahy, Wisconsin

• • •

MY FRIENDS VISITED WHEN I was recovering from my surgery. The most touching part for me was that a group of my girlfriends said they would all shave their heads with me if I needed to have chemotherapy.

Jennifer, publicity coordinator
Diagnosis of melanoma (skin cancer) at age 21 in 2004 in San Diego, California

VERY CLOSE FRIENDS STOOD by me throughout the mastectomy and breast reconstruction surgeries. My husband had left me, and my friends stepped up to the plate along with my two sisters. They saw me through all of it, and they were wonderful. I could never begin to repay them for all they did for me.

Polly, human resource administrator
Diagnosis of breast cancer at age 54 in 2005 in Port Gibson, Mississippi

• • •

MY FRIEND ADAM is one of my angels. Adam and I had not been friends for very long, but when he learned I would be having my bone marrow transplant in Boston, he told me that he would visit me every day. Adam was a nurse in a nearby hospital, and he did keep his word. During the eleven weeks I was hospitalized, he was at the hospital just about every single day to visit me. He missed one day because he thought he was getting a cold, and he felt so guilty over that. He was an incredible source of comfort, and our friendship is much stronger because of it.

Todd, oncology social worker
Diagnosis of chronic myelogenous leukemia at age 25 in 1997 and kidney cancer at age 33 in 2005 in Warwick, Rhode Island

• • •

"GRANDMA" TYPES OF FRIENDS came over to love on my children and read to them, and other people played more energetically with them than I was able to. That meant so much to me!

Laura, stay-at-home mom
Diagnosis of breast cancer at age 31 in 2006 in Hope Mills, North Carolina

"Initially, there are a lot of people around. Lots of food, friends, flowers, noise. Once people think you're okay, it stops. That was very difficult."

I OPENED UP RIGHT away and started to tell friends. Talking to people made me less afraid, and my openness made people less afraid to talk to me. The process made people treat me like me, rather than me with cancer. I could not have stood for that. I felt like I had a whole city—from work, to softball leagues, to football leagues, to my running buddy—many hands holding me up and tickling me along the way.

Jennifer, federal officer with U.S. Customs and Border Patrol
Diagnosis of cervical cancer at age 36 in 2007 in Montreal, Quebec (Canada)

• • •

> "…letting me know they were praying, asking if we needed anything. That kind of support is the best."

MY FRIEND, NANCY, LET me express my feelings as long and as often as I wanted to. One day, she met me in a parking lot and took me for a short walk. We ended up at my pastor's house. It was a good place to be.

Judi, nurse
Diagnosis of breast cancer at age 40 in 2000 in Pen Argyl, Pennsylvania

• • •

SIMPLE CALLS, LETTING ME know they were praying, asking if we needed anything. That kind of support is the best.

Candy, teacher
Diagnosis of thyroid cancer at age 31 in 2007 in El Paso, Texas.

• • •

MY HUSBAND HAS BEEN in prison since 2003, so my friend Rafael helped me. He paid my mortgage, read books to me, called me, and taught me more about my faith. He gave me the gift of time.

Alejandra, clerical worker
Diagnosis of uterine cancer at age 36 in 2005 in Torrance, California

THERE WAS A MAN who was not a close friend, but he called me every day and came to see me just to see if I had everything I needed. Every time I saw him, and even now, he hugs me and asks about my health.

John, retired
Diagnosis of esophageal cancer at age 76 in 2006 in Jamestown, North Carolina

One of the things I hear most often from survivors is how comforting it is to know that you are not alone on this journey. Whether it is a reassuring hug from a loved one on a particularly rough day, a healthy meal delivered to your dinner table by a thoughtful neighbor, or the advice and encouragement from another cancer survivor who has been where you are, those simple human connections can lessen the burden of coping with cancer.

LAURA SHIPP is the editor of *Coping with Cancer Magazine*.

References

Rauch, P. K., and A. C. Muriel. 2005. *Raising an emotionally healthy child when a parent is sick.* New York: McGraw-Hill.

Rodgers, J. 2001. *Bald in the land of big hair.* New York: HarperCollins (First Perennial edition published 2002).

5 Things To Do
for a Friend Who Lives Near You

1. **Give your friend a foot massage.** Often during treatment your body hurts. Sometimes a lot. At the same time, people may be afraid to touch you and you may feel isolated. Having someone gently massage your feet can feel heavenly. However, not everyone will be comfortable with this, so ask first. You can bring soaps, oils, and lotions along to make it even more special.

2. **Read a book or a story out loud.** As children, we loved to be read to, but at some point we grew up and no one reads to us anymore. Reading to someone evokes many nurturing memories and is highly entertaining. Be sure and pick a book or story that your friend will enjoy. Focus on something with a positive message— not too scary or too upsetting.

3. **Sit with your friend at chemotherapy or radiation or any other appointments.** Cancer makes people lonely, and it's great to have someone who cares to tag along and just offer gentle support.

4. **Bring him or her "affordable luxuries."** I like this phrase, which marketing folks use to describe things like a cup of Starbuck's coffee. Little luxuries go a long way, but don't cost a lot.

5. **Make a scrapbook.** Your friend may not be up to recording the events happening now. Step in and take pictures of his or her kids and anything else that is going on. Then, turn this into a scrapbook. If you take pictures of your friend, ask if it's okay to include them in the scrapbook. Some people don't want reminders of when they were bald, etc.

5 Things To Do
for a Long-Distance Friend

1. **Arrange for dinner to be delivered from a favorite restaurant.** Casseroles are great, and there may be neighbors pitching in with meals. However, even from a distance, you can offer a real treat by having favorite foods delivered to the door.

2. **Send him or her comfortable and stylish loungewear.** Most people consider this a luxury and often don't have really comfortable and nice clothing for wearing around the house. Now is when your friend may really appreciate something beautifully feminine or stylishly handsome and comfortable to wear.

3. **Send something great to eat.** Some Web sites offer fruit bouquets that are gorgeous and healthful with plenty of antioxidants.

4. **Send a book, CD, DVD, or magazine subscription.** Entertain your friend from afar. It's lonely and boring to go through cancer treatment. Your friend will appreciate a little diversion.

5. **Send something that is "regionally authentic" from where you live.** For example, if you live in Boston and the Red Sox are doing well, send a Red Sox hat and encourage your friend to cheer with you for your team.

CHAPTER 4

· · ·

Care and Support from the Health Care Team

In his book *Complications*, Harvard neurosurgeon Atul Gawande writes about the "practice" of medicine and how it is far less perfect than those who are ill hope for: "We look for medicine to be an orderly field of knowledge and procedure. But it is not. It is an imperfect science, an enterprise of constantly changing knowledge, uncertain information, fallible individuals and, at the same time, lives on the line. There is science in what we do, yes, but also habit, intuition, and sometimes plain old guessing. The gap between what we know and what we aim for persists. And this gap complicates everything we do" (Gawande 2002, 7).

So often my patients want more science and less uncertainty. Even though they deserve this, it's often hard to give them what they want. In the surveys for this book, I asked cancer survivors what their health care team did that really made a difference. This is an important question and one that all of us in medicine should be thinking about.

I hope that people who read this book will share this chapter with their medical team. Those of us who work in oncology need to hear more about what we are doing right and what we can be doing better. The answers survey participants gave about their medical care, not surprisingly, spanned the continuum from being extremely pleased and grateful to being quite angry and resentful.

Because this book is designed to focus on hope and healing, I specifically chose responses that highlighted what helped people the most. However, though the purpose in conducting these surveys was to provide cancer survivors with positive insights from those who have traveled this road, I am loathe to create a book that is Pollyannaish in its content—filled with nothing but positive information that doesn't reflect the real experiences of those who have cancer.

Therefore, I have included comments from survivors about what went wrong and what their health care team could have done to help them more.

Pat, a breast cancer survivor, wanted more information about the possible side effects of treatment. Many people wrote comments similar to those of Pat who said, "I think that doctors sometimes downplay the seriousness of the possible side effects of treatment. In my case, I developed chemo-induced heart failure. Would it have made a difference in my [treatment] decision? Probably not. But that diagnosis would have been easier to take had I known that it was possible, rather than being told that 'sometimes [chemotherapy] affects the heart slightly'."

Many people wrote that although their doctors were honest with them and initiated frank discussions, those conversations were difficult to understand, either because the physician presented too much information or because it was offered in an overly complicated manner. Cancer survivors often wanted to hear the statistics, but they wanted them presented in a manner that was kind, compassionate, and hopeful rather than cold, calculating, and depressing. Some people, like breast cancer survivor Kelley, had advice for oncology health professionals. Kelley advised doctors not to use the term "mortality rate."

When I talk with cancer survivors, there are recurring themes that come up—themes that also occurred in these surveys, and I think they are very important for new cancer patients to consider. Some of the themes highlighted in this chapter include experiences related to cancer staging, second opinions, and optimal healing.

The idea of accepting a "new normal" is also a recurring theme in oncology. Once someone undergoes treatment for cancer, there is no going back to a life that does not include this experience, both physically and emotionally. However, what I find in my clinical practice is that people often don't heal optimally and therefore accept more pain, fatigue, and disability than they should.

Helping survivors achieve optimal physical and emotional recovery is a major focus of my work and an incredibly important topic in cancer care. I have written several books on how to achieve optimal recovery, including *After Cancer Treatment: Heal Faster, Better, Stronger* and *Super Healing*. Recently, in fact, there has been a shift in focus in oncology to address survivorship issues as they pertain to recovery and living with the best future health possible. A recent report aptly titled "From Cancer Patient to Cancer Survivor: Lost in Transition" revealed serious problems in the health care offered to cancer survivors after treatment and made recommendations on how to improve care, including making survivorship a distinct phase of cancer treatment (Hewitt, Greenfield, and Stovall 2006).

In my office, I often hear people say how much more help they need in order to heal optimally. It would be ideal if every cancer center in the world had a survivorship center with extensive rehabilitation services. In our survey, Charose, a nurse who survived both Hodgkin disease and breast cancer, explained how focusing on physical healing improved her care: "The one thing that especially helped with the recovery after breast surgery and reconstruction was physical therapy with an excellent team that was specifically experienced with that. It made a dramatic difference with my pain and flexibility."

If you are a cancer survivor and feel that you haven't healed optimally, talk to your doctors and health care team about what might help you to recover as fully as possible. Ask them about a survivorship plan for you that ideally will include information to help you—now and in the future.

The Kindness of Strangers

People who choose to go into the field of oncology are often exceptionally kind and empathic. Survivors shared comments that revealed just how wonderful some of these folks are. Elena, whom I mentioned in the last chapter, had a diagnosis of inflammatory breast cancer. She wrote, "The infusion nursing team at my hospital have all become my dear friends (I have gone there weekly for the past four years.) In some ways, they know me better than my 'regular' friends. I can be more real and honest with them, and they have more understanding of my life with cancer than do my friends and family. I have learned that I have strengths that I never thought I had before—that I could get through the worst possible treatments and the losses of so much of my body that made me who I am, yet still survive and live a quality life."

Matt, whose brother was a bone marrow match for him after his diagnosis of chronic lymphocytic leukemia, described how sick he was after the transplant and how kind his nurses were to him and to others who came after him. He wrote, "I spent fifteen days in the hospital during the transplant. When we left, my wife gave the staff a little photo album she had made for them. It included photos of me and my donor brother, before, during, and after treatment. Not a big deal, but nice. A couple of years later, I was talking to my nurse there, and she revealed how the staff had kept that album and showed it to incoming patients, because it illustrated the steps a patient goes through and shows a guy who made it through. That was the nicest thing about the whole experience for me—that album helped ease some other person's fears."

The year after I finished medical school, I distinctly recall one of many "miracles" I have had the privilege to witness as a physician. I was working as an intern in the intensive care unit when a man (whom I'll call John) was admitted. He was extremely ill and had a rare infection—one the doctors in the intensive care unit did not think he'd survive. The physician in charge told John's wife to call anyone who might want to say goodbye to him. Family flew in from all parts of the United States to visit with John one last time. These were somber visits filled with grief over the presumed loss of a vital man in his fifties, a loving father and husband.

But the doctors were wrong. John survived. And within two weeks, he was walking around the hospital corridors, teasing the nurses and laughing about how the doctors didn't know what they were talking about.

Statistically speaking, John shouldn't have made it. The odds were so overwhelmingly against him that it truly was a miraculous recovery. I have often pondered this experience and wondered what the medical team should have told the family. Should they have given them more hope? Was it his family flying in from all over that saved him? Was this a miracle or just a case of doctors misjudging the situation or not knowing enough to predict its outcome?

Nowhere is the question of what to tell patients more important than in oncology. Of course, doctors and other health care providers are often swayed to reveal more (or less), depending on how many questions and what kind of questions patients ask. Studies show that youth, affluence, and higher education of the paient may play a role in doctors sharing more information—not necessarily as a direct result of these characteristics, but because of the fact that these qualities might be associated with people who are more assertive about asking questions. Oncology health care providers should certainly pay attention to the fact that nearly all patients want information, but some will be better at eliciting the information than others. Thus, when faced with a patient who is not asking specific questions, how much information to give is left up to the physician. The cancer survivors who shared their stories for this book had a lot to say about what their doctors should—and shouldn't—have told them.

Many people also wrote about how support groups and Internet Web sites and chat rooms were invaluable to them. Don, who had prostate cancer in his seventies, wrote, "What helped me was the Wellness Community support groups and writing poetry."

Others wrote that they tried going to a support group but didn't find it helpful, and some participants said that they didn't try that avenue because they had other sources of support. There is no right way to deal with a cancer diagnosis and its ensuing emotional turmoil; however, it's fascinating to read how people handled this experience and what helped them.

Long-time cancer survivors pointed out that there were far fewer resources available when they were diagnosed. The Internet didn't exist, there were not nearly as many support groups as there are presently, and there was often a stigma associated with cancer that did not encourage open dialogue and support. Many people were afraid to talk about it.

A Cure for Cancer

Evelyn, an executive assistant who dealt with late-stage colon cancer in her early thirties, summed up what a lot of us wished our doctors had said: "I wish my doctor had told me that he had finally found a cure for cancer."

Evelyn was not the only one who wanted to hear what will likely be true in the future—that a cure for cancer has been discovered. Though eliminating cancer altogether would be ideal (and is certainly a goal for the future), many cancer survivors would be happy just to know that the treatment they received produced a cure, and they don't have to worry about cancer anymore.

In reading the official history of the American Cancer Society published in 1987, I came across a chapter entitled "Halfway to Victory." This chapter stated, "At the present time, for all serious tumors…the relative survival rate of U.S. cancer patients for five years after diagnosis is 49 percent…In other words, American biomedical science and medicine are about halfway to the goal of controlling cancer in human beings."

Since 1987, there has been remarkable progress, but there is still much work to be done in order to "cure" cancer. Our survey participants certainly understood this, but many of them wrote about how they wished that the future was already here and that cancer was no longer something we needed to worry about. While we aren't there yet, there is reason to have hope for the future.

Keep reading and you'll hear some amazing stories about how the kindness of health care providers and other networks of support made an enormous impact on many cancer survivors as they were undergoing treatment.

• • •

THERE IS ALWAYS HOPE, and that hope is sometimes changing. It means something different for each person in any given situation. When one doctor tells you there is nothing more that can be done, he is merely saying that he has exhausted his expertise. The next oncologist may have more up his sleeve. Hope may come in the second, third, or fourth opinion, or totally evolve into a different form.

Suzanne, wife and mother
Diagnosis of colon cancer at age 31 in 1998 in Canton, Texas

• • •

I WAS THREE MONTHS pregnant with my first child. My family and friends were so supportive as were my obstetrician and urologist. During my surgery, I was awake because of the pregnancy. This terrified me, as everyone was unsure if the baby would survive, or if I would hemorrhage, etc. My obstetrician rushed in to hold my hand and tell jokes during my surgery. It really meant the world to me.

Nancy, office manager
Diagnosis of bladder cancer at age 25 in 1997 in Levittown, New York

• • •

BONNIE, THE WIG FAIRY. She was so kind. She shaved my head for the first time and gave me samples. She also taught me how to put on makeup. I did not know her before but became very close to her.

Mary, business assistant
Diagnosis of synovial sarcoma of the right forearm at age 44 in 2006 in McPherson, Kansas

ONE PERSON WHO HELPED me very much and may not even know it was the social worker at the cancer clinic where I am currently being treated. When my metastasis was first diagnosed, I was (of course) devastated. I cried every evening for weeks. My poor husband, who was grieving as well, listened every night as I talked about my feelings of fear, anger, grief, and wondering how the world would be without me in it. I went to this social worker, Jim, because I needed someone else to talk to besides my poor, weary husband. Jim greeted me with a question: "Why are you here, and how can I help you?" Tears welled up immediately. I hardly knew where to start to answer his questions. He suggested that I begin by giving my history. Ha! That was easy! I dropped into my "nurse language" as I clipped off the case presentation on myself. Not far into it, Jim stopped me. "You have used the word 'yet' three times already. Why are you using that word?" I didn't even realize I had done that. "Tell me what I said when I used that word," I countered. Jim said I had told him that I had had a brain scan and didn't have brain mets "yet." I also told him that I had not had to quit my job "yet." I don't remember what the other "yet" was. Jim suggested that I stop the sentence before using the word yet. I tried it, and it sounded so much better: "I don't have brain metastasis." See how much more positive that is? Jim taught me something I already knew, but was failing to act on. I should live in the present moment and not worry about what hasn't happened and may never happen. Jim taught me to stop the negative thought pattern I had developed. My depression lifted almost immediately! Not that I am not sad anymore. Quite the contrary. This business of living with cancer is not pretty. But it is so much more comfortable to be happy rather than sad most of the time. Jim made me realize that. God bless him.

Sandra, assistant professor of nursing
Diagnosis of breast cancer at age 54 in 2002 in Atlanta, Georgia

• • •

I WISH I HAD KNOWN to start developing partnerships with the best experts in the best teaching hospital in our region at the beginning of the journey. I also wish I had known that it is appropriate and reasonable to go anywhere in the country (or the world) to work with those few physicians specializing in my cancer.

Ric, public relations director
Diagnosis of thyroid cancer at age 50 in 1995 in Londonderry, New Hampshire

I WISH THAT the various doctors I saw in the first couple of years had had a consistent approach. The one who diagnosed my CLL [chronic lymphocytic leukemia] was a professor of internal medicine, not a hematologist. He told me that he knew of CLL patients who had lived for twenty years, taking a couple of pills a day. Another, a professor of oncology in the United Kingdom, told me when I was sixty-five and still untreated, that I should make my "biblical three-score-and-ten years all right." Yet another took a reference book from the drawer of his desk and told me that, on average, I had a life expectancy of one hundred and nine months. Only one specialist told me what I should have been told, and that was this: "CLL is a very variable disease, and patients respond very differently to treatments. I am not going to play God by making predictions of how long you will live, because the variations are enormous. You might live for five years, or you might live for fifteen or twenty years, and you might die of something else or fall under a bus!"

Colin, writer and author
Diagnosis of chronic lymphocytic leukemia at age 62 in 1998 in Roma (Italy)

• • •

THE SURGEON'S NURSE...she took the time to listen to the emotion embedded in my words. She would ask, "How are you doing?" And she did not let my answer alone tell her how I was doing. She read the emotion behind my words.

Bill, administrator
Diagnosis of prostate cancer at age 62 in 2007 in Jefferson, Wisconsin

And to my doctor:
Let evidence of
The worth of your efforts
Be in the life I live.

This Haiku was written by **SUSAN VREELAND**, a former English teacher—turned *New York Times* bestselling novelist. She is the author of *Girl in Hyacinth Blue* and *Luncheon of the Boating Party*. Susan received a diagnosis of lymphoma at age 50 in 1996.

WHEN I WAS VERY, very sick and wanted to discuss the possibility of my death, my mother refused to allow the discussion. I wish my doctor had intervened on my behalf to explain to her that although it is very difficult to discuss this with your son, it is important to him, so try to be strong and allow him to process his feelings surrounding this issue. When I was having my bone marrow transplant, there were many things that plagued me. One was that I often had difficulty sleeping at night, and it would drive me nuts. There was a night nurse who would wrap me up like a mummy (I was immunocompromised) and wheel me down to the nursery, sometimes at one or two o'clock in the morning. I don't know how she knew it would calm me and put me at peace, but seeing those newborns did it every time.

Todd, oncology social worker
Diagnosis of chronic myelogenous leukemia at age 25 in 1997 and kidney cancer at age 33 in 2005 in Warwick, Rhode Island

• • •

I WISH MY DOCTOR could have told me more about what to expect in the future and how long the remission I am currently enjoying might last.

Eileen, retired registered nurse
Diagnosis of endometrial (uterine) cancer at age 64 in 2006 in Charlotte, North Carolina

• • •

I HAVE HAD the good fortune to have a fabulous oncologist who told me—and continues to tell me—everything as I need to know it. I am very lucky that way.

Cathi, clinical social worker
Diagnosis of breast cancer at age 52 in 2003 in Waban, Massachusetts

• • •

ONE NURSE CAME into my room and, after hearing my story, prayed with and for me. That was truly an experience I will never forget. The presence of God was felt in the room!

Celestine, property manager
Diagnosis of stomach cancer at age 45 in 2006 in Rosedale, Maryland

THE FIRST THING I realized after my diagnosis was that I needed help: help with decision-making about treatment (lumpectomy, mastectomy, reconstruction); how to help my two sons—I had never been a teenager whose parent had cancer; how to help my husband—he was great, but he needed a break from hearing about everything and, of course, there were issues I did not want to discuss with him, such as body image. So the best thing I did was get an appointment with a clinical psychologist who specialized in coping with medical issues. She was such a big help to me. She helped me realize that my feelings were normal. She gave me suggestions on how to cope by using imagery, for example, and how to help my children and husband. I think it should be mandatory that every cancer patient make at least one visit to a mental health provider.

Peggy, pathologist's assistant
Diagnosis of breast cancer at age 47 in 2003 in St. Augustine, Florida

• • •

I HAVE AN AMAZING oncologist. She answered every question I had, plus some I didn't think to ask, and was always concerned and involved in my treatment and recovery.

Sarah, paralegal
Diagnosis of breast cancer at age 28 in 2000 in Miami, Florida

• • •

MY DOCTORS WERE PRETTY upfront with me. I do think they downplayed the potential side effects of treatment—probably so as not to scare or worry me. But I felt it was worse not to know what was happening. All the unknowns became major issues until I learned what was really happening.

Linda, retired
Diagnosis of breast cancer at age 54 in 2003 in Placentia, California

> "I think it should be mandatory that every cancer patient make at least one visit to a mental health provider."

OTHER KIDS WITH CANCER helped me the most. The hospital was great about pairing me as a roommate with other teenage girls being treated with cancer. Usually, they were a few cycles ahead of me. It was so incredibly helpful and heart-lifting to talk with them about shared experiences. At a time when you feel like you are the only person who understands the pain and fatigue you're going through, it is so important to be able to talk with and learn from others who are experiencing the exact same things!

Andrea, hospital administrator
Diagnosis of Ewing's sarcoma (a form of bone cancer) at age 15 in 1992 in Norfolk, Massachusetts

• • •

MY HEALTH INSURANCE CARRIER had declined providing treatment that would have been in my best interest. It was "out of plan," and they believed surgery would be the best way for me. I disagreed and asked them to reconsider, and they did allow treatment out of plan. I am so thankful that my doctor in my hometown fully encouraged me to go out of town for a new treatment. That was truly a blessing.

Laura, housecleaner
Diagnosis of esophageal cancer at age 45 in 2002 in Schenectady, New York

• • •

I FOUND COMPETENT, SUCCESSFUL, aggressive medical professionals who were willing to work hard with me in being aggressive in our approach to the cancer. The chemo treatment team was upbeat and just great to be with in a very difficult time.

David, journeyman sheet metal worker
Diagnosis of breast cancer at age 63 in 2005 in Missoula, Montana

• • •

I KEPT FOCUSING on getting better and being able to live to raise my seven-year-old daughter despite of being told by the doctors that I had six months to live.

Beth, health educator
Diagnosis of liver cancer at age 32 in 1990 in Fort Hood, Texas

I JOINED A SUPPORT group at the hospital where I was treated. It was very supportive. We also developed our own group after that one ended.

Julie, account executive in advertising/marketing
Diagnosis of laryngeal cancer at age 46 in 2002 in New York City, New York

• • •

GOING TO MY SUPPORT group helped a lot. As I met others, I listened to them and found out what they were going through, and I explained to them what I was going through. I felt better knowing that I helped someone by telling them how I handled things. Your healing treatment is meeting others who have cancer. As you meet others, you see yourself in them. They share experiences that are similar to your own—you can relate to what you are hearing. It's like you are looking at yourself in the mirror.

Rosi, student accounts office assistant
Diagnosis of colon cancer at age 52 in 2007 in Austin, Texas

• • •

> "Your healing treatment is meeting others who have cancer."

MY DOCTORS ARE AMAZING, compassionate, and patient people. I have not one complaint. It is a devastating, horrible thing to have a doctor sit you down in a little "crying room" and tell you that you have cancer, but there is hope. And if you fight your ass off, and believe, and put faith in God, it is possible to beat cancer.

Eileen, teacher
Diagnosis of breast cancer at age 43 in 2006 in Hilton, New York

• • •

THE PEOPLE IN THE LAB who drew my blood. I saw them almost every day. They became my "friends," talking about life to keep my mind off the treatment and cancer.

Sheri, actress
Diagnosis of Hodgkin disease at age 29 in 1993 in Columbia, Maryland

While I was being treated, my nurse, Latrice Haney, started introducing me to other patients, and that was when I truly began to grasp the magnitude of cancer. At the time, there were more than eight million people living with cancer. I got really angry and became interested in fighting cancer—not just my own, but cancer in general. I knew that I needed to use my experience to help others, which was how the idea for my foundation began.

LANCE ARMSTRONG received a diagnosis of advanced testicular cancer at age 25 in 1996.

I FEEL LIKE I support my hospital. (As my husband pointed out, it is pretty sad that even the folks running the parking garage know me well.)

Eileen, technology specialist
Diagnosis of breast cancer at age 34 in 1984 and acute myelogenous leukemia at age 49 in 1999 and basal cell carcinoma (skin cancer) at age 55 in 2005 in Framingham, Massachusetts

• • •

I HAD EXCELLENT DOCTORS and was sent to the right ones in the beginning. I was lucky.

Joyce, educational assistant at an elementary school
Diagnosis of breast cancer at age 41 in 1995 in Knoxville, Tennessee

• • •

MY DOCTORS WERE WONDERFUL. My treatment was coordinated via teleconference with oncologists in Seattle, Washington, and I was part of each step in the procedure. I could not have been better informed had an oncologist been present.

Ruthanne, bookkeeper
Diagnosis of breast cancer at age 51 in 1995 in Thorne Bay, Alaska

THERE IS NOTHING MY doctor possibly could have told me that would have changed anything. In fact, he was very critical of my choosing not to have chemo. I had seen a lot of others go through the process, and they were so ill for months of treatment. So I decided that if the surgery didn't fix it, I would rather enjoy the time I had left being as well as I could. This has worked for me.

Pat, retired
Diagnosis of colon and bladder cancer at age 74 in 2005 in Como (Western Australia)

• • •

MY DOCTOR WAS PRETTY upfront with me, so I felt like I understood what was going to happen. I really didn't want to know statistics or what the future might hold because I wanted to always fight like I had a good chance of survival and not get discouraged.

Patti, financial administrator
Diagnosis of ovarian cancer at age 51 in 2005 in Colorado Springs, Colorado

• • •

I JOINED A WONDERFUL support group of young women with various types of cancer. I discovered a whole community of survivors who "got" what I was dealing with, in a way that someone who hasn't heard the words "You have cancer" could not. I could ask other cancer survivors the tough questions I couldn't discuss with my family. I was dealing with a potentially fatal disease, but my husband always insisted I would be fine. But I would voice my concerns to other survivors, and they understood. I also met a woman at Look Good, Feel Better®. She made me a scarf, and I never saw her again.

Mary, administrative assistant
Diagnosis of breast cancer at age 42 in 2003 in Simi Valley, California

"My husband always insisted I would be fine. But I would voice my concerns to other survivors, and they understood."

DURING AND AFTER my diagnosis, I bought books about breast cancer. I also went to the reputable Web sites, including those of the American Cancer Society and BreastCancer.org. I communicated with other women through the message boards. I spoke directly with some women who were referred by the American Cancer Society.

Nancy, administrative assistant
Diagnosis of breast cancer at age 54 in 2006 in Fowlerville, Michigan

• • •

"I was an educated patient, because I chose to be."

THERE IS NOT an easy way to pass along bad news. My doctor was very "clinical" when he told us—no bedside manner nor any emotions shown. He seemed very cold to me about it. Maybe he was just not sure how to handle the situation.

Marla, executive assistant
Diagnosis of breast cancer at age 35 in 1994 in Jasper, Indiana

• • •

WHEN I WAS FIRST diagnosed I was thirty-four, and most of my friends didn't know how to deal with cancer, but I had a great support group at the Wellness Community that helped me through.

Julie, real estate agent
Diagnosis of thyroid cancer at age 34 in 1996 and breast cancer at age 43 in 2005 in Torrance, California

• • •

MY DOCTORS WERE GREAT, and they told me everything positive: that with determination and commitment, I could beat this thing. I didn't believe them then. But now, I am cured and the parent of a five-year-old daughter. They told me I would feel better when it was all over, and I do. They were very accurate.

Cheryl, billings account clerk
Diagnosis of Ewing's sarcoma (a form of bone cancer) at age 21 in 1987 in Malden, Massachusetts

MY FIRST DOCTOR WAS very honest, and he and I came to an agreement right from the start. From the beginning, I was a fighter, and that set the course for just how tough a battle this was going to be. He had the same spirit, and he knew I had a strong desire to survive and that I wanted to get through this as soon as possible. A bond of trust was made right in the beginning, and it continued with the transplant doctors and staff. I did not doubt their abilities, for they were the experts. The nurses and staff gave my family a lot of encouragement. They told them how proud they were of me that I was fighting so hard, and they were touched by my determination. When I was in the ICU, they took care of my family—especially my younger son who would sometimes sleep in the family room of the ICU.

Susan, homemaker
Diagnosis of acute myelogenous leukemia at age 50 in 2003 in Medina, Ohio

• • •

THE TIMING OF MY diagnosis and treatment was awesome! A new cancer center had been opened only a few months before, and several medications had just been released to help with nausea and to treat the pathology of my tumors.

Cynthia, administrative assistant
Diagnosis of breast cancer at age 55 in 2003 in Highland Lakes, New Jersey

• • •

THE DOCTOR AND NURSE, as well as my surgeon took the time necessary to answer my questions. My oncologist made a pros and cons list to help determine which would be the most helpful: lumpectomy or mastectomy.

Jan, retired hospice chaplain
Diagnosis of breast cancer at age 55 in 2006 in Wichita, Kansas

• • •

I HAVE NEVER ASKED the tough questions like, "How long do I have to live?" One of the nurses is so caring and so encouraging that I look forward to seeing her at my chemo just to bring me around.

Audrey, disabled
Diagnosis of lung cancer at age 51 in 2007 in Baltimore, Maryland

MY DOCTORS (medical oncologist, radiation oncologist, and surgeons) told me everything that was going to happen. I was an educated patient, because I chose to be. I was an active participant in my treatment. My doctors worked for me; they were "my staff."

Jerri, state employee
Diagnosis of breast cancer at age 48 in 2006 and endometrial (uterine) cancer at age 50 in 2008 in Standish, Michigan

• • •

I THINK MOST CLL "lymphomaniacs" will tell you that they wished their doctor had not told them it was an old man's disease and that they would die of something else, not CLL. Me too. Other than that, the doctors have been good and have listened to me, as well as communicated with me.

Teri, retired kindergarten teacher
Diagnosis of chronic lymphocytic leukemia at age 51 in 1999 in Fort Langley, British Columbia (Canada)

Faith in God. Trust in my doctors, nurses, and technicians. Love and caring from my wife, Anne, family, and friends.

RETIRED SENATOR EDWARD W. BROOKE was the first African American to be elected by popular vote to the United States Senate in 1966 as a Republican from Massachusetts. In 2002, at the age of 82, he received a diagnosis of breast cancer and less than two weeks later, underwent a double mastectomy. He chronicles his cancer journey in the book *Bridging the Divide*.

WHEN I WAS TOLD I had cancer, the first doctor was a very uncaring person. The only thing he could tell me was that I was fat and that I had cancer. He did not even tell me where the cancer was. The only problem he seemed concerned with was my weight. He did not say "large"; he just kept saying "fat." Later, I had a wonderful nurse practitioner. Every time I went to her, she let me talk until all my fears were gone.

Lovey, homemaker
Diagnosis of uterine cancer at age 52 in 2000 in Cadiz, Kentucky

I WISH MY DOCTOR had had the knowledge and courage to tell me where they specialized in treating myeloma. He really needed information on hand for patients, such as that from the International Myeloma Foundation and the Multiple Myeloma Research Foundation. After receiving my diagnosis and going out to the lobby, I looked at the cancer handouts. There was nothing for myeloma patients! If I had had any other kind of cancer, there seemed to be pamphlets filled with helpful information. I felt lost and alone. Plus, it was late on a Friday afternoon. The booklet he handed me was discouraging, but it had the American Cancer Society number on the back. We went to my mom's house, and I called the number the moment we walked in the door. They told me about the Multiple Myeloma Research Foundation. I called them, and the rest is a survival story!

Kathryn, homemaker
Diagnosis of multiple myeloma at age 39 in 2001 and basal cell carcinoma (skin cancer) at age 45 in 2007 in St. Charles, Missouri

• • •

THE BEST THING I did was to join the Cancer Survivors Network chat room and meet other survivors and caregivers.

Marie, retired
Diagnosis of ovarian cancer at age 59 in 2004 in Lebanon, Ohio

I was fortunate enough to have an incredible medical team and, of course, the love and support of my family and friends.

SHARON OSBOURNE became Ozzy Osbourne's manager in 1979 after he was fired from Black Sabbath and began his solo rock career. Sharon is a colon cancer survivor.

THE DAY I WAS DIAGNOSED, I received a call from the American Cancer Society. They sent me information, reassured me, and told me that they were there with anything I needed.

Kathleen, retail manager
Diagnosis of breast cancer at age 48 in 2007 in Washington Township, New Jersey

I CAREFULLY FOLLOWED MY doctor's orders and advice. I did not launch into doing extensive research about my cancer and the various treatments offered, as some have chosen to do. I felt sure that God had put me in my doctor's hands, and so I trusted him and God to work my situation for good.

Barbara, homemaker
Diagnosis of breast cancer at age 38 in 1986 in Conway, Arkansas

• • •

EVERY TIME THE NURSE is going to put some needle in me, I zone out. I pinch the side of my thigh and concentrate only on that feeling or I press down on my thumb and focus only on that. I have bad veins, and the nurses will take three or four jabs at me, so I need to zone out. I don't like needles; it works for me.

Yvonne, paralegal
Diagnosis of colon cancer at age 48 in 2004 in San Antonio, Texas

• • •

I HAVE A WONDERFUL doctor who takes time to listen, and he talks to me like he has no other patients waiting.

Mariann, receptionist
Diagnosis of bladder cancer at age 50 in 2002 and endometrial (uterine) cancer at age 50 in 2003 in West Haven, Connecticut

• • •

MY ONCOLOGIST WAS BRUTALLY blunt; I never felt she hid anything from me. At our first appointment, she said, "I see why you have so many dead relatives." I could have fallen over. My primary doctor and plastic surgeon for reconstruction have always been positive and treat me as someone who will be alive in the future. Not everyone does that.

Luanne, registered nurse
Diagnosis of breast cancer at age 45 in 2007 in Morris, Illinois

> "One of the nurses is so caring and so encouraging that I look forward to seeing her ..."

I WISHED THE ONCOLOGIST had treated me like a patient with breast cancer, rather than a breast cancer patient. I wished that he had taken the time to listen to me, answer my questions, and show interest and compassion. So I fired that one and found another.

Debbie, hospice nurse
Diagnosis of breast cancer at age 52 in 2004 in Phoenix, Arizona

• • •

I REMEMBER FOUR or five very dark days when my wife came down with cold symptoms and, because of my white cell count, they would not let her visit me. A very perceptive nurse on staff came in to talk to me one morning and said, "I think maybe you just need a literal shoulder to cry on. Am I right?" She was right. I bawled for twenty minutes. And when it was all over with, I truly felt "recharged" and recommitted to coping.

Jerry, computer software instructor
Diagnosis of acute myelogenous leukemia at age 43 in 2003 in Anoka, Minnesota

• • •

> "I just wish my doctor had held my hand and said, 'I know this is awful, but you will be okay.'"

I JUST WISH MY doctor had held my hand and said, "I know this is awful, but you will be okay."

Cheryl, homemaker
Diagnosis of breast cancer at age 49 in 2006 in Garland, Texas

• • •

I CAN'T THINK OF anything that any of my doctors should have told me that they didn't. They were all very straightforward, telling me what was going to happen each step of the way and answering any question I or my husband put to them.

Judy, retired accounting clerk
Diagnosis of lung cancer at age 64 in 2004 in Norwalk, California

THE STAFF WHO WORK in physicians' offices need to remember that just their tone of voice can make an impact on someone—good or bad.

Laura, unemployed psychiatric social worker
Diagnosis of breast cancer at age 43 in 2006 in Avon, Connecticut

• • •

MY ONCOLOGIST IS VERY supportive as well, and I trust him implicitly. So, I have everything I need to keep fighting. I am truly blessed.

Barbara, retired art therapist
Diagnosis of pancreatic cancer at age 72 in 2006 in Golden, Colorado

• • •

I AM SURE MY doctor told me what he knew, but I am not sure I listened closely enough.

John, retired
Diagnosis of prostate cancer at age 57 in 1995 and chronic lymphocytic leukemia at age 65 in 2003 in Jacksonville, Florida

• • •

THE DOCTOR WHO FOUND my cancer—whenever I got really sick from my treatment and ended up in the hospital, he would make me laugh, not just any old laugh but hysterical laughing. He and his nursing staff were loving and caring, but I thank God that he's always been the funniest guy I know.

Lisa, unemployed
Diagnosis of lung cancer at age 42 in 2007 in Colebrook, New Hampshire

• • •

IN 1989, MY SURGEON said they didn't expect I would still be here many years later. The doctors tell me I am their miracle, as I have beaten the odds.

Lorraine, emergency service dispatcher
Diagnosis of melanoma (skin cancer) at age 33 in 1985 and thyroid cancer at age 52 in 2004 in Skaneateles, New York

I do not ask most of my patients to make a decision regarding treatment on their first visit. It is a lot of information to process, and they often need to discuss it with their family and friends. I often find that it takes two to three visits before we can make a treatment plan. I consider this decision-making process to be an interactive process where my patient's wishes are a part of the equation, along with the research evidence available and my clinical experience. Evidence-based health care should always include the patient's wishes and values.

KARIN HAHN, MD, MSC, MPH, is a medical oncologist and is medical director of the Breast Survivorship Clinic at The University of Texas M. D. Anderson Cancer Center, and chief of medical oncology at the Lyndon B. Johnson General Hospital in Houston, Texas.

IT'S WHAT I WISH my doctor had not told me that counts. I was told I had bone cancer one year after breast cancer treatments, and it turned out to be nothing. I was told I must have had a recurrence when, in fact, I didn't. Doctors need to be more sensitive in their approach to people. They need to treat the "whole" person and deliver only positive and factual news to them. Ask for a CT scan or MRI first to confirm it.

Buffy, self-employed
Diagnosis of breast cancer at age 58 in 2005 in Bobcaygeon, Ontario (Canada)

• • •

IT IS GREAT TO make sex jokes and embarrass your doctors (especially the interns—my husband and I had great fun with that—they are all so innocent!).

Jennifer, federal officer with U.S. Customs and Border Patrol
Diagnosis of cervical cancer at age 36 in 2007 in Montreal, Quebec (Canada)

I'VE LEARNED A LOT more about cancer, radiation, and different treatments. See, when no one in your family has ever had cancer, you only hear about it from other people talking about it, or by watching TV. And you just can't relate because no one near you has had such a problem. When you receive the diagnosis and begin the research, the nightmare brings you into a different reality than the one you lived before you heard the doctor tell you for the first time, "Mrs. F., you have thyroid cancer." Then life stops for a second, and everything starts going in slow motion. It took a couple of times to tell myself I had cancer, and I still didn't understand how it happened.

Candy, teacher
Diagnosis of thyroid cancer at age 31 in 2007 in El Paso, Texas

> "Having a caring and supportive medical staff to help me gave me hope."

• • •

MY DIAGNOSIS was a complete shock; it was picked up on my very first mammogram at age thirty-eight. I was going to wait and have my first mammogram at age forty because, at the time, there was no family history of breast cancer, and I had been doing monthly self-exams for years. I never felt a lump. Then my mother called me a month before I was diagnosed to tell me that she had been diagnosed with breast cancer and that I should go for a mammogram immediately, which I did. When a person is diagnosed with breast cancer, I think the first thing that runs through your mind is that you are going to die. At least, that's what I thought. I never knew any breast cancer survivors. The woman who coordinated my surgery was awesome. She was the person who recommended me to Reach to Recovery®. She was very helpful and was always there to answer questions or listen to my concerns. We walk together each year for the Susan G. Komen walks. My Reach to Recovery® volunteer was also very helpful; she made me feel that I was not alone and that the feelings I was experiencing were normal. I also took the advice of my doctors and took it easy the first few weeks of recovery. Having a caring and supportive medical staff to help me gave me hope.

Lisa, administrative assistant
Diagnosis of breast cancer at age 38 in 2000 in Owings Mills, Maryland

THE NURSES WERE REALLY great during my chemo and radiation. I was impressed by how compassionate they were. I believe I would not have come through as well without them.

Sheila, legal secretary
Diagnosis of breast cancer at age 65 in 2006 in Walnut Creek, California

• • •

MY DOCTOR NEVER SAID the word cancer. He said, "I don't have good news for you. You will need surgery and chemotherapy. Depending on your surgery, you may or may not need radiation." He also respected my request to give me the results after my daughter's fourth birthday party. I wasn't able to find a support group when I needed it. I felt a lot of the leg work was left for me to do, and it is just one of those things that takes a lot of time to research.

Judi, nurse
Diagnosis of breast cancer at age 40 in 2000 in Pen Argyl, Pennsylvania

• • •

MY DOCTOR WAS EXCELLENT. He told me the biggest "battle" would be the one that goes on in my head. And that cancer could be considered as treatable as most chronic illnesses now. He made me feel it was beatable! He also told me not to be a victim. My breast care nurses were always there when I needed them most—at the end of a phone when I called them or when they called me "just to check" on me. It was a secure and safe feeling that they were there for me.

Pearl, nurse
Diagnosis of breast cancer at age 32 in 2004 in Glasgow (Scotland)

• • •

MY DOCTOR WAS PRETTY straightforward with us. He was very caring and even prayed with us during our first visit. He promised that I would get through the treatments and be able to have more children.

Carlyn, administrative assistant
Diagnosis of Hodgkin disease at age 30 in 2004 in Willow Spring, North Carolina

> It is difficult to tell a patient she has cancer. I approach each case by trying to understand the patient as a person.
>
> **DAVID NATHANSON, MD**, is a breast surgical oncologist and director of Breast Care Services at the Henry Ford Health System in Detroit, Michigan. He is also the author of *Ordinary Miracles: Learning from Breast Cancer Survivors*.

MY DOCTOR GAVE ME a soft, cuddly, and beautifully dressed breast cancer bear about twelve inches tall. I sat her on a small chair in my great room, and everyone asked about her. Then, before I knew it, everyone was giving me stuffed, cuddly bears! My daughter sent me a black bear called Flip-Flop that had a long body that I used to comfort any place that hurt. I also used him as a pillow and under my arm where all of the lymph nodes were removed. Now he sits on the top of my bear chair with all of the other bears that are a constant reminder to me of all those who cared enough to come visit me and help make my days a little brighter.

Pam, retired dental hygienist
Diagnosis of breast cancer at age 57 in 2005 in Lakeland, Florida

• • •

I SEARCHED THE INTERNET but had trouble finding information about my cancer. I was too young and did not relate to the older women featured in the brochures.

Alejandra, clerical worker
Diagnosis of uterine cancer at age 36 in 2005 in Torrance, California

> Today, I wish I had known more about my tumor type. There wasn't as much known then. The more information you have, the better.
>
> **NANCY BRINKER,** received a diagnosis of breast cancer at age 37 in 1985. She had founded the Susan G. Komen for the Cure in 1981 in memory of her sister and best friend.

WHEN I FIRST GOT word about a positive diagnosis, I went on the Internet and looked around at the information. At that point, I knew the cancer had metastasized to the lymph, and there was some suggestion that it was also in the spine and maybe the brain. When I looked at the material, I saw pictures of what looked like my situation and saw the survival figure of 17 percent. I felt fine; how could this be me? Then I realized that the information there was based on epidemiological studies, and being a researcher with training in statistical analysis, I knew that these numbers were a mixture of information from all over the country and from people being treated in all sorts of medical facilities. I was not being treated in a remote community hospital. I was in Boston, and being treated at a major teaching hospital with the best resources and expertise in the world.

Anne, psychologist
Diagnosis of breast cancer at age 50 in 2005 in Boston, Massachusetts

References

Gawande, A. 2002. *Complications: a surgeon's notes on an imperfect science.* New York: Picador (Henry Holt and Co.).

Hewitt, M., Greenfield, S. and E. Stovall, eds. 2006, *From cancer patient to cancer survivor: lost in transition.* Washington, DC: The National Academies Press.

5 Things
Your Oncologist Should Tell You

1. **You have treatment options.** You and your oncologist are a team. Together you should understand your diagnosis and treatment options. This doesn't mean that you know as much about cancer as your oncologist, but it does mean that you are an intelligent person who should be told what your options are for your body.

2. **You may be a candidate for clinical research trials.** It's important for oncologists to include clinical research trials in their discussion about treatment options. Not everyone will want to participate, and certainly not everyone will meet the criteria for any given study, but it's important to get information about the trials in which you may be eligible to participate.

3. **You may be at risk for other cancers.** Though no one wants to hear this, it's important in some cases to know other types of cancer for which someone may be at risk. They may need screening tests to monitor their cancer risk and have the opportunity to catch the disease very early. Or even eliminate the risk (e.g., a woman at high risk for ovarian cancer might be screened for it or elect to have her ovaries removed).

4. **It will take a long time after cancer treatment for you to heal.** People expect to feel better far sooner than the true recovery process really takes. Having your doctor share this with you upfront will help you to have realistic expectations and not wonder why it's taking you so long to heal.

5. **New research is on the horizon.** I call this the "all of a sudden phenomenon" in medicine. There are thousands of studies ongoing at any given time. Then, all of a sudden, the results will be released and it will change the way we treat patients. No one can possibly know what is going on in every study in every part of the world. So, there is a lot of the "all of a sudden phenomenon" going on all the time. Maybe all of a sudden there will be something to help you. I hope so!

CHAPTER 5

• • •

What Helped My Children Cope

NBC correspondent Betty Rollin, whose breast cancer was diagnosed in 1974, summed up how hard it is on children and families when one member is seriously ill. She wrote, "Disease may score a direct hit on only one member of the family, but shrapnel tears the flesh of the others" (Rollin 1998, 122).

No doubt, one of the kindest things you can do to help people who are going through a serious illness like cancer is to do something for their children. My family and friends knew this when I was going through cancer treatment. People did many things that, to this day, I still remember with gratitude. I couldn't possibly describe them all, but here are a few examples of how others helped nurture my children during this time.

My youngest daughter was three years old when my cancer was diagnosed. Her "blankey" was a huge comfort to her; however, it was getting tattered and worn. My friend Alison took the blanket home with her and quickly patched it up with a beautiful fabric that closely matched the original. Alison knew that my daughter would need her blanket back right away, so she bought everything ahead of time and literally kept it for only a couple of hours. My daughter was thrilled to have her blanket back in wonderful condition, and I was so grateful to my friend for that incredibly kind gesture.

Many people brought us meals and included special desserts for the children. Colleagues from work sent a box of Halloween gifts and decorations that the children loved. A grandson of one of my patients worked for a toy company, and he sent a box of toys for my children during the holidays. They loved the toys, which kept them busy for weeks.

No matter how old you are, having a parent with cancer is extremely difficult. As the survey participants conveyed, what others do to help can make a tremendous difference.

Before I get to the survey participants' stories, I want to share with you some suggestions from my friend and colleague, pediatric psychiatrist Paula Rauch, for helping children cope when their parent is going through cancer treatment: maintain familiar routines, protect family time, do fun things together, and communicate openly with them. Dr. Rauch also has this great suggestion:

> I think the idea of appointing a "Captain of Kindness" is great. The Captain of Kindness is the person to whom a parent sends the well-wishers when they are looking for ways to be helpful. For example, a mom is in the supermarket with her seven-year-old child and another mom comes up and asks, "Can I do anything to help?" The mom with the illness or with an ill partner can simply respond, "People have been great. Jane Jones is organizing the help and kindness." Then, the well-wisher can follow up with Jane Jones (or not.) The Captain acts as a buffer so the parent doesn't have to ask for things friends may not be able to do. The Captain does the time-consuming task of organizing meals or rides, etc., so the parents can focus their time on their children. Those delivered meals, for example, can be arranged by the Captain to be left in a cooler outside the family's door and the dishes picked up the next day from the same cooler. That way, the children don't have to share their evening family time with the well-wishers.

Dr. Rauch has other tips for families and children who are coping with illness (see page 112), and so do many cancer survivors who participated in this book. I was delighted to review the surveys and discover how many people understood the importance of reaching out to the children of cancer survivors. Even adult children need support during this time, and the stories of how loved ones supported the offspring of those affected by cancer are truly heartwarming.

My children were young at the time my cancer was diagnosed, but many people who responded to the surveys had adult children. I thoroughly enjoyed reading about how adult children gave and received support during a difficult time. Many respondents who didn't have children still shared stories about how children eased their journey.

I hope that you enjoy reading this chapter. It's one of my favorites.

• • •

THE FIRST QUESTION my children asked was, "Are you going to die?" I told them that I didn't know and that even the doctors couldn't tell us at that time. My husband and I tried (successfully) to make their lives as normal as possible. We did not require them to be caregivers. We made certain that they did not miss their after-school activities. We told them that while my job was to get better, their job was to do well in school. We were totally honest with our children. First of all, they can tell if you are not telling them something. Also, I spent a lot of time on the phone, and they could definitely overhear anything I was saying to other people. I didn't want them to learn about anything from my inadvertently telling another adult about it. My son also saw a therapist (social worker) a year or two later, which helped him tremendously.

Elena, arts administrator
Diagnosis of inflammatory breast cancer at age 44 in 1999 in Silver Spring, Maryland

• • •

MY ELDEST SON PREPARED his son for the fact that I was bald, like my son. I didn't know this and put on a wig for my visit with them. When they arrived my son said, "Mom, I prepared him all week about your hair." Then he told me to sneeze, and when I did, he pulled off my wig. My grandson laughed so hard. When he was finished, he looked at my daughter who has long black hair and said, "Sneeze, Aunt Jen!" She laughed and said, "Oh no, my hair doesn't come off!"

Jo Ann, retired
Diagnosis of breast cancer at age 60 in 2006 in Lanoka Harbor, New Jersey

• • •

JUST RECENTLY, MY HUSBAND told me that my son (then ten years old) was running back and forth while I was sleeping, putting his soldiers around me and on me. He had put on his cape and mask saying, "I am going to fight the cancer, so my mommy won't get sick anymore!"

Bernadette, cardiovascular technician
Diagnosis of breast cancer at age 48 in 2001 in Oxnard, California

BEFORE MY SURGERY, I decided to get my hair cut. It was a spur of the moment thing in the middle of the mall, something I never ever did! I was with my youngest daughter who decided she would also get a trim. She has the most gorgeous head of hair and generally gets hysterical when it's touched. The mall beautician had decided on her own that my daughter should have shorter hair and also put layers in it, even though she had been specifically told not to. My daughter went ballistic, crying hysterically and carrying on to the point where I wanted to get up and leave her there. She continued this behavior all the way home (this is a twenty-two-year-old woman!). I was really getting annoyed, and I finally told her so. Through her sobs she managed to say, "You don't understand, Mom! I wanted to save my hair for you if you needed it...now it's too short." At that point, I cried with her. Her thoughtfulness was the most special thing to me. I don't think anyone could have beaten that! The weekend before my surgery she invited me to her apartment for a pajama party. She waxed my legs and gave me a foot massage and pedicure, and we ate everything bad that we could find. We laughed and cried into the wee hours of the night. We watched funny movies and ate ice cream. It was the most precious night of my life.

Kathie, nurse and social worker
Diagnosis of kidney cancer at age 53 in 2005 in Kingston, New York

• • •

> "My two-year-old child knew just when to give me a hug and say, 'Mommy, I love you.'"

I WANT TO SHARE an epiphany that I had one day while praying for my children. The Lord reminded me that He loved my children more than I did. He assured me that if He decided my time was up, He would take care of my kids. I found such peace with this thought, as I had come to terms with what death would mean for me; I was just torn up thinking about leaving them without a mother. I realized that God uses all things to the good of those who love Him, and I turned my kids' destiny over to Him and His will.

Sherri, elementary school teacher
Diagnosis of endometrial (uterine) cancer at age 42 in 2004 in Bruceville, Indiana

I THINK THE MOST special things were done by my kids. My two-year-old child knew just when to give me a hug and say, "Mommy, I love you." My fifteen-year-old daughter watched the youngest with no questions or complaints. My thirteen-year-old daughter was visiting with my mom when I received my diagnosis. I had sent her with $100 for spending money. She took that money and found another $240 in change around my mom's house, then called me and asked me how much money I would need to have surgery. She wanted to pay for it so that I could live. I don't think I realized how important my life was until that phone call.

Rochelle, manicurist
Diagnosis of melanoma (skin cancer) at age 34 in 2007 in Las Vegas, Nevada

• • •

WE WERE COMPLETELY HONEST with our seven-year-old daughter. We called her in and told her that I was sick and would have to undergo surgery. She said okay and then asked if she could go out and play. In an hour, she returned and asked me if I was going to die. I told her everyone dies, but I hoped I would not for a long time. From that moment forward, we raised her to be independent. Because of my poor prognosis, we wanted her to be able to care for herself if something happened to me. Today, she is a very compassionate young woman, with a heart for cancer patients. A seventh-grade teacher, she currently has a student in her class with cancer. She has said she knows better how to help the student and her family since she herself has gone through this process with me.

Beth, health educator
Diagnosis of liver cancer at age 32 in 1990 in Fort Hood, Texas

• • •

MY DAUGHTER WAS JUST entering adulthood, and we had some residual "issues" from her adolescence. As soon as my cancer was diagnosed, all those issues became far less important for both of us. Now, we try harder to understand each other and to forgive when it's necessary. We have a very close, comfortable adult–adult relationship, rather than a parent–child relationship. We accept our differences.

Sandra, assistant professor of nursing
Diagnosis of breast cancer at age 54 in 2002 in Atlanta, Georgia

> **"Tell them what to expect, and tell them it's not their fault. Reassure them in all ways."**

MY DAUGHTER WAS TOO young to know that I was sick, let alone sick with cancer. However, the consequences were still very negative. At that age, all she wanted was to be carried around but, after my surgery, I had a lifting restriction for six weeks, and I couldn't carry her. She would get really angry because of that and, unfortunately, she detached herself from me because she felt rejected. After I recovered, it took a considerable amount of time to regain her affection. I don't think I have fully regained it, and I wish I could reason with her and explain why all that happened...alas, she's still too young for that.

Federico, cancer chemical biologist
Diagnosis of testicular cancer at age 32 in 2006 in Brookline, Massachusetts

• • •

MY SON WAS VERY quiet, as he is with everything. He fell apart when my hair fell out. It was the only time I saw him cry. I feel the need to do something good within the cancer community, now that I am in remission. I believe my son would prefer to move on.

Ann, homemaker
Diagnosis of breast cancer at age 47 in 2003 in Mechanicsburg, Pennsylvania

• • •

I AM THANKFUL EACH day that it was me and not one of my children who had this burden. I tried to keep things as normal as possible around the house, almost to a fault. I never let them see me without my wig. I always remained upbeat and didn't allow them to see me not feeling well (although I truly was fortunate and did feel good!). In some ways I might have sheltered them too much from it but, ultimately, they seemed to handle it fine.

Joyce, legal secretary
Diagnosis of breast cancer at age 44 in 2006 in South Amboy, New Jersey

WHEN I EXPLAINED THAT I had lymphoma, my three children offered hugs and seemed to be supportive. I truly don't know what they were thinking inside, but they were always upbeat. Then, one night I was kissing my youngest child goodnight and assured him I would beat this cancer. He burst into tears and asked if I was going to die. I then realized that he never associated the word lymphoma with cancer. Once I used the "C" word, he was devastated.

Midge, accountant
Diagnosis of non-Hodgkin lymphoma at age 52 in 2005 and breast cancer at age 54 in 2007 in Westford, Massachusetts

My children were one, three, and five years old when I was diagnosed with cancer. I've been in and out of treatment ever since. My children are now well-adjusted and happy young adults who have learned how to thrive when life is not what you expect or want. They have shared with me what helped them most and what they advise any parent with cancer: "Tell your children the truth and include them in the crisis because the greatest gift you can give your children is not protection from the world, but the confidence and tools to cope and grow with all that life has to offer."

WENDY S. HARPHAM, MD, is a doctor of internal medicine, a long-term lymphoma survivor, and the author of several books, including *When a Parent Has Cancer* and *Happiness in a Storm*.

MY ADVICE FOR CHILDREN coping with a parent's cancer diagnosis is to be honest with them. Use the "C" word. Tell them what to expect, and tell them it's not their fault. Reassure them in all ways.

Jennifer, psychotherapist
Diagnosis of breast cancer at age 39 in 2004 in Pennington, New Jersey

I AM PROUD of the fact that my adult children were strong and loved and well adjusted, and when the time came, they had the strength to deal with a crisis.

Matt, carpenter
Diagnosis of chronic lymphocytic leukemia at age 51 in 2003 in Bath, New York

• • •

MY DAUGHTER WAS THE ONE who took me to the hospital for my surgical procedures, to the medical team meeting, to the appointment to have my head shaved and put on the wig. She came to stay with me after my first chemo, to make sure I wasn't alone until we figured out how I would cope. She would call to make sure I was okay…or just to share a silly story to make me smile. She "took care of me," so to speak.

Pat, office manager
Diagnosis of breast cancer at age 53 in 2001 in Canton, Michigan

• • •

MY CANCER WAS FIRST diagnosed when my oldest child was six months old. When my recurrence was diagnosed, my youngest was six months old. The first time, it only affected my oldest son briefly. He was six months old at the time of surgery and eight months old when I received radiation and had to be isolated from him for a week. He briefly didn't want to go to me, but within one hour of my return home he was back to normal. The second time, my oldest had a really hard time with it. While I was receiving radiation treatment and had to be in isolation, he stayed with grandma and grandpa. Every time I called, he would cry and cry, saying he wanted Mommy and wanted to go home. Now, even a month later, I can't even walk outside to get the mail or retrieve something from the car without him screaming and crying. We are having major separation anxiety issues with him now. My youngest (who is the same age that my oldest was the first time) has had no repercussions from it. My mom kept my kids the second time around and just tried to keep them busy and distracted. I thought I had done everything possible to make it easy on my children, but it was still very, very hard.

Nicki, homemaker
Diagnosis of thyroid cancer at age 20 in 2005 in Union, Missouri

THE VISITS AND THE MEALS that were provided impressed my grown sons. It made them aware of how many people cared about me.

Debra, administrative assistant
Diagnosis of ovarian cancer at age 51 in 2007 in Chicago, Illinois

• • •

I WANTED TO SHOW my children that everyone will experience a difficult time and that you can accept this and still have a great time.

Peggy, pathologist's assistant
Diagnosis of breast cancer at age 47 in 2003 in St Augustine, Florida

• • •

> "My four-year-old niece referred to my wig as 'hair in a box.'"

MY CHILDREN WERE FOURTEEN and ten years of age when my cancer was diagnosed—both are boys, and they don't show a lot of emotion. They knew I was going to have some minor surgery, but I didn't provide any details until I was home from the hospital. I didn't want to cause any stress for them, and since I didn't know the questions to ask, I didn't think they would either. I needed them to see that I was okay after the surgery. I did sit down with them throughout the treatment, especially before undergoing radiation, to let them know that Mommy was going to be tired and not to worry if they saw me lying down for naps. I didn't really notice any negative impact on either of my children. My youngest did come into my room when I rested to check in and see if I needed anything. My cancer was diagnosed during baseball season, and they were both playing. So friends and family would pick them up and take them to games and practices. They would also swing by to take them for dinner or to get ice cream, so I could rest. It was really great not having to worry about driving them around or them missing things.

Kelley, massage therapist
Diagnosis of breast cancer at age 36 in 2006 in Rochdale, Massachusetts

THAT IS THE WEIRD part. I was really emotional when my cancer was first diagnosed. I would cry a lot. I really dreaded telling my children that I had cancer. When I tearfully told them about my cancer, it didn't seem to faze them. They just went on like before. They never said much about it, even when I lost my hair. The neighborhood friends would come over, and I didn't wear a wig when I was in the house, and they never said anything about my bald head. It was like life was still normal. To this day, I have never asked my children what they felt like. I don't usually discuss the cancer journey. It is in my past.

Joyce, educational assistant at an elementary school
Diagnosis of breast cancer at age 41 in 1995 in Knoxville, Tennessee

• • •

> "My then nine-year-old son wanted to know everything about it..."

MY NIECES AND NEPHEWS were as much a part of my disease and treatment as if they had been my own children. I have a favorite picture of my infant nephew in my arms, and our hair matches in style and color! My four-year-old niece referred to my wig (which I did not like and only wore twice) as "hair in a box." The children I taught used to ask me if they could "feel my hair," when I wore hats to cover the baldness.

Kathleen, teacher
Diagnosis of Hodgkin disease at age 40 in 1997 in Lisbon, Connecticut

• • •

THE GREATEST IMPACT was on my grandchildren who, being very young, were scared. I was able to convince each of them that I was not going to die and that we would do all the things we had planned as soon as I was out of treatment. They loved the game of wearing masks when they visited and took them to school for show and tell. At one point, they brought part of their first grade class to me so I could be show and tell. Today, my grandchildren are active participants in Relay for Life®.

Ruthanne, bookkeeper
Diagnosis of breast cancer at age 51 in 1995 in Thorne Bay, Alaska

AFTER MY SURGERY, my daughter came to the hospital every morning in time to talk to the doctors when they did their rounds. I was too wiped out for the first week to take in much of what they said. She asked all the right questions and was very patient in explaining to me what my options were and making sure I was being well cared for.

Pat, retired
Diagnosis of colon and bladder cancer at age 74 in 2005 in Como (Western Australia)

• • •

MY THEN NINE-YEAR-OLD SON wanted to know everything about it, asked a lot of the hard questions, and was very aware of all that was going on. Now he's in a PhD program in medical biology, planning to do cancer-related research as a career.

Janet, elementary school teacher
Diagnosis of colon cancer at age 42 in 1993 in Philadelphia, Pennsylvania

• • •

IT WAS A WHOLE new world for all of us. Mom was spending days on the couch; Mom was losing her hair. My children handled it easier than did my husband! We just took it day by day. The Reach to Recovery® coordinator gave my eight-year-old daughter a book called *Our Mom Has Cancer*. It is one of her most prized possessions.

Mary, administrative assistant
Diagnosis of breast cancer at age 42 in 2003 in Simi Valley, California

• • •

MY CHILDREN WERE VERY young; I don't think they fully understood the whole thing. I do remember getting up one night and not putting on a turban or my wig, and I scared my son. He actually jumped away from me! Years later, my daughter gave a witness of her faith, which centered around my cancer diagnosis and how she wasn't sure what was going on but that she just kept praying.

Marla, executive assistant
Diagnosis of breast cancer at age 35 in 1994 in Jasper, Indiana

MY TEENAGE CHILDREN are now much closer to my husband, and we have a family bond that is wonderful.

Julie, real estate agent
Diagnosis of thyroid cancer at age 34 in 1996 and breast cancer at age 43 in 2005 in Torrance, California

• • •

[SOMEONE WHO REALLY HELPED me was] my eight-year-old grandson—his innocence and guarded care of me during my treatment. He has been my inspiration, and I am the only grandmother he has known. During his first eight years, we rode bikes, skated, went hiking, and spent endless hours at the parks. During the one year when I was not able to do those things, I promised him that I would once again do those things with him, and I have. He was with me when the staples were pulled out of my stomach, and his strong faith in me and God has kept me going.

Rose, government contractor
Diagnosis of stomach cancer at age 60 in 2002 in Centreville, Virginia

• • •

"My survivor goal was that I would see my son graduate from high school."

MY SURVIVOR GOAL was that I would see my son graduate from high school. The day I started treatment in the hospital was the first day of his senior year of high school. Although I was still sick when he started college, having that goal had mentally kept me going. Both my sons spent a lot of time at the hospital in addition to attending high school and college classes. They became dependent on each other. At that time they could have gotten wild, but they were responsible and did the best they could. The difficulties in their lives made them stronger. They grew up quickly. Nothing was normal.

Susan, homemaker
Diagnosis of acute myelogenous leukemia at age 50 in 2003 in Medina, Ohio

MY AUNT PROVIDED ENOUGH money for full-time child care for our youngest child. I suffered extreme short-term memory loss and depression with anxiety. I would forget I put something on the stove to cook, etc. I was in no shape to properly care for him. It was such a blessing knowing he was in a safe environment.

Danielle, financial service specialist
Diagnosis of melanoma (skin cancer) at age 30 in 2000 in Ramstein (Germany)

"We live with cancer, and it is not so scary anymore."

• • •

AT FIRST [MY CHILDREN] were very upset. My daughter clammed up and would not cry. My son did cry and moved into our bedroom; for about a year, he slept on the floor next to me and would hold my hand. He was afraid I was going to die right away. As time went by and we all grew stronger from the cancer education, we involved our kids in the good news of promising new drugs and other hopeful things. We also got them involved in Relay for Life® and other positive activities related to fundraising and awareness for cancer research. They discovered others living with cancer. During their teenage years, I found that being honest about the cancer let my kids handle it the best way for them. We live with cancer, and it is not so scary anymore. I think they are better-behaved teenagers because of it. Both [of my children] have excelled in school and sports and have grown into mature young adults.

Kathryn, homemaker
Diagnosis of multiple myeloma at age 39 in 2001 and basal cell carcinoma (skin cancer) at age 45 in 2007 in St Charles, Missouri

• • •

MY DAUGHTER WAS JUST maturing into a young woman when I lost my breasts to cancer. I cannot even begin to understand all that [my experience] did to her emotionally. However, she handled it beautifully and is today a strong and lovely young woman—both inside and out.

Barbara, homemaker
Diagnosis of breast cancer at age 38 in 1986 in Conway, Arkansas

Children need to know that they did not do anything to cause their parent to have cancer. They also need to know that it is not contagious, and they cannot catch it from you or anyone else. Many children have scary thoughts about cancer that may actually be worse than the reality of the situation. It is vitally important for parents to talk honestly with their children and use language that each age group can identify with.

ELYSE CAPLAN was 34 years old when her breast cancer was diagnosed. She has watched her three sons—the oldest was age 8 at the time—grow into successful and compassionate men. Elyse oversees educational programming for Living Beyond Breast Cancer.

AS SOON AS I found out my diagnosis, I called a friend who is a child psychiatrist and asked her when I should tell my son. Her answer was, "Immediately."

Laura, unemployed psychiatric social worker
Diagnosis of breast cancer at age 43 in 2006 in Avon, Connecticut

• • •

MY DIAGNOSIS IMPACTED my seven-year-old son so much. I did not have the energy to take him out like I used to. And the money was not abundant like before. There were no private lessons or luxuries like before. He missed me and wrote me poems and songs about my illness. Some were very touching and clearly revealed his feelings of despair and loneliness. He often expressed his fear that I would die. He became afraid of the dark and afraid to be left alone even in the daytime. I made certain family members took my son out of the house for drives or on trips to the zoo—it doesn't have to be expensive to take the children out for some entertainment. I also made time for him with me; we did homework together and read in bed. I made time for him no matter what—every day, even if only for a couple of hours.

Yvonne, paralegal
Diagnosis of colon cancer at age 48 in 2004 in San Antonio, Texas

MY HUSBAND HAD TO travel the day after one of my surgical procedures. I was fine being home alone, but my son came to my house that evening to sleep in my guest room. It was just such a loving thing to do.

Barbara, nurse
Diagnosis of breast cancer at age 58 in 1995 in Stoneham, Massachusetts

• • •

WHAT GOT ME THROUGH that most difficult time was the day my daughter called to tell me she and her husband were expecting a baby. I was tickled to be having a grandbaby and was able to stop focusing on my own problems and prepare for the most joyous event of my life. I shopped for nursery furniture, and then I began to look for baby clothes when we found out she was a girl. What a special gift she is and always will be.

Cheryl, homemaker
Diagnosis of breast cancer at age 49 in 2006 in Garland, Texas

• • •

DON'T SUGARCOAT. Kids— even youngsters—are smarter than that. But there is also no reason to dwell on the negative. Your kids need the power that comes from positive thinking just as much as you do. You can give that to them without being phony about it.

Jerry, computer software instructor
Diagnosis of acute myelogenous leukemia at age 43 in 2003 in Anoka, Minnesota

> **"Don't sugarcoat. Kids are smarter than that."**

• • •

NO KIDS. I was thirty-eight years old when my cancer was diagnosed, and we were about to start our family. We found an experimental fertility-preserving treatment. I have finished treatment, and we have begun to work with a fertility doctor. We are beginning to see what God has in store for us now.

Karen, real estate broker
Diagnosis of breast cancer at age 38 in 2001 in Loganville, Georgia

> ## "My daughters had a special treat for me each time I went in for chemo..."

MY DAUGHTERS had a special treat for me each time I went in for chemo treatments: a scrapbook, a book with letters of support from each family member, a video message of support from friends and family members, a love necklace handmade by family members, a photo album of reasons to fight the cancer, a special T-shirt. My daughter delivered each item to the office before I arrived, and the nurses and doctors were always anxious to see what was waiting for me before I started my treatment. I felt so loved and supported and special.

Karen, medical assistant
Diagnosis of breast cancer at age 43 in 2001 in Cincinnati, Ohio

• • •

MY GROWN DAUGHTER was scared for her life, as well as mine. She didn't want to lose her mom or get breast cancer down the road. She now gets regular mammograms.

Buffy, self-employed
Diagnosis of breast cancer at age 58 in 2005 in Bobcaygeon, Ontario (Canada)

• • •

THE MOST MEMORABLE [part of the experience] was the way my adult sons, who live far away, kept calling me every day. One time my oldest son talked to me for an hour and a half when I was in terrible pain. It helped immensely.

Sigrid, registered nurse
Diagnosis of endometrial (uterine) cancer at age 72 in 2006 in Oceanside, California

• • •

MY ADULT SON WORRIED a lot. He lost about as much weight as I did.

John, retired
Diagnosis of esophageal cancer at age 76 in 2006 in Jamestown, North Carolina

THEIR BIGGEST FEAR, other than possibly losing their mom, was that Mom would be without her hair. As I was starting chemo treatments, I went out and bought a wig and allowed them to play with it so they would be comfortable with it.

Lorraine, emergency service dispatcher
Diagnosis of metastatic melanoma (skin cancer) at age 33 in 1985 and thyroid cancer at age 52 in 2004 in Skaneateles, New York

• • •

AT FIRST, my son was scared. But then he wrote to me while he was in basic training, saying that he knew I was going to make it, because I was a tough lady. My daughter cried hysterically. But after the day I told her, it was like everything was the same as it ever was.

Lisa, unemployed
Diagnosis of lung cancer at age 42 in 2007 in Colebrook, New Hampshire

• • •

WE PRAYED TOGETHER WHEN we got home from learning about my cancer diagnosis (their daddy was deployed at the time), because I wanted them to see from the beginning the truth of our situation. They weren't scared of the word cancer. They had never heard of it. But I just told them we were really going to need God's help, and my unborn son needed God to keep him safe and help him grow healthy and fat.

Laura, stay-at-home mom
Diagnosis of breast cancer at age 31 in 2006 in Hope Mills, North Carolina

• • •

THE BIGGEST BLESSING is my daughter. The doctors believe I had had cancer for two years [at diagnosis], which means I had it the entire time I was pregnant. My daughter helped me to realize that I had to fight and endure the pain and exhaustion so that I could see her grow up.

Carlyn, administrative assistant
Diagnosis of Hodgkin disease at age 30 in 2004 in Willow Spring, North Carolina

> "My daughter helped me to realize that I had to fight and endure the pain and exhaustion so that I could see her grow up."

MY DAUGHTER TOOK THREE weeks off when I had my bilateral mastectomy. My son even stripped my many drainage tubes when I was too weak to do it myself. He and my daughter brought me home from surgery to the new house that I had built, but had not yet lived in. Later that first night when I could not get comfortable or even lie in my bed, they went to a store and brought me a new recliner to sleep in. That was truly a "special delivery."

Pam, retired dental hygienist
Diagnosis of breast cancer at age 57 in 2005 in Lakeland, Florida

• • •

I WANTED A THIRD child, but now can't have one. At first when I heard babies cry, it would upset me. It's not so bad now—maybe someday I will hold my grandchildren and spoil them.

Alejandra, clerical worker
Diagnosis of uterine cancer at age 36 in 2005 in Torrance, California

• • •

MY CANCER had a tremendous impact on my children. My son developed fears, including a fear of death, and had problems with separation anxiety. My daughters were each affected differently. My youngest is convinced she, too, will get breast cancer. However, she believes she will make it through as I did. My oldest daughter took the scientific route. She was going through puberty and wanted to know the medical facts about cancer. I believe my children are proud of me and have a deeper compassion for me and for others. As a family, we participate in the various walks to raise money for cancer research, and they are always proclaiming, "That's my mom; she is a breast cancer survivor!"

Shelly, program coordinator for adults with disabilities
Diagnosis of breast cancer at age 32 in 2004 in Concord, New Hampshire

My kids were fifteen and thirteen at the time of my diagnosis, and they were by far the most upset of any of my close set. My son was playing football, and his team and coach all signed a football and sent it home to me. Several of the other football parents called me one night from the only game I missed due to chemo. The assistant coach's mother had had breast cancer when he was in high school, and he spent a lot of time talking my son through the ordeal. My daughter's friends and their mothers went crazy with the food and flowers and homemade cards; they sort of took me on as a fall project.

HALA MODDELMOG received a diagnosis of breast cancer at the age of 45 in 2001. She is the president and CEO of Susan G. Komen for the Cure.

Reference

Rollin, B. 1998. *Last wish*. New York: Public Affairs™. (First published in 1985. First Public Affairs Edition, 1998.)

by Dr. Paula Rauch

10 Tips
to Help Children and Familes

1. Turn off the telephone during meal time (until bedtime), and make that period a family time that is focused on the children.

2. Have an adult friend who volunteers to help build the grade school projects that require lots of adult assistance.

3. Obtain a journal that a child can leave next to a parent's bed with "Things I want you to know" in it. The child can write in the journal and ask for a parent's response or simply request that the parent read it.

4. Remember to tell children who will be doing drop off and pickup from school and who will be staying with them when they get home.

5. Schedule two weeknights to be family dinner nights for busy teens.

6. At bedtime ask about a child's favorite thing of the day, worst thing that happened that day, and thing he or she is most proud of doing that day.

7. Organize a special event such as an overnight mini-vacation at a nearby motel with a pool.

8. Send the children and family gift certificates for local restaurants that offer a delivery service.

9. Sit down with a family member or friend and organize favorite family photos to place in a scrapbook; personalize each snapshot with a sentence or two about the pictured moment.

10. Purchase gas cards to help with the transportation expenses.

Paula Rauch, MD, a child psychiatrist, is director of the Parenting at a Challenging Time (PACT) Program at the Massachusetts General Hospital Cancer Center in Boston and co-author of the book Raising an Emotionally Healthy Child When a Parent Is Sick.

5 Things
to Tell Your Children about Your Cancer

1. **It's not your fault.** Cancer is never anyone's fault, even if there are risk factors that could have been avoided. Blaming oneself is never helpful, and it's important to tell children that cancer is a group of diseases that some people get for reasons that are not entirely clear.

2. **It's not their fault.** Children believe that they have enormous power and influence—superpowers. They may mistakenly believe that they somehow had the ability to cause your cancer. Reassure them that it's not their fault.

3. **People can't catch cancer from other people.** Explain that cancer is not like a cold that can be transmitted from person to person. Most kids are not old enough to go into explanations about genetics. Keep it simple, and explain that you can't catch cancer.

4. **Your doctors are smart and are working hard to help you.** No matter what type of cancer you have, or what stage, the message should always be that you are getting the best help possible. If you aren't getting the kind of help you need, then work toward that goal. Your message should be honest, of course.

5. **You are still the same mom or dad who loves them—cancer doesn't define you.** Put cancer in its place. Don't let your kids believe that a disease defines their parent.

CHAPTER 6

• • •

Balancing Work and Family

When I received my cancer diagnosis, I took some time off from work to undergo treatment. When the worst of the treatment was over, I went back to work, but I still needed to heal. For many months, I was very fatigued and did not function like I usually do. I vacillated between whether to tell people how I was feeling versus just "toughing it out." I had three young children at home who needed constant care and attention. In addition to my work and family commitments, I knew I needed to devote time to helping my body recover from the cancer treatments. I never reached the point where I thought everything was perfectly balanced. But I did the best I could under very difficult circumstances.

Katherine Russell Rich, writer and editor, chronicled her experience with breast cancer in *The Red Devil: A Memoir About Beating the Odds*. Kathy received a diagnosis of breast cancer at age thirty-two and had a recurrence of cancer in her bones five years later. She underwent a bone marrow transplant in 1995, two years after the recurrence. For the past several years, Kathy has been a popular speaker at a publishing course that I direct at Harvard Medical School. As I have gotten to know her, I am extremely impressed by how this young single woman has dealt with her cancer.

In Kathy's memoir, she described what it's like to live in two time zones: one that focuses on cancer and the other, which is the regular, real world. When I asked her to elaborate on this, she explained, "There was cancer time and real-life time when I was sick, and existing in both realms was like being in two time zones at once. In one, I was supposed to be concerned with the day-to-day stuff of life: IRAs and remembering to get the dry cleaning and sitting through meetings at work. In the other, I kept getting clobbered by life and death questions: Did I truly believe in God? What about mortality? Why are we on the earth?"

Because Kathy has fought cancer for so long, she has been through several job changes. How cancer has affected her career has changed over time. She shared this: "I remember feeling like cancer was this unwieldy, demanding, unbridled part-time job that kept interfering with my real work. The first time I was sick, I had a boss who was a cancer-phobe, and that made it really hard—I got the distinct impression that it would be best to downplay the illness on the job. But the illness was often so huge, it wasn't possible to live a double life, and so it constantly felt like I was doing the wrong thing. In my next job, my boss was great about letting me do whatever I needed to. With that pressure lifted, I became incredibly grateful to have absorbing work I could throw myself into—that I had somewhere to channel my energies."

Nearly two decades after her initial diagnosis, I asked Kathy about what it means to her to be a survivor, and this is what she told me: "I've had the illness so long that by now, I'm not sure I think of myself as a cancer survivor. Cancer's become just one part of the vast fabric that's been my life so far. In fact, I kind of balk at this point at defining myself by the illness—I've worked so hard to stay alive, that would seem to undermine the effort if I did."

I was impressed with the stories that survivors shared about the impact of their diagnosis on their careers and families. In every chapter of this book, there is evidence of the far-reaching effects of how what others did not only helped the survivor, but also helped his or her loved ones. However, there is one story that I thought was really meaningful to share with people who might reach out and help a colleague at work—perhaps someone they don't even know well. Julie, an advertising and marketing executive in New York City, is a laryngeal cancer survivor who was diagnosed in her forties. Since the larynx is in the neck, people undergoing treatment for this kind of cancer typically have problems with eating and swallowing. In order to make sure she took in enough calories, Julie had a feeding tube for seven months. She wrote about how her parents, who were in their mid-seventies, would drive a long distance to be with her for all of her appointments. Her mother fretted that she wasn't eating enough and was constantly urging her to eat more. As she lost weight, her parents worried. She knew that they felt like breaking down and crying, but were stoic for her sake.

Julie lives alone, and in addition to her brother and parents, whose support and presence she valued tremendously, she also wrote about her colleagues at work, especially her boss, who made an enormous impact on her ability to get through the difficult treatments. Julie wrote, "I was given seventeen weeks off, and my nurse practitioner told me to take all the time I needed [and not return to work too soon]. My boss sent me gifts (books, slippers, flowers, etc.) every week. She sent a pillow with everyone's photo and a folder with notes from my coworkers. She called me all the time. The gifts that my boss sent to me really touched my mother. She couldn't believe the kindnesses they showed me."

I think this is a powerful story, because it shows how kindness has a ripple effect and touches the lives not only of the people who are direct beneficiaries of the act of kindness, but also the lives of their loved ones. Everything you do to help someone going through cancer also helps those they love. I experienced this time and again when what others did to help me had an incredibly positive impact on my husband and children who live with me, as well as my brother, sister, and mother who live on the opposite coast.

A cancer diagnosis does change the balance between work and family. It was wonderful to read about how many people had kind bosses and coworkers who eased the cancer burden for a colleague who was going through treatment.

• • •

FORTUNATELY, I WORK for a most understanding employer, and needing time off for surgery and recovery has not been an issue at all. Now that I am back at work, my employer has let me know that if I need to leave early because of post-surgery issues, for clinic follow-ups, or whatever, I am not to worry about any of it...take what I need to recover and regain health.

Bill, administrator
Diagnosis of prostate cancer at age 62 in 2007 in Jefferson, Wisconsin

"We are just now digging ourselves out of the hole cancer put us in."

MY HUSBAND CAME to every treatment. He talked to doctors when I was the sickest. And he listened to me break down when I hit a really low spot a few days after each chemo infusion. When I thought I couldn't go on, he kept telling me I could do it. He cut back on his time at work to help me and to spend time with our son. Every evening, he and our son would go to the pool for a swim. It provided relief for my son from seeing his mom look so sick and thin. In the end, my husband's biggest sacrifice was his job. Despite all the laws in the world [to protect workers], his company staged a campaign to incrementally edge him out. Before my cancer, he had been one of the top performers in his division. From the point of my diagnosis on, after he had spoken to management about cutting back his hours at the office for the next few months, small changes were made that eventually made it impossible for him to succeed. Within one month, they moved his backup employee to another job and eliminated the position altogether. They reduced his sales territory and increased his quota. The list is endless. Finally, he left that position and moved on to another company. Employers need to know this: Cancer is expensive, and a lot of things aren't covered by insurance, such as the salary for the cleaning lady we hired during my treatment. It is cruel and unjust to treat employees in the callous manner in which my husband was treated. My husband's salary went down by 50 percent for three years consecutively, thanks to someone's clever plan to get rid of a cancer liability. We are just now digging ourselves out of the hole cancer put us in. So, in the end, my husband made a huge sacrifice. I couldn't have made it through the treatment without him. He gave up a lot for me.

Ann, homemaker
Diagnosis of breast cancer at age 47 in 2003 in Mechanicsburg, Pennsylvania

• • •

"Be gentle with yourself; think as positively as possible."

I TOOK QUITE a bit of time off work, and I just hung out at home. I spent the afternoons sitting in the sun on the patio reading or napping. My husband works from home, so he was always there for me. We were able to spend a lot of time together.

Leslie, programmer analyst
Diagnosis of pancreatic cancer at age 51 in 2006 in Prescott, Arizona

YOU CANNOT BALANCE WORK, family, and treatment. I took off six months, ran my business to ruin, and decided I would reboot my life later.

Suza, self-employed
Diagnosis of mantle cell lymphoma at age 41 in 2005 in Johannesburg, Gauteng (South Africa)

• • •

WHEN MY HUSBAND'S UNION voted to strike, he decided to retire a year earlier than planned because he was concerned about our insurance, and he was concerned that he would not be able to take care of me and take me for treatments if he had to find work until the strike was over. I was too weak to work or to drive. So when I needed to go into work for a few hours at the library to help my supervisor with administrative duties, such as monthly report and pay period closing, he drove me and sat and read while he waited. Until I regained my full strength, he would take me to work and wait or come back for me when I called.

Linda, genealogy associate at a historical library
Diagnosis of breast cancer at age 59 in 2006 in Sulphur, Louisiana

• • •

TO GET ME THROUGH treatment, I did a couple of key things. During my first round of treatment, which included chemotherapy and radiation, I began to walk up to two miles per day at the local YMCA, took time off work, and spent at least one day each week with friends. We simply gathered and went out to a local restaurant to talk about life and enjoy each other's company. The exercise made all the difference—both for my mental outlook and for easing the recovery from surgery. As a husband and father, it was very difficult to focus on me, but that was critical. I spent time with my wife while the kids were in school by enjoying trips to the grocery store or the local coffee shop. Anything to break the pattern each day. During six months of adjuvant treatment, I did return to work, but also took vacations with my family and took it slow. I lowered my personal expectations for delivering on anything other than my family's needs.

Mike, management professional
Diagnosis of rectal cancer at age 38 in 2006 in Rochester, New York

I TOLD A FEW key people at work who needed to understand if I was out of the office on certain days but, generally, I did not tell my colleagues or my patients. I found this actually helped—I wasn't constantly being asked how I was and forced to focus on my illness, my patients weren't worrying about me, and I wasn't being overlooked for professional opportunities because I might be "too tired" or have "too much going on."

Anne, psychologist
Diagnosis of breast cancer at age 50 in 2005 in Boston, Massachusetts

Once you have been able to cope with the disease, it is very probable that you can resume your ordinary activities—including work. Only a small percentage of cancer survivors, probably less than 10 percent, have persisting difficulties in returning to work.

JOS VERBEEK, MD, PhD, is an occupational physician and researcher. He has studied how cancer affects survivors' ability to return to work. Dr. Verbeek works both at the Finnish Institute of Occupational Health and the Coronel Institute of Occupational Health in Amsterdam, The Netherlands.

I HAVE A VERY hectic schedule with full-time work, a long commute, and three children. From the moment my cancer was diagnosed, I decided that I was going to treat this disease like it was just one more thing in my life to manage and that it would not overtake my life. I was fortunate to be able to work throughout my treatment, only taking days off for my chemo. I would come home exhausted and go to bed early, but I found that working kept me from sitting around and feeling sorry for myself.

Midge, accountant
Diagnosis of non-Hodgkin lymphoma at age 52 in 2005 and breast cancer at age 54 in 2007 in Westford, Massachusetts

TRY TO KEEP WORKING as much as you can; otherwise, this disease is so demanding it makes one too self-centered. Often, I need to lose myself and escape into something meaningful that goes beyond me and this insipid, sullen monster of an illness.

Kyle, pastor
Diagnosis of kidney cancer at age 60 in 2004 in Johnstown, Pennsylvania

• • •

I WAS MY OWN worst enemy, and I found myself living on the computer, looking for the worst news possible. I cured that by going to work...it really helped the depression and getting back into a normal life.

Kathie, nurse and social worker
Diagnosis of kidney cancer at age 53 in 2005 in Kingston, New York

• • •

I CONTINUED WORKING FULL-TIME as a secretary. Having this outlet allowed me to focus many hours a day away from me. I also found that talking frankly to a few colleagues freed up my mind and relieved some of the pressure from all of the nagging questions I carried around. Being able to talk openly about my situation had a healing effect on me.

Linda, administrative assistant
Diagnosis of breast cancer at age 55 in 2006 in Superior, Colorado

> "Try to keep working as much as you can...this disease is so demanding..."

• • •

I MADE A CAREER change and am now working with the American Cancer Society with other survivors and fighting back against cancer. I have been much more active in politics and making a difference in the time I have, no longer waiting for a more convenient time to volunteer.

Elizabeth, American Cancer Society volunteer coordinator
Diagnosis of breast cancer at age 44 in 2002 in Des Moines, Iowa

I CHOSE TO GO to counseling about eighteen months after completing my treatment. I had a sort of breakdown at work. I am a nurse, and I was crying beside unconscious patients, hoping they wouldn't wake up and see me crying. I wasn't coping at work or with my work colleagues. So, I chose to reduce my work hours to part-time and I began a course of counseling.

Pearl, nurse
Diagnosis of breast cancer at age 32 in 2004 in Glasgow (Scotland)

• • •

MY WIFE WOULD NOT allow me to wallow in self-pity. She kicked my ass right out there to work and play and be fully alive in every way.

Matt, carpenter
Diagnosis of chronic lymphocytic leukemia at age 51 in 2003 in Bath, New York

• • •

I WAS TOLD I would not likely survive. Yet within a few hours of hearing that, I never again considered that possibility and beat those 90 percent mortality odds against me. I delved deeply into my work and became a "workaholic," which kept me sane and looking forward. I became so completely driven that I have worked sixty to eighty hours a week most of my life since. I went ten years without any vacation after my cancer.

Ronald, business owner and entrepreneur
Diagnosis of testicular cancer at age 20 in 1975 in Dover, New Hampshire

• • •

> "Having financial security makes an enormous difference."

I TOOK TIME OFF from work. I do housecleaning and wasn't able to do that kind of work after my treatments. I had time to recover. My advice is to be gentle with yourself; think as positively as possible. Take this time to sit with family and talk; bond again.

Laura, housecleaner
Diagnosis of esophageal cancer at age 45 in 2002 in Schenectady, New York

A LITTLE OVER a year after my diagnosis, a coworker in the corporate office also received a cancer diagnosis. I was able to really help her cope with her journey because I had been there. We established an unparalleled bond.

Pat, office manager
Diagnosis of breast cancer at age 53 in 2001 in Canton, Michigan

• • •

I RECEIVED LETTERS and notes from people who work in my industry, telling me that I was in their thoughts—I still have most of them. My staff from work made every attempt to keep me in the loop, to let me know that I was still part of the team and they were keeping things going until I got back. They never let on (until much later) that they often wondered if I would be back.

Eileen, technology specialist
Diagnosis of breast cancer at age 34 in 1984 and acute myelogenous leukemia at age 49 in 1999 and basal cell carcinoma (skin cancer) at age 55 in 2005 in Framingham, Massachusetts

• • •

MY FAMILY RECEIVED a lot of support that I wasn't aware of at the time. The U.S. Navy was very supportive to us and to my father as well.

Randy, respiratory therapist
Diagnosis of Hodgkin disease at age 6 in 1965 in Ewa Beach, Hawaii

• • •

I HAVEN'T FIGURED OUT how to balance work yet. I haven't advanced that far. As for family, let them in. Let them take control. As hard as it is, that is what will make the recovery better. Let someone help you. Ask someone to help you.

Rochelle, manicurist
Diagnosis of melanoma (skin cancer) at age 34 in 2007 in Las Vegas, Nevada

> "Let friends and family help you. They want to... so give them something to do."

I CONTINUED TO WORK full-time, even through chemotherapy, when I had to take toxic drugs for ten months.

Sheri, actress
Diagnosis of Hodgkin disease at age 29 in 1993 in Columbia, Maryland

• • •

I HAD A MOST wonderful boss. Sometimes I just felt like crying, and he would just sit and hug me. He was the tower of strength.

LaDonne, retired
Diagnosis of kidney cancer at age 40 in 1978 in Mundelein, Illinois

• • •

FOCUS ON YOURSELF FIRST. Enjoy your family next, when you are having a good day. If you are able to take some time off work, do so. Let friends and family help you. They want to do that, so give them something to do. I would always have a "to do" list on my kitchen table. Anyone who stopped by and wanted to help would just look on the list and pick one or two things to do for me. It was great. It helped me, and it made them feel like they were helping. When you go back to work, take it slow. My life is now in the right order: family, friends, then work. I enjoy spending time doing big things, time doing small things, and time doing nothing. I enjoy dropping everything and running out the door to get an ice cream cone or take the dog for a quick walk. When it is my time [to go], I will have no regrets, as I am truly living my life.

Beth, health educator
Diagnosis of liver cancer at age 32 in 1990 in Fort Hood, Texas

• • •

IF A PERSON'S GOAL is to survive and get on with life, then the order should be treatment, family, then work. Make sure that family and friends will take care of each other and help you deal with the treatment plan. For the sake of the family, try to allow them to have (as nearly as possible) a normal daily life. Do not ask others to do for you what you can do for yourself.

David, journeyman sheet metal worker
Diagnosis of breast cancer at age 63 in 2005 in Missoula, Montana

My whole life stopped during my year-plus of cancer treatment. I hadn't really been on a career trajectory at that point, but I had to quit my temp job as a customer service representative. My treatment gave me a year or so to think about "What if?" while I was lying on the bed, anemic, watching shadows move across the walls. What would I really like to do with the rest of my life, assuming I was going to have the chance? I always knew I loved writing, but I never had had the nerve to put anything out in the public domain. After a year of fighting insurance companies, handling my treatment, and dealing with stares and comments on my baldness, I had enough nerve to do pretty much anything. I worked as a magazine editor for a couple of years, then moved into advertising copy writing. After a few years, though, I realized that I needed something deeper and more meaningful—that I couldn't spend my precious time selling somebody else's soapsuds. That's when I took the plunge and launched Planet Cancer to help other young adults from feeling the same isolation I had felt going through my own treatment, surrounded by patients my grandparents' age. It was the best thing I've ever done, and I've never looked back.

HEIDI ADAMS received a diagnosis of bone cancer (Ewing's sarcoma) of her left leg at age 26 in 1993. After undergoing treatment, she founded and is now the executive director of Planet Cancer, a community of support and advocacy for young adults with cancer in their 20s and 30s.

I LOOK AT LIFE much differently. I used to define myself by my work position. Now I see myself and other people as people. I learned that, in many ways, the burden that cancer caregivers carry is heavier than that of the cancer patient. As the cancer patient, I knew there was a protocol to follow and how I felt after treatment. The caregiver stands there on the sideline, trying to figure out what he or she can do to help, often not knowing.

Greg, disabled
Diagnosis of mantle cell lymphoma at age 57 in 2005 and acute myelogenous leukemia at age 60 in 2008 in Orland Park, Illinois

• • •

I WAS PLANNING a women's conference at the time of my diagnosis. One of the women who was assisting me put postcards out at the conference and told the attendees that if they wanted to send me a note, she would mail them to me since I couldn't attend the conference. About two weeks after the conference, I began receiving three or four postcards in the mail each day. This went on for a month! What an encouragement and blessing!

Patti, financial administrator
Diagnosis of ovarian cancer at age 51 in 2005 in Colorado Springs, Colorado

• • •

GOING TO MY EMPLOYER and my supervisor to tell them what I was dealing with and asking them to be understanding of the fact that I would need to take time off, even though I knew the Family Medical Leave Act would protect me. In that situation, it would have been helpful to have an advocate to speak on my behalf.

Nancy, administrative assistant
Diagnosis of breast cancer at age 54 in 2006 in Fowlerville, Michigan

• • •

I DID BECOME SELF-CENTERED and realized that I needed to take exceptional care of myself. The first thing I did was to take a leave of absence from my stressful job.

Julie, real estate agent
Diagnosis of thyroid cancer at age 34 in 1996 and breast cancer at age 43 in 2005 in Torrance, California

MY EMPLOYER MADE SURE that I knew they would support me if and when I needed treatment. Having financial security makes an enormous difference. It removes an enormous worry.

Kelly, financial services executive
Diagnosis of chronic lymphocytic leukemia at age 50 in 2003 and basal cell carcinoma (skin cancer) at age 53 in 2007 in Arlington, Virginia

• • •

MY COMPANY WAS GREAT in allowing me to work part-time, which allowed me to have day-to-day interaction with my coworkers. I drove myself to my chemotherapy and radiation therapy appointments, as I did not want to give up on doing things for myself. I also continued to have both body and facial massages. When I lost all my hair, I wore wigs, which gave me the incentive to continue to look healthy versus looking sick.

Rose, government contractor
Diagnosis of stomach cancer at age 60 in 2002 in Centreville, Virginia

• • •

I TOOK MY SISTER-IN-LAW'S advice (she's had lymphoma twice): "Don't be anyone's hero." I wasn't going to be Superwoman. If I was sick, I stayed home (luckily I had very understanding employers). I've learned not to take work so seriously. And to make sure I enjoy my work and coworkers. I always was a perfectionist. Today, I can relax a little.

Carmela, technical writer
Diagnosis of endometrial (uterine), bladder, and ovarian cancer at age 48 in 2005 in Clinton Township, Michigan

• • •

I WORKED DURING the early treatment phase of my first episode of cancer. My colleagues were more than helpful and supportive, and I took all the help I could without feeling like I was imposing on them.

Bryna, management development consultant
Diagnosis of tongue cancer at age 35 in 1985 in Brockton, Massachusetts

Work and family were my salvation. Work kept me busy and took my mind off the chemo. I missed only three days, and that was for the mastectomy. Fatigue was my culprit. Some days, I didn't feel like doing as much as usual. My students and coworkers at Oklahoma University were amazing, a tremendous support group. My wife, Becky, only worked part-time that year, and it allowed her time to baby me, a treat I didn't resist. She understood when I needed to go to bed as soon as I got home, when I needed a more palatable menu, or when I just needed a little TLC. My family's love sustained me.

JACK WILLIS taught journalism at the University of Oklahoma and is the author of *Saving Jack*. He received a diagnosis of breast cancer at the age of 64 in 2005.

I WAS A KINDERGARTEN teacher in an inner city school. I felt I couldn't quit work, so I arranged to have my chemo over the summer. I worried about what would happen if I had to continue on with chemo over the fall, how I would operate with substitute teachers and the children, but it proved a moot point as the oncologist stopped the chemo after three rounds (and I have been in remission ever since). So I did not have to miss any school for chemo, and life went on!

Teri, retired kindergarten teacher
Diagnosis of chronic lymphocytic leukemia at age 51 in 1999 in Fort Langley, British Columbia (Canada)

• • •

I HAD CANCER, and I work for the American Cancer Society—that's a tough combo. It's been several years now, and the prognosis for my type of cancer is very good.

Allie, Director, Distinguished Events; American Cancer Society
Diagnosis of thyroid cancer at age 46 in 2003 in Fair Haven, New Jersey

I GOT MAD! From the beginning, it was a fight, and I was absolutely going to win. My business partner dissolved our partnership while I was in chemo. Talk about, "What else could happen?" Turns out it was the best thing that could have happened. The cancer fight and having to change my work made me step out of my comfort zone. Now I'm totally a risk taker. I recently opened my own company!

Karen, real estate broker
Diagnosis of breast cancer at age 38 in 2001 in Loganville, Georgia

• • •

I LEFT MY JOB in a hospital after fifteen years. I'm home in the morning when my son leaves for school, and I'm waiting at the door for him when he gets off the bus. I might not be bringing home a paycheck, but my son's smile when he sees me in the doorway is more payment than I will ever need.

Laura, unemployed psychiatric social worker
Diagnosis of breast cancer at age 43 in 2006 in Avon, Connecticut

• • •

I WENT BACK to work housekeeping as soon as I could, and I think the exercise helped me to stay a little more in shape, and it kept me mentally busy as well.

Jennifer, housekeeper
Diagnosis of breast cancer at age 40 in 2004 and skin cancer at age 41 in 2005 in Craig, Colorado

• • •

WHILE IN TREATMENT, do what you normally do as much as you can. It gives normalcy to the experience and prevents one from "curling up in a little ball." I was able to take chemotherapy and then go to work. The treatment was part of my day's process, not all of it.

John, retired
Diagnosis of prostate cancer at age 57 in 1995 and chronic lymphocytic leukemia at age 65 in 2003 in Jacksonville, Florida

> "I finally realized that my one and only job was to fight cancer."

WORK WILL GET DONE without you. If possible, take the time off to concentrate on yourself. Allow yourself to heal fully, without guilt.

Linda, purchasing agent
Diagnosis of breast cancer at age 47 in 2007 in Antioch, California

• • •

I FINALLY REALIZED that my one and only job was to fight cancer. Not to do the dishes, not to continue seeing patients, not to read the medical literature, not to catch up on things left undone because of our busy schedules. Just to fight cancer.

Deborah, physician
Diagnosis of breast cancer at age 47 in 2007 in Overland Park, Kansas

• • •

WHEN YOUR CANCER is diagnosed, there is a weird dichotomy: on one hand, the world stops; on the other, you move through the blood tests, the scans, the doctors' appointments, the reading, and it seems as if you wake up the next day and your uterus is gone. You need to slow down. You need to involve your family. You need to scale back work (or take as much time off as you can). You need to allow yourself the time and the rest to cope. Focus on you. It is better to get out and exercise (when you can) for a few weeks rather than rush back to work as soon as you can walk. You need to take the time to get better, before you face the added demands of work. This goes for family demands as well. Get help with your children and with household chores. Let someone else cook. Spend your time reading or playing with the kids, not doing their laundry. All of this will make you feel stronger, more quickly.

Jennifer, federal officer with U.S. Customs and Border Patrol
Diagnosis of cervical cancer at age 36 in 2007 in Montreal, Quebec (Canada)

Reference

Rich, K. R. 1999. *The red devil: a memoir about beating the odds.* New York: Three Rivers Press.

CHAPTER 7

• • •

How I Changed My Diet

I was speaking at a conference at M.D. Anderson, a large cancer center in Houston, Texas. During the conference, a participant asked the panel members whether breast cancer survivors should avoid eating soy products. Soy products may contain some estrogen-like compounds, and the concern is that these compounds may promote tumor growth in people who have cancer that responds to the presence of estrogen (estrogen receptor–positive tumors). The oncologist gave a thoughtful response in which she recommended that people with estrogen receptor–positive tumors avoid eating soy products as much as possible, but not to worry about eating a little bit. This is an important point in discussing nutrition and cancer because, with few exceptions, anything in the diet that really impacts someone's health status must be eaten in fairly large quantities and somewhat consistently. This is true for both a positive and a negative impact. For example, a diet high in fruits and vegetables appears to have a positive impact on helping prevent many health problems, including some types of cancer. However, the occasional apple or carrot won't likely help. The opposite is also true. If you drink soy milk and have soy with most meals, this might be a problem if you have an estrogen receptor–positive tumor. However, if you occasionally have some soy, it's extremely unlikely to be a problem.

In other books I have written, I have discussed the best ways to fortify your body after a cancer diagnosis (see page 144). In this book, I want to share what other cancer survivors have done regarding their diets. Very briefly, here's what I tell cancer survivors when they need some guidelines for their diet. First, something you eat will only be a problem if you eat a lot of it and eat it consistently. So, if you are worried about whether to eat a specific food, just limit how much of it you eat and don't eat it every day. Second, eating fruits and vegetables is very good for you, so try to eat at least five or more servings each day. Third, worrying about your diet is worthwhile only if you make positive changes and get into the habit of eating healthier meals and snacks.

When my cancer was diagnosed, I found myself worrying a lot about my diet. I began analyzing everything I ate. Knowing that there is a relationship between diet and some cancers made me worry even more. I definitely made some changes to my diet, including making a conscientious effort to eat more fruits and vegetables every day. Because I cook for my family, this changed their diet, too.

At first, my children grumbled about the changes, but then they became accustomed to seeing a colorful plate full of fresh fruits and vegetables. One night, when I was particularly tired, I ordered pizza and served it with a glass of milk. My youngest daughter eyed her plate and asked, "Where's the rest of the food?" What she was really asking me was, "Where are all the colorful fruits and vegetables?" I realized that I had achieved a measure of success in converting my family to a healthier diet if my youngest child was actually asking me for fruits and vegetables.

My children wrote two children's books for the American Cancer Society called *Our Mom Is Getting Better* and *Our Dad Is Getting Better*. *Our Mom Is Getting Better* is a book for children about how families meet the challenges of having a parent with cancer, and it is based on our real experiences. *Our Dad Is Getting Better* is a companion book that has much of the same content, but has a fictional dad who is recovering from cancer. When my youngest daughter was ready to draw the illustration that is used in both books about how our family changed our eating habits, my other two kids scurried around the kitchen, piling on the counter all of the nutritious foods we had in the house. Soon, the counter was covered with colorful fruits and vegetables, so my daughter simply drew what was in front of her. Seeing all of the different types of fruits and vegetables that I had encouraged my children to eat day after day really hit home for me. The efforts I had made had helped not only me, but also my kids, achieve better health through nutritional changes.

Consider this: What we eat is more about habit than anything else. If children become accustomed to eating lots of fruits and vegetables, they come to expect it as part of the structure of their lives. It may take many tries to get them to eat a new food, so don't be discouraged. Just keep putting it on their plates. When children get used to seeing a colorful plate, even though they may complain about their diet on occasion, they'll likely miss these nutritious foods if you don't serve them. Adults, too, eat what they feel comfortable with and what they are used to consuming. We all have dietary habits that are surprisingly consistent over time. This means that the more you fill up your plate with fruits and vegetables, the more habitual it will become and the more comfortable you will feel eating these foods over time.

Certainly a cancer diagnosis can be a catalyst for one to take stock and make lifestyle changes that promote good health. However, undergoing cancer treatment is incredibly stressful, so this may not be the perfect time to make changes. In this chapter, you'll read what many survivors have done when faced with decisions about whether and how to change their diets.

• • •

I WAS A VEGETARIAN when my cancer was diagnosed, but now I eat much healthier overall and avoid alcohol and second-hand smoke like the plague.

Eileen, teacher
Diagnosis of breast cancer at age 43 in 2006 in Hilton, New York

• • •

I CAN'T EAT a lot of what I used to—my body doesn't like it too much. I try to eat a lot more fruit, but can't afford it most of the time. I did start drinking green tea.

Kimatha, medical laboratory technician
Diagnosis of kidney cancer at age 42 in 2001 in Edinburgh, Indiana

• • •

I WISH DOCTORS PROVIDED more consistent information on the value of nutrition, but that is a training deficit in the medical world that I believe is beginning to change. For now, it requires extra effort and personal research to investigate and evaluate.

Beth, massage therapist
Diagnosis of breast cancer at age 39 in 2006 in Tempe, Arizona

I THINK THAT EXERCISE and eating healthy are very important, although I have to be honest in saying that I don't always do so.

Joyce, legal secretary
Diagnosis of breast cancer at age 44 in 2006 in South Amboy, New Jersey

• • •

"If I can't have what I want and like, what's the point of it all? Why bother?"

I TURNED TO YOGA and reverted to (primarily) a vegetarian diet. Having grown up in India in the 1980s, I rarely ate meat or food with a lot of preservatives, or any kind of food with high-fat content. I am a Chitpavan Brahmin from the state of Maharashtra, and our staple diet is quite healthy. However, when I came to the United States for graduate school in 1991, my lifestyle radically changed. I began to consume a lot of high-fat food, meat, beer, etc.

Jitendra, software engineer
Diagnosis of non-Hodgkin lymphoma at age 28 in 1994 in Cleveland, Ohio

• • •

I DRANK AN AWEFUL-AWEFUL every day to help put on weight. My mother went to Newport Creamery and got me a coffee-mint Aweful-Aweful every day (on advice from my physician). I went for walks around the neighborhood to help build my strength and drank the milkshakes to help put on weight. My mother's home cooking helped a great deal with that as well when my taste buds started to return.

Todd, oncology social worker
Diagnosis of chronic myelogenous leukemia at age 25 in 1997 and kidney cancer at age 33 in 2005 in Warwick, Rhode Island

• • •

AT FIRST, I ATE everything and started gaining weight. Then I went back to my regular healthy diet and have gotten back to my "fighting" weight.

James, retired police officer
Diagnosis of lymphoma at age 66 in 2007 in Sheridan, Wyoming

IT'S BASICALLY THE SAME diet, except that now I have to chew my food carefully (my salivary glands were affected, and I don't have as much saliva). If I eat quickly and don't chew the food (especially steak), I have problems swallowing.

Julie, account executive in advertising/marketing
Diagnosis of laryngeal cancer at age 46 in 2002 in New York City, New York

• • •

I'D LIKE TO REPORT that I've now adopted a healthy diet, consisting only of fish, chicken, and occasional lean meats, together with vegetables and fruit, whole grains, nuts and the like, but it's not true. I do eat all those things, but I also eat all of the sweets and desserts I have always loved—candy, cookies, chips, cake, pie, sweet rolls, pancakes, and bacon. Hell, I'm sixty-seven years old and have endured cancer. If I can't have what I want and like, what's the point of it all? Why bother? Ha!

Mike, retired real estate developer and cattle rancher
Diagnosis of colon cancer at age 66 in 2006 in Red Lodge, Montana

After reviewing the diagnosis and treatment options with my patients, I want them to understand their own important role in recovery through behavior modification that incorporates diet and regular exercise. Simple life changes are the way to start—there is no magic to it. *Get moving and eat well.* Eat real food, not processed food. Shop the perimeter of the grocery store to avoid more highly processed foods. Try to reduce saturated fat. Eat mostly plants, and eat a rainbow of colors. Colorful foods are naturally higher in the micronutrients the body needs. Don't be afraid to cook; fresh food is always best. I recommend hormone- and pesticide-free food.

ANITA JOY HILLIARD, MD, is a radiation oncologist at the Alan B. Pearson Regional Cancer Center of Centra Health in Lynchburg, Virginia.

I PAY VERY CLOSE attention to nutrition, exercise, and cutting down on my alcohol intake. I believe I have to do everything I can do to prevent a recurrence or a new cancer.

Cathi, clinical social worker
Diagnosis of breast cancer at age 52 in 2003 in Waban, Massachusetts

• • •

I HAVE ELIMINATED CERTAIN types of food even though they were an insignificant part of my diet before cancer. I am much more mindful of eating only for need and not for desire. This has helped me lose nearly thirty pounds since my cancer was diagnosed. Dropping red meats and fried foods has not been a problem. And I am discovering new foods and methods of preparation that I enjoy.

Bill, administrator
Diagnosis of prostate cancer at age 62 in 2007 in Jefferson, Wisconsin

• • •

NOW I EAT BROCCOLI and blueberries!

Peggy, pathologist's assistant
Diagnosis of breast cancer at age 47 in 2003 in St. Augustine, Florida

• • •

AT MY ONCOLOGIST'S DIRECTION, I stopped eating red meat. I began to drink more water, rather than soda and coffee. Also, I buy chicken that is farm-raised with no steroids, hormones, or antibiotics. It is an ongoing battle to eat healthy and try to stay away from sweets, but I do my best.

Sarah, paralegal
Diagnosis of breast cancer at age 28 in 2000 in Miami, Florida

• • •

I DO NOT CONSUME anything with added sugar or white flour. I never eat red meat. I eat more vegetables and fruit and drink more water.

Laurie, medical assistant
Diagnosis of breast cancer at age 43 in 2006 in Sacramento, California

I BECAME A GRANDMOTHER during that time, and my daughter has made the choice to feed her girls healthy, organic foods. My daughter has inspired me to eat whole foods, not processed, crap foods. I am taking small steps toward eating healthier. I will achieve this goal.

Laura, housecleaner
Diagnosis of esophageal cancer at age 45 in 2002 in Schenectady, New York

• • •

SHORTLY AFTER THE END of all of my treatments, I began to gain back the weight I had lost, but I kept gaining. Finally I put myself on Weight Watchers and lost the extra thirty-five pounds I had gained. I still try to watch what I eat. I also have to watch what I eat and how much I eat because the radiation damaged my stomach muscles, so food doesn't digest properly. If I eat more than a very small amount, it comes right back up. Not pleasant, but one more thing I have learned to deal with.

Eileen, technology specialist
Diagnosis of breast cancer at age 34 in 1984 and acute myelogenous leukemia at age 49 in 1999 and basal cell carcinoma (skin cancer) at age 55 in 2005 in Framingham, Massachusetts

• • •

I HAVEN'T CHANGED MY diet yet. I am still all new to this, but I will change it. I want to be around to see my girls graduate, get married, and have kids of their own. That won't happen at three hundred pounds!

Rochelle, manicurist
Diagnosis of melanoma (skin cancer) at age 34 in 2007 in Las Vegas, Nevada

• • •

I AM TRYING TO eat healthier and follow a more plant-based diet. It's hard!

Evelyn, executive assistant
Diagnosis of colon cancer at age 33 in 2004 in Boston, Massachusetts

> "Still eating the same and not exercising very much. I will tomorrow, though."

I FOUND THAT EATING bland foods like oatmeal and grits helped keep any feelings of nausea away.

Cynthia, administrative assistant
Diagnosis of breast cancer at age 55 in 2003 in Highland Lakes, New Jersey

Unfortunately, many cancer survivors turn to dietary supplements believing they will improve health and prevent further cancers. What many people don't realize is that dietary supplement laws are very lax in the United States. Many supplements are contaminated or don't provide what they claim on the label. Another problem is that research studies regarding supplements are still in the infancy stages. Most of the studies show positive results in a laboratory setting, but the effect can be quite different in humans. In fact, some studies had to be halted because the number of cancer cases in those taking the supplement actually increased. What has become very clear from all the research is that cancers and many other diseases can be reduced by these guidelines: losing weight, eating five to nine servings of fruits and vegetables daily, including more whole grains and less refined starches and sugars in the diet, cutting back on dietary fats, and doing daily exercise.

ALICE RICHER is a registered dietitian and co-author of *Understanding the Antioxidant Controversy — Scrutinizing the "Fountain of Youth."* She works with cancer survivors at one of Spaulding Rehabilitation Hospital's outpatient centers in Framingham, Massachusetts. Alice is also the team dietitian for the major league soccer team, the New England Revolution.

I HAD JUST EARNED my black belt in Korean Tae Kwon Do. Not only was it about physical strength but about spiritual strength as well. I ate extremely well prior to my diagnosis. I was in training with my martial arts.

Sheri, actress
Diagnosis of Hodgkin disease at age 29 in 1993 in Columbia, Maryland

• • •

I EAT MORE SALAD and less meat. I eat more fish and fruit. I drink wine. I choose good bread. I eat yogurt—this is my dairy intake because I have never liked milk. I drink less coffee but have not given it up entirely. I did not want my life to become dedicated to eating and drinking and every thought to be around health.

> "Eat a good breakfast daily. It really helps through the day."

Pat, retired
Diagnosis of colon and bladder cancer at age 74 in 2005 in Como (Western Australia)

• • •

ACTUALLY, I HAD BEEN improving my diet already with less sugar, less diet pop, more organic foods. I have always gardened, and we have fresh vegetables from there. I also cook most of our meals, and we don't eat out very often. I do have my splurges, though, and still love sugar.

Charose, nurse
Diagnosis of Hodgkin disease at age 17 in 1972 and breast cancer at age 51 in 2006 in Omaha, Nebraska

• • •

I AM AVOIDING SOY as much as possible. My husband and I are eating more natural products and fewer processed foods. I am drinking more water and green tea and less soda.

Jan, retired hospice chaplain
Diagnosis of breast cancer at age 55 in 2006 in Wichita, Kansas

> ## "I've moved to a much healthier diet—less alcohol, more fruits and veggies, more whole grains, no red meat."

I LOST MY CRAVINGS for chocolate! Godiva chocolate doesn't even tempt me anymore.

> **Nancy, administrative assistant**
> *Diagnosis of breast cancer at age 54 in 2006 in Fowlerville, Michigan*

• • •

ALL THE ANTIOXIDANT FOODS found their way into my pantry and fridge. Good-bye McDonald's!

> **Kathleen, retail manager**
> *Diagnosis of breast cancer at age 48 in 2007 in Washington Township, New Jersey*

• • •

STEROIDS HAVE CAUSED SIGNIFICANT weight gain, so I've moved to a much healthier diet— less alcohol, more fruits and veggies, more whole grains, no red meat.

> **Deborah, physician**
> *Diagnosis of breast cancer at age 47 in 2007 in Overland Park, Kansas*

• • •

I AM MORE AWARE of warnings of [foods] that can cause cancer, but I haven't changed my diet as much as I should.

> **Teri, retired kindergarten teacher**
> *Diagnosis of chronic lymphocytic leukemia at age 51 in 1999 in Fort Langley, British Columbia (Canada)*

• • •

I GAVE UP ALCOHOL.

> **Yvonne, paralegal**
> *Diagnosis of colon cancer at age 48 in 2004 in San Antonio, Texas*

I TRY TO DRINK protein shakes instead of hitting the local burger joint, but it's difficult some days.

Karen, real estate broker
Diagnosis of breast cancer at age 38 in 2001 in Loganville, Georgia

• • •

SUPPLEMENTS.

Cheryl, homemaker
Diagnosis of breast cancer at age 49 in 2006 in Garland, Texas

• • •

I WISH I COULD say that I've transformed into a health food fanatic and exercise freak, but I haven't. Still eating the same and not exercising very much. I will tomorrow, though.

Laura, unemployed psychiatric social worker
Diagnosis of breast cancer at age 43 in 2006 in Avon, Connecticut

• • •

I DRINK MORE WATER to try to flush things out.

Jennifer, publicity coordinator
Diagnosis of melanoma (skin cancer) at age 21 in 2004 in San Diego, California

• • •

I DON'T EAT ANY sugar or red meat, and I eat lots of fruits and almonds.

Luann, stay-at-home mom
Diagnosis of colon cancer at age 50 in 2003 in Charleston, West Virginia

• • •

EAT A GOOD BREAKFAST daily. It really helps through the day.

Tracey, radiation oncology information analyst
Diagnosis of breast cancer at age 37 in 2002 in Villa Park, Illinois

I TRIED TO EAT healthy, but there were days I ate the unhealthy stuff! I had a horrible diet during my treatment. I ate continually, and most of it was not healthy food. Meat, fresh fruits, and vegetables all tasted terrible during chemo.

Linda, purchasing agent
Diagnosis of breast cancer at age 47 in 2007 in Antioch, California

• • •

I ALWAYS ATE PRETTY well. I now eat even better. I get a minimum five to ten fruits and veggies (more often seven to ten) five days a week.

Jennifer, federal officer with U.S. Customs and Border Patrol
Diagnosis of cervical cancer at age 36 in 2007 in Montreal, Quebec (Canada)

• • •

I AM A HEART patient as well, and while I had cancer, I was put on a high-calorie diet, which was three hundred and sixty degrees from my former diet. I'm back on the heart diet now.

John, retired
Diagnosis of esophageal cancer at age 76 in 2006 in Jamestown, North Carolina

• • •

I HAVE CHANGED my diet and how I look at food in general. I try to eat only organic foods. I eat less red meat. I stay away from artificial colors and preservatives. I try to limit the amount of junk food that is brought into the house.

Lisa, administrative assistant
Diagnosis of breast cancer at age 38 in 2000 in Owings Mills, Maryland

• • •

I TAKE ALL MEDS on time every day.

Candy, teacher
Diagnosis of thyroid cancer at age 31 in 2007 in El Paso, Texas

There isn't a "one size fits all" diet during chemotherapy. Even small adjustments to an eating pattern may help manage treatment-related side effects such as constipation, diarrhea, or nausea. Find credible resources; toss the rest. An oncology dietitian can help sort through the vast amount of flashy information in a credible, honest, and open way.

TARA MARDIGAN is a registered dietitian and senior nutritionist at the Dana-Farber Cancer Institute in Boston, Massachusetts. She is also the team nutritionist for the Boston Red Sox.

I PURCHASED VITAMINS and a juicer and became a vegetarian. It goes back and forth. I am no longer juicing or a vegan. I do know what a healthy diet is. When I eat well, I eat better than most of the people around me.

Judi, nurse
Diagnosis of breast cancer at age 40 in 2000 in Pen Argyl, Pennsylvania

• • •

I WEIGHED NEARLY FOUR hundred pounds when my cancer was first diagnosed, which in itself was totally unhealthy. I now weigh about one hundred and fifty pounds because I have a lot of trouble swallowing, but I do drink supplemental shakes to maintain my weight.

Kathy, babysitter
Diagnosis of tongue cancer at age 38 in 1997 in Niles, Illinois

• • •

I AVOID BUFFETS more often now!

Todd, oncology social worker
Diagnosis of chronic myelogenous leukemia at age 25 in 1997 and kidney cancer at age 33 in 2005 in Warwick, Rhode Island

Ways to Improve Your Diet

1. Aim to eat at least five servings of colorful fruits and vegetables each day.

2. Talk to your doctor or dietitian about how much protein you need.

3. Choose whole grains instead of processed grains and flours (an easy way to think of this is to "go brown").

4. Limit the amount of refined sugar in the diet, and choose nutrient-dense foods instead.

5. Eat a low-fat diet.

6. Avoid nicotine completely, and limit alcohol as much as possible.

7. Consider taking a multivitamin that provides 100 percent of the Recommended Dietary Allowances (RDA) for essential nutrients established by the U.S. Food and Nutrition Board of the National Academies/Institute of Medicine (never exceed the tolerable upper intake levels [UL] for any of them). Ask your doctor or dietitian whether you need to take calcium and vitamin D supplements.

8. Discuss with your doctor all supplements you are taking or plan to take.

CHAPTER 8

• • •

How I Changed My Exercise Routine

The role of exercise is becoming increasingly important in cancer care to help people stay physically and emotionally strong during and after treatment. New research has indicated that some cancers, for example, breast and colon, might be less likely to recur in someone who is physically active.

I was talking to a breast oncologist about the many things people recommend for cancer survivors—some of them clearly ridiculous. He told me, "If people are willing to make just one change, exercise will likely have the greatest impact." By "greatest impact," my colleague meant that exercise will not only help survivors through their treatments, but have beneficial effects long afterward. Physical activity can make it easier for patients to tolerate toxic cancer therapies and to heal more quickly from the treatments. Exercise can also help prevent the major disease threats to people: heart disease, stroke, and cancer.

If you have cancer, ask your doctor whether exercise can impact your prognosis by helping prevent cancer recurrence. Research on the benefits of exercise in cancer prevention or recurrence is evolving, so by the time you read this, there may be new, important studies to consider. Even if exercise won't change your prognosis, it can help tremendously with other aspects of your health.

Of course, for a variety of reasons, not every cancer survivor is able to exercise. Moreover, exercising during treatment is another thing you'll want to talk over with your doctor to determine whether it is safe to exercise and how best to do it. Whenever you begin to exercise, checking in with your doctor is a good idea, even if you haven't been through cancer or treatment.

Here's a simple tip that I give people to get started: Obtain a pedometer and use it for one week to count how many steps a day you are taking. Then, set a goal to walk up to 10,000 steps per day. Not everyone can do this, which is why you'll want to check in with your doctor. However, 10,000 steps a day is the goal for average, healthy adults. Remember to start by simply determining how many steps you are taking now. Having a baseline is important, because from there you can track your progress. Reasonable goals during treatment will widely vary. It might be unwise to exercise at all during treatment—your doctor can tell you. After the worst of the cancer treatments are over, then most people can increase the number of steps a day they take by about 250 to 500 over the course of a week. So, if you start out at an average of 2,000 steps per day, then the next week you might want to aim for 2,250 or 2,500 steps. Symptoms such as shortness of breath or chest pain or anything else that seems worrisome should be immediately reported to your doctor.

Later in this book, I discuss healing in a bit more detail. It's unfortunate that even though many people truly want to feel better, they often don't put things that will help them heal at the top of their "to do" list. Exercise will help facilitate physical and emotional recovery, so if you are physically able to exercise and your doctor approves it, consider making physical activity a daily priority. It may not be easy, but it does become less difficult with time and practice.

During a visit to Lynchburg, Virginia, I gave a series of talks to the health care providers at Centra Health. When I arrived, I had a couple of hours to drop off my luggage and relax before my first meeting. My friend and host for the day, orthopedic surgeon Jim Dunstan, asked me, in typical Southern gentleman fashion, what I wanted to do with the time I had before the meeting. He suggested we go sightseeing or take a long walk and, of course, I chose the walk. A couple of days later, in a speech I was giving at the meeting, I emphasized how exercise has to be a priority, even when you'd rather do something else. I confessed to the audience that I had waived an opportunity to see their hometown in favor of physical activity. I added that I hoped such choices would allow my health to flourish, so that someday I could return and really take in that beautiful part of Virginia.

You'll read more about the importance of exercise from the survivors who responded to the surveys. My advice is simple: Don't fret over whether you are doing enough physical activity. Your health status will change over time, and your physician can guide you. Often, people will exercise in fits and starts and then gradually incorporate exercise into a part of their regular routine. In short, if you are a cancer survivor, don't sweat the exercise issue, but do realize that it *will* help you feel better.

• • •

MY DOCTOR TOLD ME if I could walk from my house to his office, he would buy me a cup of coffee. (It's a five-minute walk). I joined a gym and began walking every day. Now, I walk five miles every day.

Carrie, information management specialist
Diagnosis of breast cancer at age 44 in 2002 in New York City, New York

• • •

AS SOON AS I was able, I started exercising and getting in shape. I've never felt better in that respect. I have also signed up to do a 5K race, which is something I have never done before. I've been training for it, and even though it's not really a competition (it's a cancer fundraiser), it has motivated me to try something new while supporting a great cause.

> "I joined a gym and began walking every day."

Federico, cancer chemical biologist
Diagnosis of testicular cancer at age 32 in 2006 in Brookline, Massachusetts

• • •

I AM A RUNNER. I started to get in shape and was in training before I received my cancer diagnosis. Being in shape made the surgery much easier. After surgery, physical activity was essential. I was out walking and moving as soon as I could. It helped the constipation, the swelling, and the pain. It helped me sleep. It helped my muscles return to normal. Most of all, it helped my head. Physical activity has huge psychological benefits.

Jennifer, federal officer with U.S. Customs and Border Patrol
Diagnosis of cervical cancer at age 36 in 2007 in Montreal, Quebec (Canada)

I TOOK UP GOLF a week before receiving my diagnosis—went through chemo and the beginner's course. You do what you can, when you can.

Suza, self-employed
Diagnosis of mantle cell lymphoma at age 41 in 2005 in Johannesburg, Gauteng (South Africa)

• • •

I WALKED AROUND my neighborhood as much as I could. I began working right after my last chemo treatment, which helped me get back into a routine.

Carlyn, administrative assistant
Diagnosis of Hodgkin disease at age 30 in 2004 in Willow Spring, North Carolina

• • •

> "After surgery, physical activity was essential. I was out walking and moving as soon as I could."

I WALKED EVERY DAY. After my recovery, I took self-defense lessons with my son. I also took motorcycle lessons and joined a health spa. I still can't do all of those activities, but I sure try!

Alejandra, clerical worker
Diagnosis of uterine cancer at age 36 in 2005 in Torrance, California

• • •

THE SIDE EFFECTS of the medicines made it difficult to take the long hikes that I had depended on. I learned to push to exercise in every way that I could—yoga, swimming, and machines at the "Y." I respect my body more, but I am also less prone to invest myself in it. I have never been this out of shape, but I know that I am doing the best I can, so it is okay.

Kyle, pastor
Diagnosis of kidney cancer at age 60 in 2004 in Johnstown, Pennsylvania

I WAS A WALKER before my diagnosis, so the faster I could get out to the park and take my walks, the better I felt. Actually, the first time I made it down the block to the corner—five houses down—I cried because I made it that far. I was so happy!

Dorinda, retired teacher
Diagnosis of ovarian cancer at age 50 in 2005 in Edison, New Jersey

• • •

I WALK A LOT more. I got a puppy, and he keeps me fit because I walk him a lot. He has the role of keeping Mum fit and getting her out and about.

Pearl, nurse
Diagnosis of breast cancer at age 32 in 2004 in Glasgow (Scotland)

Exercise is the key to feeling well. Fat cells make estrogen, and estrogen is a growth factor for some types of breast cancer. There is no need to join a fitness club; just start walking. Simple, deliberate efforts to become more active go a long way in restoring and maintaining your body. Exercise is also an important way to combat the depression that often accompanies a diagnosis of cancer.

ANITA JOY HILLIARD, MD, is a radiation oncologist at the Centra Alan B. Pearson Regional Cancer Center in Lynchburg, Virginia.

MY WIFE is a physical therapist and owns her own clinic. She made me go there many times to work out and build my strength. I started skiing cross-country within a couple of months after the transplant, and that got me out and going. Exercise is the only thing that works for me. Well, a little whiskey can take the edge off.

Matt, carpenter
Diagnosis of chronic lymphocytic leukemia at age 51 in 2003 in Bath, New York

> **"Being in motion and working the whole body brings me a sense of well-being and fitness that is invaluable."**

I HAVE BEGUN RUNNING and now run three to five times a week, for thirty-five minutes. I'm in better shape now than before I had cancer.

Cathi, clinical social worker
Diagnosis of breast cancer at age 52 in 2003 in Waban, Massachusetts

• • •

I GOT PHYSICALLY ACTIVE just as soon as the surgeon gave me the go ahead. Being in motion and working the whole body brings me a sense of well-being and fitness that is invaluable. My major activity now is to rebuild my fitness and endurance for cycling. I am working with a trainer from the sports medicine clinic at the hospital where my surgery was done.

Bill, administrator
Diagnosis of prostate cancer at age 62 in 2007 in Jefferson, Wisconsin

• • •

I EXERCISE A LITTLE less with one lung.

Bill, retired
Diagnosis of colon and lung cancer at age 63 in 2004 in Niceville, Florida

• • •

I STILL HATE EXERCISING...but I am trying to be more physically active.

Evelyn, executive assistant
Diagnosis of colon cancer at age 33 in 2004 in Boston, Massachusetts

• • •

I TRY TO WALK three times a week with my dog.

Kelley, massage therapist
Diagnosis of breast cancer at age 36 in 2006 in Rochdale, Massachusetts

MY PERSONAL TRAINER HELPED me regain my muscle strength. He was great. I feel better now than I did before.

Peggy, pathologist's assistant
Diagnosis of breast cancer at age 47 in 2003 in St. Augustine, Florida

• • •

ONE OF THE SIDE effects I am dealing with is shortness of breath. So far they haven't determined whether it is a cardiac problem or a pulmonary problem. As a result, I can no longer climb more than a very short flight of stairs, and walking up hills (even slight inclines) is taxing. Despite this, I walk on a treadmill every morning for thirty minutes.

Eileen, technology specialist
Diagnosis of breast cancer at age 34 in 1984 and acute myelogenous leukemia at age 49 in 1999 and basal cell carcinoma (skin cancer) at age 55 in 2005 in Framingham, Massachusetts

• • •

I WAS ALREADY EXERCISING, but did attend weight-training classes through our cancer center after recovery. I did learn to exercise properly and loved the camaraderie of being with other survivors, but because of time constraints, I'm continuing my exercise at home. I think I am even more committed to my exercise program now and definitely have better muscles.

> **"I'm in better shape now than before I had cancer."**

Charose, nurse
Diagnosis of Hodgkin disease at age 17 in 1972 and breast cancer at age 51 in 2006 in Omaha, Nebraska

• • •

MORNING WALKS with my dog were wonderful for my well-being.

Mary, administrative assistant
Diagnosis of breast cancer at age 42 in 2003 in Simi Valley, California.

I DON'T WORK OUT as much as I did before cancer...but I have started walking more with my newly adopted Maltese. It has helped my legs, as well as my breathing, to get stronger. My last surgery was a doozy!

Celestine, property manager
Diagnosis of stomach cancer at age 45 in 2006 in Rosedale, Maryland

• • •

I HAVE RECENTLY STARTED working out at a women's exercise facility that is owned by a woman who is a cancer exercise specialist. She has been helpful in guiding me into an exercise program that I can build upon to give me more strength and energy.

Patti, financial administrator
Diagnosis of ovarian cancer at age 51 in 2005 in Colorado Springs, Colorado

I often tell people that exercise is not chemotherapy, but can be just as important. People can use exercise to "build up their battery so that they can hold a day's charge longer." This allows them to live more, tolerate more, and do more, before their energy for the day runs out. Frequently, I am asked to recommend an exercise program to help people tolerate or sometimes even qualify for more chemotherapy—an important reason to exercise indeed.

KI Y. SHIN, MD, is a rehabilitation doctor (physiatrist) and an associate professor at The University of Texas M. D. Anderson Cancer Center.

I WALK MORE, but not nearly enough.

Pat, retired
Diagnosis of colon and bladder cancer at age 74 in 2005 in Como (Western Australia)

I AM STILL UNDERGOING chemotherapy and will be on another regimen for a year. However, being physically fit before I started the treatment was extremely helpful with my healing from the surgical procedures...so the doctors have told me.

Nancy, administrative assistant
Diagnosis of breast cancer at age 54 in 2006 in Fowlerville, Michigan

• • •

I'D LIKE TO REPORT that I now exercise daily, but I don't. I've always hated exercise and could never do it for very long. During my recovery and toward the end of my chemotherapy, I did begin walking every day down my unpaved ranch road to the highway and back again, a three-mile roundtrip. But after several weeks, I started skipping a day here and there, and then I stopped altogether. I am just too lazy. I hate exercise. Still I know I should. I should build up my muscle mass so I'll have an energy reserve if and when I get sick again. So I will. I promise. But I've promised before and not followed through. We'll see.

Mike, retired real estate developer and cattle rancher
Diagnosis of colon cancer at age 66 in 2006 in Red Lodge, Montana

• • •

I BECAME A DEVOUT exerciser—five days a week for two hours a day. I went from getting hardly any exercise to getting about ten to twelve hours a week. My sister calls them my psycho workouts!

Eileen, teacher
Diagnosis of breast cancer at age 43 in 2006 in Hilton, New York

• • •

I TRIED TO KEEP as normal a schedule as possible. I am normally very active, so I pushed myself as far as I could. I was inspired by Lance Armstrong's work, and I believe trying to live as normally as possible is key to recovery. Only during the worst of chemo did I have to throttle back on the most strenuous exercises.

James, retired police officer
Diagnosis of lymphoma at age 66 in 2007 in Sheridan, Wyoming

> # "...I believe trying to live as normally as possible is key to recovery."

YES, I EXERCISE every day.

Melody, medical secretary
Diagnosis of breast cancer at age 39 in 2004 and lung cancer at age 42 in 2007 in Jessup, Maryland

• • •

IT'S SOMETHING I KNOW is important in keeping me healthy, and I plan to start a regimen soon!

Danielle, financial service specialist
Diagnosis of melanoma (skin cancer) at age 30 in 2000 in Ramstein (Germany)

• • •

I TRIED TO DO some physical exercise to build up body strength and I walked a lot, even in the hospital. They called me the "road runner" because I walked many laps around the hospital floor to build up strength.

Bryna, management development consultant
Diagnosis of tongue cancer at age 35 in 1985 in Brockton, Massachusetts

• • •

ONE OF THE LITTLE things I did that made everyday life easier (after spending six weeks flat on my back) was to join a health club. I decided that I was going to get myself as strong as I possibly could but on my terms. This was enormously empowering to me, because I could start very slowly and gradually work my way up. So, rather than spending a lot of time worrying about the grim prognosis I had been given, I could actually focus on positive goals—even if they were at first quite modest. It made me feel a lot more positive and made me easier to live with. The "two in five" prognosis I was given for surviving the first year without a relapse scared the hell out of me, and I chose not to dwell on it.

Jerry, computer software instructor
Diagnosis of acute myelogenous leukemia at age 43 in 2003 in Anoka, Minnesota

A FRIEND GOT ME a dog so that I could get out and walk—even when I really didn't want to—and that made a big difference.

April, disabled
Diagnosis of breast cancer at age 34 in 1999 in Wichita, Kansas

• • •

I AM MORE MOTIVATED to work out.

Cheryl, homemaker
Diagnosis of breast cancer at age 49 in 2006 in Garland, Texas

• • •

I TRY TO GET out each day at work to walk around downtown. I am now in training to do a five-mile walk in my town for breast cancer.

Brenda, government clerk
Diagnosis of breast cancer at age 58 in 2006 in Madison, Tennessee

• • •

> "I wanted to be able to walk in my favorite park as soon as possible..."

FOR YEARS MY HUSBAND, who was seventy-one at the time, and I, then sixty-four, had been very much into walking and eating a healthy diet. Although it didn't prevent my getting cancer, I really believe that being in good physical condition went a long way toward my healing so fast. I wanted to be able to walk in my favorite park as soon as possible, so I worked hard every day in building my strength to reach that goal. Today, I'm as strong as I ever was.

Judy, retired accounting clerk
Diagnosis of lung cancer at age 64 in 2004 in Norwalk, California

• • •

I GET TIRED EASILY, so I don't do much exercise.

Luann, stay-at-home mom
Diagnosis of colon cancer at age 50 in 2003 in Charleston, West Virginia

During or after cancer treatment, set short-term and long-term goals. Setting realistic and attainable goals over time can aid in your recovery. This may offer you something to strive toward and look forward to each day, month, and year. Once you achieve a goal, savor it and then set a new goal. The sense of accomplishment that comes with achieving your goals can feel very empowering, satisfying, and healing.

> **ELYSE CAPLAN** oversees Living Beyond Breast Cancer's educational programming. She was 34 years old in 1991 when her breast cancer was diagnosed. She underwent a modified radical mastectomy and came home from the hospital on her oldest son's eighth birthday.

WAS NIL—REMAINS NIL. I did purchase a really cool pair of lightweight sneakers, though.

Laura, unemployed psychiatric social worker
Diagnosis of breast cancer at age 43 in 2006 in Avon, Connecticut

• • •

I HAD ATTENDED a Curves [fitness program for women] exercise studio three to four times a week for five years prior to my diagnosis. I tried to go back twice, but came down with a high, unexplained fever and had to stop. But I hope to go back one of these days.

Sigrid, registered nurse
Diagnosis of endometrial (uterine) cancer at age 72 in 2006 in Oceanside, California

• • •

I WALK THREE MILES with my husband every night. I never exercised before cancer because I was very thin and not very athletic.

Fran, postmaster
Diagnosis of breast cancer at age 42 in 1999 in LaVergne, Tennessee

IT'S BECOME FAR MORE sporadic. Prior to cancer, I competed in two marathons and was very, very active. During this year, the chemo and surgical procedures have interrupted my exercise routine, although I still try to walk the dog every day.

Deborah, physician
Diagnosis of breast cancer at age 47 in 2007 in Overland Park, Kansas

• • •

I DO KNOW I am in better shape than most fifty-year-olds, and everyone thinks I am in my thirties (really!).

Randy, respiratory therapist
Diagnosis of Hodgkin disease at age 6 in 1965 in Ewa Beach, Hawaii

The race is run one step at a time.

NANCY BRINKER is a breast cancer survivor and founder of Susan G. Komen for the Cure in memory of her sister, Susan Goodman Komen.

CHAPTER 9

• • •

What I Did to Relieve Stress

I write a lot about survivorship issues for consumer health Web sites. One day I was responding to a young woman who wrote that she had a psychiatric diagnosis of bipolar disorder and was causing her mother, a cancer survivor, a lot of stress. The reader's question was, "Will I make my mom's cancer come back?" That was a valid inquiry and one with which scientists and doctors have been grappling for years.

Does stress cause cancer? To date, the answer from the research is no. Stress alone does not seem to be a significant risk factor for cancer. That doesn't mean that stress is good for us. In fact, when it comes to physical recovery, such as healing wounds from surgery, stress can slow things down a bit. Too much stress also makes one feel emotionally battered. Yet, there is no way to navigate a cancer diagnosis without a tremendous amount of stress. It's just part of having a serious illness.

Much of the stress that goes along with a cancer diagnosis is related to the uncertainty that accompanies it. At first, there is the period of uncertainty surrounding the diagnosis itself, when patients must wait for the results of tests and biopsies. Then, there is the uncertainty of which treatment will work best and the decision of how aggressive to be—usually there is more than one therapy approach. The prognosis, too, is fraught with uncertainty. Doctors can only offer expert opinions about this in most cases.

How is it possible to deal with so much uncertainty and such a devastating diagnosis—even if the prognosis will ultimately be good? Psychologist Susan Jeffers writes about this issue in her book *Embracing Uncertainty*. Dr. Jeffers encourages people to consider the unknown as an adventure, to "train ourselves to be adventurers instead of worriers" (Jeffers 2003, 18). That can be difficult with a cancer diagnosis, but it is a worthwhile thing to try. Dr. Jeffers also writes, "Nowhere has it been proven that a rich, joyous, abundant life cannot exist in the presence of uncertainty" (Jeffers 2003, 5).

I've never met anyone with a recent cancer diagnosis who had a rich, joyous, and abundant life during that period. Instead, every cancer diagnosis is the beginning of a personal and family crisis. Over time, however, the shock fades. And, as many survivors reported in their surveys, it is possible to go on to have a rich, joyous, and abundant life.

Stress plays a role in everyone's life and can be particularly problematic for cancer survivors, not only when their cancer has just been diagnosed, but months or even years later. Being proactive about doing things to decrease stress is the best way to manage it. We know that activities such as meditation or exercise can help diminish stress.

At the end of this chapter, see my list of things people can do to relax.* If you are a cancer survivor, try adding some of these things to your day to help you decompress. If you are a friend or family member of a cancer survivor, you can encourage and even participate in some of these activities.

The survey participants had a lot of great ideas about managing stress. Read on to see what they did to avoid feeling overwhelmed.

• • •

I DID NOT PRACTICE any stress-reduction techniques at any time during my treatment or since. Stress comes from worry or fear, and neither has ever solved a problem. So I just don't worry about anything. To be sure, I think about everything in order to plan and resolve problems as they come up, but I don't worry and I don't experience stress.

Mike, retired real estate developer and cattle rancher
Diagnosis of colon cancer at age 66 in 2006 in Red Lodge, Montana

---

*A variety of complementary and alternative therapies that helped contributors deal with the effects of cancer and cancer treatments are mentioned in this chapter. These therapies are discussed in a book entitled *The ACS Complete Guide to Complementary & Alternative Cancer Therapies, Second Edition*. The book is available in bookstores and online at **www.cancer.org/bookstore**.

PRIOR TO MY DIAGNOSIS, I lived a very stressful life. I worked extremely hard, constantly traveling all over the world as a consultant. I had numerous other commitments because I could never could say no to anything, and I was constantly under pressure to meet deadlines. My diagnosis helped me get my life in perspective and determine what was most important. Fortunately, I was in a position after a lifetime of work not to have to worry too much about money, so I decided to take only the assignments that really interested me, to live day by day and only do things I knew I would enjoy.

Colin, writer and author
Diagnosis of chronic lymphocytic leukemia at age 62 in 1998 in Roma (Italy)

• • •

I HAVE LISTENED to meditation tapes and had massages for relaxation. They have helped tremendously. They help the most when my mind is going a million miles a minute. They help me focus and calm my entire body.

Beth, massage therapist
Diagnosis of breast cancer at age 39 in 2006 in Tempe, Arizona

• • •

MY MEDITATION PRACTICE and yoga helped more than anything else.

Leslie, programmer analyst
Diagnosis of pancreatic cancer at age 51 in 2006 in Prescott, Arizona

• • •

I CALLED Y-ME WHEN I could not sleep and attended a support group for awhile.

Luanne, registered nurse
Diagnosis of breast cancer at age 45 in 2007 in Morris, Illinois

• • •

I TOOK A MEDITATION class that CancerConnection held, and it helped me relax better. I took a guided imagery class that helped me as well.

Rosi, student accounts office assistant
Diagnosis of colon cancer at age 52 in 2007 in Austin, Texas

I GOT LOTS OF REST. [During my cancer treatment], I learned that even though my eyes were not tired, my body was. So I would rest every afternoon for two hours. Most of the time, I did not sleep; I would listen to soft music, read, or talk with someone, but I would still be on the couch resting. Music therapy helped me relax. My dear friend brought a CD player and CD of my favorite Christian artist to my room as soon as I was out of the ICU. It not only helped control my stress, but also my blood pressure. I still use this technique.

Beth, health educator
Diagnosis of liver cancer at age 32 in 1990 in Fort Hood, Texas

• • •

I WRITE IN MY journal. This is an excellent way to rant, rave, and explode over things that bother me. My journal is not pretty or flowery; it is me. I know it is safe to let out all the tension and anger that has built up over time. My journal allows me to express a lot of what I used to keep pent up inside—now I use my writing as a release for my feelings. I don't want to sound as if all my journaling is negative, but it does serve as a stress-reduction release.

Greg, disabled
Diagnosis of mantle cell lymphoma at age 57 in 2005 and acute myelogenous leukemia at age 60 in 2008 in Orland Park, Illinois

• • •

> "Stress comes from worry or fear, and neither has ever solved a problem."

I THINK ABOUT how lucky I am to have a good wife and son, good friends, and a good oncologist. I usually end up having a pleasant sleep.

James, retired police officer
Diagnosis of lymphoma at age 66 in 2007 in Sheridan, Wyoming

• • •

I FOUND THAT HOT bubble baths helped a lot.

Joyce, legal secretary
Diagnosis of breast cancer at age 44 in 2006 in South Amboy, New Jersey

I USED A RELAXATION tape. My son put a lot of my favorite songs on my MP3 player so I could take it to treatments.

Cathy, retail district manager
Diagnosis of pancreatic cancer at age 45 in 2005 in Columbus, Ohio

• • •

I WAS TOO ILL to be stressed. I just gave in to the misery and let the whole system re-boot itself. Slowly, I climbed out of the ditch.

Suza, self-employed
Diagnosis of mantle cell lymphoma at age 41 in 2005 in Johannesburg, Gauteng (South Africa)

• • •

MUSIC. IT CAN TAKE you anywhere you want to go.

Kimatha, medical laboratory technician
Diagnosis of kidney cancer at age 42 in 2001 in Edinburgh, Indiana

• • •

YOGA BREATHING, FOCUSED MEDITATION, and prayer. They have helped me avoid a lot of pain medication.

Kyle, pastor
Diagnosis of kidney cancer at age 60 in 2004 in Johnstown, Pennsylvania

• • •

"[During treatment], I learned that even though my eyes were not tired, my body was. So I would rest every afternoon for two hours."

I HAD REFLEXOLOGY and Reiki before each chemo session. This was offered free at the hospital where I underwent chemotherapy.

Pearl, nurse
Diagnosis of breast cancer at age 32 in 2004 in Glasgow (Scotland)

I'VE LEARNED TO PRACTICE mindful meditation daily, especially during times of stress. Mindful meditation is a technique that I can use anywhere, anytime. And I do.

Ric, public relations director
Diagnosis of thyroid cancer at age 50 in 1995 in Londonderry, New Hampshire

• • •

I STARTED DOING YOGIC meditation and deep-breathing exercises. It calmed my mind, brought on only positive thoughts, and gave me a perception of strength.

Jitendra, software engineer
Diagnosis of non-Hodgkin lymphoma at age 28 in 1994 in Cleveland, Ohio

Taking time to relax and de-stress is more than just taking care of you. It provides you with the emotional energy to be able to be there for family and friends, even when you are not 100 percent. And, there is no better boost to one's psyche than being able to be there for others when you both expected the opposite. That "give and take" allows you to feel better about asking for the things you need when things get tough. I like to reassure patients that no one expects anything more of them than who they are. The mantra should be this: no heroics—recognize your limitations, relax, politely educate others if necessary, and feel good about caring for yourself.

KAREN SOMMER, MSN, RN, AOCNP, is an oncology nurse practitioner with the Lance Armstrong Foundation Adult Survivorship Clinic and Perini Family Survivors' Center at Dana-Farber Cancer Institute in Boston, Massachusetts.

I LEARNED HOW TO DO meditation, particularly self-hypnosis. Whatever works for each individual...I just found it to be helpful occasionally to get into a very relaxed state. This would allow all of my worry to disappear, even if only for a short while.

Todd, oncology social worker
Diagnosis of chronic myelogenous leukemia at age 25 in 1997 and kidney cancer at age 33 in 2005 in Warwick, Rhode Island

• • •

I AM A BIG believer in an afternoon nap.

Matt, carpenter
Diagnosis of chronic lymphocytic leukemia at age 51 in 2003 in Bath, New York

• • •

WALKING OR RUNNING in the woods or near the ocean are my best stress-reduction techniques.

Cathi, clinical social worker
Diagnosis of breast cancer at age 52 in 2003 in Waban, Massachusetts

• • •

I FOUND THAT BEING able to use meditation and yoga helped calm the "galloping fear" that comes along with this disease.

Bill, administrator
Diagnosis of prostate cancer at age 62 in 2007 in Jefferson, Wisconsin

• • •

I TOLD MY MOM that if she kept complaining about how bad her life was—by the way, she has a great life— I would not visit her any longer. I had to rid myself of the stress that accompanied my visits with her. She complains because she has to sweep up leaves that fall in her back yard after a windstorm, as if that's the worst thing ever. Well, she should try chemo!

Linda, retired
Diagnosis of breast cancer at age 54 in 2003 in Placentia, California

WORRY IS MY MIDDLE name...I sometimes wrote in a journal. Or I just cried whenever I wanted to, and that made me feel better. I kept in contact with all my friends, and talking with them really helped.

Evelyn, executive assistant
Diagnosis of colon cancer at age 33 in 2004 in Boston, Massachusetts

• • •

"I just found it to be helpful occasionally to get into a very relaxed state. This would allow all of my worry to disappear..."

BEFORE SURGERY AND DURING my chemo treatment, I always practiced deep breathing—actually, I do that before every test and appointment. It's very calming. During chemo, I also did visualization. I would close my eyes and do deep breathing, kind of meditating, and then I would visualize the chemo moving through my body like a white light, making all the darkness (cancer) disappear. I would visualize my body like a chalkboard covered with letters, numbers, and other figures; the chemo acted as an eraser, wiping everything clean. That's the teacher in me. Again, these visualizations were calming, and they also helped me view the chemotherapy as a positive thing, even though going through chemo was so challenging.

Kathi, retired special education teacher
Diagnosis of breast cancer at age 49 in 2003 in Wrightstown, Wisconsin

• • •

I HAVE TAKEN ADVANTAGE of complementary therapies offered by the hospital and by a friend who does reflexology. This takes time each week, but these are special times for me when I relax and allow myself to be pampered a bit. I have learned to let other things go and to focus on helping myself get well.

Patti, financial administrator
Diagnosis of ovarian cancer at age 51 in 2005 in Colorado Springs, Colorado

DURING TREATMENT, I LISTENED to a relaxation and visualization audiotape. I would close myself in a quiet room, close my eyes, and listen. It definitely helped me relax and feel that I was doing something to help myself get better, since most of the rest of my treatment was beyond my control. I would regularly visualize the cancer leaving my body. I would consciously turn unpleasant, depressing thoughts into positive experiences. For instance, if I started to imagine my funeral, I would force myself to turn the setting into a celebration of my becoming disease free and having all of my friends and family there, celebrating my health rather than mourning me.

Janet, elementary school teacher
Diagnosis of colon cancer at age 42 in 1993 in Philadelphia, Pennsylvania

• • •

I HAVE A TYPE-A personality with a stressful work and volunteer life. I actually enjoy a fair amount of stress; without it, I'm bored.

Jerri, state employee
Diagnosis of breast cancer at age 48 in 2006 and endometrial (uterine) cancer at age 50 in 2008 in Standish, Michigan

Two things got me, my wife, and my family through my diagnosis and treatment: hope and laughter. Hope showed us the strength in dreaming of better days to come. Laughter reminded us all that life continued and incredible moments can be found and shared in the darkest of places.

STEVE MAZAN is a comedian who often performs on CBS's *The Late Late Show with Craig Ferguson*. Steve had a diagnosis of intestinal and liver cancer in 2005 at age 35.

TO PASS THE TIME, I crocheted, and that seemed to calm me and bring me peace.

Danielle, financial service specialist
Diagnosis of melanoma (skin cancer) at age 30 in 2000 in Ramstein (Germany)

I WAS IN THE HOSPITAL for a long time, and there was a music ministry there. Volunteers would come play the keyboard, guitar, or harp. There was also a woman who did hand and leg massage.

Susan, homemaker
Diagnosis of acute myelogenous leukemia at age 50 in 2003 in Medina, Ohio

• • •

THIS IS A BIGGIE for me…relaxing during and after chemo and even daily. I find reading, listening to music or audio books, and crocheting all take my mind off the fact that I have an incurable disease.

Marie, retired
Diagnosis of ovarian cancer at age 59 in 2004 in Lebanon, Ohio

As director of Art for Recovery for the past twenty years, I believe that art has the power to heal: it can soften the realities of the patient experience such as loss of control, isolation, pain, anxiety, and deep feelings of vulnerability. Our patients tell us how good it feels to do something creative, whether it is art making, writing, composing a song about illness, or participating in an Open Art Studio for patients and medical staff. This is an opportunity to express fear, hope, anger, and dreams and to not only share your life story, but to bear witness to the stories of others who are also coping with illness. The expressive arts build a community—teaching the outside what the inside is feeling.

CYNTHIA PERLIS is the director for Art for Recovery at the University of California at San Francisco's Helen Diller Family Comprehensive Cancer Center.

I'M NOT MUCH of a pill taker, but if there is ever a time in your life when you need medication to help you relax, it's when you have cancer. Xanax and Ativan helped get me through the worst times. I think I would have lost my mind otherwise. Today, I don't need any of it, but I did then.

Carmela, technical writer
Diagnosis of endometrial (uterine), bladder, and ovarian cancer at age 48 in 2005 in Clinton Township, Michigan

• • •

LISTENING TO PRETTY MUSIC, nice big roaring fires, walks with my dog in the cool fresh air, anything to bring me peaceful feelings.

Allie, Director, Distinguished Events; American Cancer Society
Diagnosis of thyroid cancer at age 46 in 2003 in Fair Haven, New Jersey

• • •

SOFT MUSIC WITH HEADPHONES accompanied by slow, deep breathing. And I like the hum of a fan, as well as the air circulation [it provides]. People think I'm crazy, but I use the fans in the dead of winter.

Jerry, computer software instructor
Diagnosis of acute myelogenous leukemia at age 43 in 2003 in Anoka, Minnesota

• • •

I VISITED A REIKI practitioner for the first time. It helped me with self-understanding, relaxation, and decision-making.

Barbara, nurse
Diagnosis of breast cancer at age 58 in 1995 in Stoneham, Massachusetts

"I would visualize my body like a chalkboard covered with letters, numbers, and other figures; the chemo acted as an eraser, wiping everything clean."

> ## "I made it a point to wake up earlier, put on some of my favorite violin music, get my coffee, my book, and head back to bed for a stress-free half hour..."

NORMALLY, I WOULD JUMP into my day by turning on my computer as soon as I got up at 5:30 in the morning. The doc said to "de-stress," so I made it a point to wake up earlier, put on some of my favorite violin music, get my coffee, my book, and head back to bed for a stress-free half hour before I took on my day. I also stopped listening to crazy radio shock jocks, and even eliminated the pop-up, sensational news from my Yahoo Web site. I did not bury my head in the sand, but I did control the stress input!

Robin, college professor
Diagnosis of breast cancer at age 50 in 2006 in Costa Mesa, California

• • •

I HAVE LEARNED to walk away when upset.

Jocelyn, social worker
Diagnosis of breast cancer at age 43 in 2006 in Macedon, New York

• • •

I DID ACUPUNCTURE and massage every week...this really allowed me to relax and fight the beast.

Chris, oncology nurse
Diagnosis of breast cancer at age 35 in 2005 in Yardley, Pennsylvania

• • •

I FOUND THE PRACTICE of meditation. I taught myself to relax and calm my body and, most important, my mind, which was in dire need. Even though three years have passed, I continue to practice meditation as often as I can and recommend it highly. I plan to spend the rest of my life practicing meditation.

Judy, retired accounting clerk
Diagnosis of lung cancer at age 64 in 2004 in Norwalk, California

TO STAY CALM, I play music and meditate. Watching TV is also very relaxing to me, as well as working on my plants and walking my little dog. I walk my dog in the park quite often.

Brenda, government clerk
Diagnosis of breast cancer at age 58 in 2006 in Madison, Tennessee

• • •

BREATHING, STRETCHING...just letting things go. I don't let people waste my time or my energy.

Karen, real estate broker
Diagnosis of breast cancer at age 38 in 2001 in Loganville, Georgia

• • •

I DID YOGA at Gilda's Club. That helped a lot with stress reduction and body image.

Judy, chaplain
Diagnosis of colorectal cancer at age 48 in 2003 in Cudahy, Wisconsin

• • •

> "Breathing, stretching... just letting things go. I don't let people waste my time..."

WHENEVER I FELT OVERWHELMED, I took time to relax. I knew that calming down and resting was more important than getting certain work done. I needed to focus on me at that moment. So for the first time in my life, I put myself ahead of everyone else.

Mary Anne, word processor
Diagnosis of melanoma (skin cancer) at age 26 in 2007 in Dixon, California

• • •

MEDITATION AND YOGA. I am addicted.

Jennifer, publicity coordinator
Diagnosis of melanoma (skin cancer) at age 21 in 2004 in San Diego, California

DEEP BREATHING HELPS RELEASE the stress that accumulates in my neck and shoulders.

Polly, human resource administrator
Diagnosis of breast cancer at age 54 in 2005 in Port Gibson, Mississippi

• • •

I SPENT A SIGNIFICANT amount of time knitting. The meditative power of knitting gifts for others was amazing. The world would be a much better place if everyone had two sticks and a piece of string.

Deborah, physician
Diagnosis of breast cancer at age 47 in 2007 in Overland Park, Kansas

• • •

AS I LOOK BACK over the few years prior to receiving my cancer diagnosis, I realize I was under a lot of stress because my best friend, my oldest son, and my mother all died within months of each other in the same year. I was under tremendous stress, and I did not eat properly. I have changed my way of eating and do not allow things to bother me for long periods.

Marguerite, retired deacon
Diagnosis of breast cancer at age 60 in 1993 in Cheltenham, Maryland

• • •

MY ONLY WAY TO DEAL with stress is through prayer. Other techniques don't work for me; in fact, they stress me out more. Relaxation tapes and exercises don't work for me. I don't meditate, but I do pray and think about good things.

Buffy, self-employed
Diagnosis of breast cancer at age 58 in 2005 in Bobcaygeon, Ontario (Canada)

• • •

I IMAGINED THE ONCOLOGIST'S office as a place of healing. I imagined the chemotherapy as being divinely therapeutic.

Judi, nurse
Diagnosis of breast cancer at age 40 in 2000 in Pen Argyl, Pennsylvania

Baby Steps. I coped by looking at my treatment as baby steps. Thinking about the upcoming year of surgery, chemotherapy, and radiation left me overwhelmed and panicked and caused anxiety and insomnia. So I began to focus only on the week ahead. I would tell myself, "Okay, let's just get through this week's treatment and then deal with next week." It really helped me stay calm to tackle one day at a time.

HEATHER WARRICK (AKA CANCER PRINCESS), received a diagnosis of breast cancer at age 24 in 1994. Her cancer has recurred nine times, and she now lives with cancer as a chronic condition. Heather works as the manager of Health Programs for the American Cancer Society.

EXERCISE AND LAUGHTER (can I stress the laughter enough?) are my only stress relief techniques.

Jennifer, federal officer with U.S. Customs and Border Patrol
Diagnosis of cervical cancer at age 36 in 2007 in Montreal, Quebec (Canada)

• • •

LEARNING TO RELAX is extremely hard for me still! [My advice is to] increase your endorphins. So laughter or having a good sense of humor is great. Read, read, read, and pray, pray, pray. Surround yourself with good people with good energy.

Alejandra, clerical worker
Diagnosis of uterine cancer at age 36 in 2005 in Torrance, California

• • •

I TOOK YOGA for awhile. That was a great stress reliever.

Lisa, administrative assistant
Diagnosis of breast cancer at age 38 in 2000 in Owings Mills, Maryland

A FRIEND WOULD DO Reiki with me when she came over. It was very relaxing and calming to me. I would simply lie there while she moved her hands over my body to take away the bad energy. She was amazing. I would listen to her prayers as she removed the energy. Her voice was truly relaxing to me.

Carlyn, administrative assistant
Diagnosis of Hodgkin disease at age 30 in 2004 in Willow Spring, North Carolina

• • •

I THINK ABOUT CANCER and start to feel a panic, but then I remind myself that even if it returns, I have a plan to deal with it next time. So I find comfort in having a plan.

Jennifer, housekeeper
Diagnosis of breast cancer at age 40 in 2004 and skin cancer at age 41 in 2005 in Craig, Colorado

At The Wellness Community we see people living with, through, and beyond cancer every day—all types of cancer. We believe that fighting for survival; asking questions and seeking answers; and uniting mind, body, and spirit in the battle for survivorship not only creates an enhanced quality of life while fighting the disease, but can also enhance recovery.

JAY LOCKABY is the executive director of The Wellness Community in Southwest Florida.

Reference

Jeffers, S. 2003. *Embracing uncertainty: breakthrough methods for achieving peace of mind when facing the unknown.* New York: St. Martin's Press. First published in Great Britain by Hodder and Stoughton, a division of Hodder Headline.

Stress Busters

Listen to music, talk radio, audio books, or a relaxation tape.

Meditate or pray.

Watch television (choose an upbeat show).

Read a book or magazine.

Sit down and talk with someone, in person or on the phone.

Perform deep breathing and relaxation exercises.

Play a game on the computer or with a friend.

Play a musical instrument.

Crochet, macramé, knit, needlepoint, or sew.

Make a craft or jewelry.

Carve wood.

Make a scrapbook.

Do a jigsaw or crossword puzzle.

Draw or paint a picture.

Write a letter, e-mail, journal entry, or poem/short story.

Sit in a comfortable place with a warm drink (decaffeinated and nonalcoholic is best).

Lie down and take time to reflect.

Go for a scenic drive.

Sit outside or take a walk someplace where you can enjoy nature.

Go for a manicure, pedicure, massage, or other spa treatment.

Exercise.

CHAPTER 10

· · ·

How Being Spiritual Helped

In her memoir, *Flying Crooked*, breast cancer survivor Jan Michael wrote, "Other people went to counselors. I went to church…I like the way it puts me into perspective, makes my health relative" (Michael 2005, 7).

The notion that spirituality is good for our health has good science to support it. Whereas the terms spirituality and religion are often used synonymously, they really have different meanings. Stephen Kliewer (2004) explored these differences in an article he wrote for the *Journal of Family Practice* entitled "Allowing Spirituality into the Healing Process." He relied on his own research, as well as that of others, for these descriptions: "*Spirituality* is defined as a search for what is sacred or holy in life, coupled with a transcendent (greater than self) relationship with God or a higher power or universal energy (Larson 1997). *Religion* is seen as focusing more on prescribed beliefs, rituals, and practices, as well as social institutional features (Zinnbauer 1998) and on the undertaking of a spiritual search using specific means or methods (i.e., rituals or behaviors) within an identifiable group."

Studies show that people who attend religious services tend to have better health and that prayer seems to cause chemical changes in our bodies that may help boost our immune systems. Nonreligious spiritual practices, such as communing with nature, also seem to be beneficial. There are many possible explanations for these research results. For example, people who go to church may be more attentive to things overall, like eating well, exercising, and avoiding nicotine and excess alcohol. Prayer may work in a manner similar to that of meditation by lowering blood pressure and heart rate and facilitating the release of chemicals that promote immune function. Another explanation, of course, is divine intervention.

I have written about the science of spirituality in my other books, and I often include this topic in talks that I give to cancer survivors. Because people have very strong views about spirituality and religion, this is always a tricky subject. So when I speak or write about it, I am careful to stick to the science, which is really quite fascinating. Nevertheless, even the mention of this topic gets some people upset. I vividly recall a participant's response at one particular breast cancer conference where I mentioned the research on the effects of spirituality and health. I noted that spirituality can entail many things, and it doesn't have to involve formal religious practices. During the question and answer period, a young woman stood up to exclaim how she was "sick and tired of hearing about God." She added that she wasn't spiritual at all and thus resented the well-wishers who said that they were praying for her.

I appreciated her comments and wondered how many other people going through cancer felt that way. I'm not sure of the answer, though studies show that the vast majority of Americans (well over 90 percent) believe in God or a higher power. Another young breast cancer survivor named Laura, who filled out a survey for this book, wrote that her faith in God helped her tremendously when her cancer was diagnosed in 2006. She said, "I was five months pregnant with my son and, from the first moment the words came out of the doctor's mouth, I felt the Lord holding me up. Every fearful thought or worry that came into my mind was nearly immediately replaced with a verse or part of a hymn or a reassurance of His care and plan to carry us through. I spent a lot of time reading the Bible. At first I also read about cancer and treatments and diet and statistics, but then I stopped. I savored every moment with my husband and daughters and the family and friends who came out to visit and help, and I relished my son as he grew inside me and the obstetrician continued to pronounce him 'healthy' at each appointment."

When I reviewed the surveys, I included as many points of view as possible. Not surprisingly, most people reported that praying helped them. Many others wrote that going to church, synagogue, or other religious places was beneficial. Quite a few people noted that even though they weren't particularly religious, they appreciated the prayers of others. Read on and consider what these survivors have to say about whether and how spirituality helped them as they went through treatment.

• • •

SPIRITUALITY DID HELP ME. It made my mind stronger by allowing me to concentrate on my fight.

Jitendra, software engineer
Diagnosis of non-Hodgkin lymphoma at age 28 in 1994 in Cleveland, Ohio

• • •

MY SPIRITUALITY IS WHERE I found the most profound help. Friends of like faith supported me with prayer. I felt a strength beyond understanding and had little, if any, fear of what was ahead. Spirituality was a vital help for me in recovering. Knowing that all good or bad things in life can be looked at as given by God, and knowing that He will bring you through. Meditating on scriptures brings peace to one's soul.

Laura, housecleaner
Diagnosis of esophageal cancer at age 45 in 2002 in Schenectady, New York

• • •

PRAYER, PRAYER, AND MORE PRAYER. You have to believe in something or someone to help you get through the cancer ordeal.

Debra, administrative assistant
Diagnosis of ovarian cancer at age 51 in 2007 in Chicago, Illinois

• • •

MY BREAST CANCER was first diagnosed in 1982. Then, I received a diagnosis of inflammatory breast cancer in 1995 and, in 1996, was told I had cancer of the left lung and chest wall. In 1996, I had cancer in my right breast, with recurrences in 1998, 1999, and 2000. I now have breast cancer on the chest wall. God was and still is with me every step I take on this journey with cancer. When I had cancer in my lung, He healed me because, when they did the surgery, there was no evidence of cancer in my lung. Same with the chest wall. God wanted me here for a purpose, and if it is [contributing to] this book or being an example to how to live with cancer, then I will do it.

Susan, retired preschool teacher
Diagnosis of breast cancer at age 37 in 1982 in Graham, Washington

ALTHOUGH I AM JEWISH by birth, I do not observe any religious rituals or beliefs. I did regularly see a "hands-on healer"—a wonderful woman who would bring me such peace through the calm placement of her hands. Although I didn't totally believe that she was healing my body through her hands, I did believe that laying on of her hands brought my body and soul true peace and calmness.

Elena, arts administrator
Diagnosis of inflammatory breast cancer at age 44 in 1999 in Silver Spring, Maryland

• • •

FAITH. MY MOTTO DURING my entire cancer experience was and still is "Faith and Humor." I even had this tattooed with the colon cancer ribbon on my ankle. I went to Las Vegas and had it (the tattoo) done two days after my chemo doc said I was cancer free. I knew I was a survivor from the day my cancer was diagnosed. The Lord made it very clear to me that this road was not going to be easy, but that I would make it to the end.

Susan, housewife
Diagnosis of colorectal cancer at age 43 in 2006 in Mobile, Alabama

• • •

"I knew I was a survivor from the day my cancer was diagnosed."

I COMPLETELY TRUSTED GOD through the entire process. I prayed and sang hymns of joy and praise unto God. I stayed positive and never gave in or accepted any negativity from any doctor, nurse, or anyone else! I educated myself on my type of cancer. I stayed on top of my doctors and every report they had on me. I asked loads of questions every time someone walked into my room with a needle; and if I agreed with them, I allowed them to stick me. I also questioned the need for every medicine and every procedure. I got a lot of respect from the hospital staff because of this.

Celestine, property manager
Diagnosis of stomach cancer at age 45 in 2006 in Rosedale, Maryland

WE ARE VERY ACTIVE in [practicing] our Catholic faith. Our church community has been, and continues to be, helpful to us in so many ways—from prayer to practical things like housecleaning and meals. One group of women has been meeting weekly for over a year to say the Rosary for my health. Another group paid for me to take a trip to Lourdes, France, for a week. I was treated like a queen! For a whole week, I was cared for, fed, bathed in Lourdes water, and prayed over. It was amazing. To say that I am humbled and grateful for these people is an understatement of my feelings.

Sandra, assistant professor of nursing
Diagnosis of breast cancer at age 54 in 2002 in Atlanta, Georgia

• • •

I WENT TO MY SYNAGOGUE to talk to my rabbi. When I got there, she had just received a breast cancer diagnosis, and she had just returned from seeing my doctor. Small world!

Carrie, information management specialist
Diagnosis of breast cancer at age 44 in 2002 in New York City, New York

• • •

MY CHURCH FAMILY gave me a "Hat Party." It was like a wedding or baby shower would be, with a cake (in the shape of a hat) and finger foods. They gave me gifts, such as hats, earrings, scarves, pins, and money. We laughed and talked.

Angie, volunteer and cancer advocate
Diagnosis of vulvar cancer at age 31 in 1998 and breast cancer at age 36 in 2003 in Anderson, South Carolina

• • •

I AM A FIRM believer in prayer. It calms me and gives me peace in times that I am spinning with emotions. It gives me someone to tell everything—however I want to say it—rather than picking the things that are appropriate for the person I'm talking to or working to say what I mean without seeming ungrateful or selfish or rude. I believe God knows me and understands what I need.

Beth, massage therapist
Diagnosis of breast cancer at age 39 in 2006 in Tempe, Arizona

I CAME BACK TO GOD. I felt there was a purpose for me. I am presently working on my master's degree in divinity studies.

Iris, artist
Diagnosis of liver cancer at age 50 in 2007 in Sante Fe, New Mexico

• • •

I AM NOT a religious person (I guess that's the scientist in me), but I do believe in a greater good that brings people together. Call it a Zen state or whatever, but finding some sort of inner peace can go a long way.

Federico, cancer chemical biologist
Diagnosis of testicular cancer at age 32 in 2006 in Brookline, Massachusetts

• • •

BEFORE CANCER, WHEN I prayed I would always say "thank you" for this or that and was always appreciative of what I had. I always asked God to watch over others and really never asked for anything for me. When I got sick, I did have to ask Him to help me get through my illness. I thought it was okay to ask for this.

Lynne, Web coordinator
Diagnosis of breast cancer at age 43 in 2006 in Rome, New York

• • •

MY MOTHER IS RELIGIOUS and brought [to me] one churchman after the other and one pressure group after the other. No thanks.

Suza, self-employed
Diagnosis of mantle cell lymphoma at age 41 in 2005 in Johannesburg, Gauteng (South Africa)

• • •

GOD IS THE BEST support system a person can have. The peace I get when I read the Bible. It is really a very good book to read. I had never taken time before to know that.

Kimatha, medical laboratory technician
Diagnosis of kidney cancer at age 42 in 2001 in Edinburgh, Indiana

I FOUND MYSELF USING prayer to cope with pain, to provide insight, transcendence, and even humor. Hymns, scriptures (especially those from memory) and, when I was up to it, reading really helped. My faith has deepened, and I live more in the present and value each moment and each relationship. I am a better pastor, friend, father, and my counseling skills have been honed by my experience, so I can listen differently from before.

Kyle, pastor
Diagnosis of kidney cancer at age 60 in 2004 in Johnstown, Pennsylvania

As I listen to cancer patients I find they consistently refer to a person or object or idea for which they are grateful. A sense of gratefulness takes patients outside of their situation, which has the possibility of consuming each moment of their lives. Gratefulness gives the cancer patient a glimpse of the world beyond the treatment regimen that may otherwise define their days.

ALAN WRIGHT is an oncology chaplain at the Baylor University Medical Center in Dallas, Texas.

ALTHOUGH I AM NOT a Catholic, many Catholic friends said novenas for me.

Kenneth, career transition teacher for Navy retirees
Diagnosis of kidney cancer at age 64 in 1999 in San Diego, California

• • •

MY FAITH GIVES ME daily comfort and contentment. When I can't sleep at night because I am worried, I pray the Rosary, which helps tremendously.

Kelly, financial services executive
Diagnosis of chronic lymphocytic leukemia at age 50 in 2003 and basal cell carcinoma (skin cancer) at age 53 in 2007 in Arlington, Virginia

I SAW HOW MUCH my parents hurt for me and how scared they were of losing me. Knowing that God loves me even more than they do, I knew He was with me every step of the way. I read scripture, sang, listened to Christian music, and prayed (and prayed, and prayed...). When I was suffering the most, I would imagine that my bed was the hand of God, I always felt better as I felt Him hold me up and carry me through the pain or sadness.

Sherri, elementary school teacher
Diagnosis of endometrial (uterine) cancer at age 42 in 2004 in Bruceville, Indiana

• • •

I HAVE BECOME OPEN to spiritual insights and beliefs. I now ask for help from the Universe instead of trying to manage everything myself. Before breast cancer, I thought that was all very hippie-ish and just not me at all!

Pearl, nurse
Diagnosis of breast cancer at age 32 in 2004 in Glasgow (Scotland)

• • •

I PRAYED THE ROSARY nightly. I learned to be more patient and to let go of things over which I have no control. Before cancer I had to be in charge—I was making the plans—I was taking control. Now I take care of my family and myself and let go of those little things that don't really matter—the dust on the furniture will still be there tomorrow. I put more things in God's hands. I tell people that family, good medicine, and faith got me through the surgery and nine months of treatment.

Dorinda, retired teacher
Diagnosis of ovarian cancer at age 50 in 2005 in Edison, New Jersey

• • •

I AM NOT a particularly religious person, but my family is, and I did find it comforting when people told me that they were praying for me or that I was in their prayers. It was also comforting to receive little medals or prayer cards.

Todd, oncology social worker
Diagnosis of chronic myelogenous leukemia at age 25 in 1997 and kidney cancer at age 33 in 2005 in Warwick, Rhode Island

RELIGION HAD NO PART for me. A lot of well-meaning people said they were praying for me, I always thanked them and [did so] from my heart, but it is not for me.

Matt, carpenter
Diagnosis of chronic lymphocytic leukemia at age 51 in 2003 in Bath, New York

• • •

IF ONE CONSIDERS GRATITUDE and love of the world to be spiritual thoughts, then I guess I felt very spiritual.

Cathi, clinical social worker
Diagnosis of breast cancer at age 52 in 2003 in Waban, Massachusetts

• • •

I HAVE HAD the good fortune to travel extensively and have lived overseas several times. The contact with other cultures has helped broaden my perspective on life. Drawing on spiritual insights from these varying cultures helped me deal with the emotional challenge of this disease.

Bill, administrator
Diagnosis of prostate cancer at age 62 in 2007 in Jefferson, Wisconsin

• • •

> "Drawing on spiritual insights from...varying cultures helped me deal with the emotional challenge..."

I STOPPED ATTENDING CHURCH (Protestant) at the age of twelve when we moved to Massachusetts. As I've grown older, I've become more of a spiritual person. Whether some of that is due, in part, to having experienced cancer I'm not certain.

Lindy, hospice volunteer
Diagnosis of breast cancer at age 35 in 1984 and radiation-induced sarcoma at age 55 in 2004 in Lexington, Massachusetts

MINDFULNESS. PRACTICING LIVING EACH day in the moment and enjoying just that one day...each day.

Shelly, program coordinator for adults with disabilities
Diagnosis of breast cancer at age 32 in 2004 in Concord, New Hampshire

• • •

I JUST BELIEVED that what will be will be. If anything, I became more anti-religious...no caring God would do this. And the argument that He only gives you things you can handle is crap. I had too many religious zealots telling me not to go through treatment but that they would "pray" for me.

Linda, retired
Diagnosis of breast cancer at age 54 in 2003 in Placentia, California

• • •

I APPRECIATED QUIET TIMES with nature, contemplating life and life cycles.

Kirsten, distribution assistant
Diagnosis of colon cancer at age 49 in 2006 and endometrial (uterine) cancer at age 50 in 2007 in Buford, Georgia

Keep the faith, Baby. My positive attitude, my spirit, my will to live, made a world of difference. I knew things could always be worse. I had to hold on to something to give me hope, and I held onto God.

JACK WILLIS received a diagnosis of breast cancer at age 64 in 2005. He taught journalism at the University of Oklahoma and is the author of *Saving Jack*.

I HAVE ALWAYS BELIEVED that all things happen for a reason. That God has a plan and somehow my cancer figured into that plan.

Pat, office manager
Diagnosis of breast cancer at age 53 in 2001 in Canton, Michigan

I VALUED THE PRAYERS and good thoughts of others, and I prayed for strength, healing, and hope. I attended church and spoke with my pastor about my cancer, and his support was helpful. But on a day-to-day basis, it was more spirituality— meditating and personal communication with my higher power.

Kathi, retired special education teacher
Diagnosis of breast cancer at age 49 in 2003 in Wrightstown, Wisconsin

• • •

I DEFINITELY THINK that prayer has helped. With my second diagnosis, three different doctors reviewed a first round of films from scans and thought the cancer had recurred in the lymph nodes. When it came time for treatment and a final scan, after several weeks of prayer, the cancer wasn't in the lymph nodes; it was only in the thyroid bed where it had originated. Also, a lot of people were praying about some moles that the doctors thought "at best" would be "precancerous." Of five of them, only one was precancerous; the rest were totally normal.

Nicki, homemaker
Diagnosis of thyroid cancer at age 20 in 2005 in Union, Missouri

• • •

BEFORE CANCER, I REALLY wasn't a spiritual person. That all changed. I truly believe in guardian angels; I know mine helped me.

Kelley, massage therapist
Diagnosis of breast cancer at age 36 in 2006 in Rochdale, Massachusetts

• • •

MY RABBI WOULD VISIT; however, truthfully, I didn't find his visits comforting. I still question how a god can let people suffer from things like cancer or Alzheimer's.

Eileen, technology specialist
Diagnosis of breast cancer at age 34 in 1984, acute myelogenous leukemia at age 49 in 1999, and basal cell carcinoma (skin cancer) at age 55 in 2005 in Framingham, Massachusetts

> ## "I have always believed that all things happen for a reason."

I DO BELIEVE IN GOD, but with this, I found I needed to believe in myself first. Somewhere along life's path, I had lost that. I learned that I have to make myself happy. I would make everyone else happy at my own expense, and now I am teaching myself that my family and I come before anything and anyone else.

Rochelle, manicurist
Diagnosis of melanoma (skin cancer) at age 34 in 2007 in Las Vegas, Nevada

• • •

I'M NOT PARTICULARLY RELIGIOUS or even spiritual. I believe in the here and now, in being good to people, and we'll see how it all turns out after we're gone. I'm sixty-seven years old, I've had a great life, and I don't fear death one bit. Sure, I'd like to squeeze another twenty years out of this old body, but if I died tomorrow it would not be a disaster. I've shared these sentiments freely and openly with my family and friends and, consequently, it is not at all difficult for us to talk about it whenever the subject comes up.

Mike, retired real estate developer and cattle rancher
Diagnosis of colon cancer at age 66 in 2006 in Red Lodge, Montana

• • •

PRAYING REALLY WORKS.

James, retired police officer
Diagnosis of lymphoma at age 66 in 2007 in Sheridan, Wyoming

• • •

I REDISCOVERED GOD and prayer. God saved me. He used my sister as an instrument. If not for her, I would not have gotten a mammogram and the tumor would probably have spread. He definitely guided her.

Eileen, teacher
Diagnosis of breast cancer at age 43 in 2006 in HIlton, New York

NO MATTER HOW DIFFICULT and alone I felt, it became apparent to me that God and the men and women of my church were extremely supportive and expressed their love and care for my wife and me. The churchmen held a "Talking Stick Circle" (borrowed from native culture) where each man talked about his relationship with me and what it meant to him; in turn, I did the same with each of them. It was very moving for all of us.

David, journeyman sheet metal worker
Diagnosis of breast cancer at age 63 in 2005 in Missoula, Montana

• • •

MY FAITH WAS STRENGTHENED. I realized, too, that there is some reason for me to be where I am at this time and place. That I was meant to help others face some of the realities of the journey I faced.

> "God saved me. He used my sister as an instrument... He definitely guided her."

Greg, disabled
Diagnosis of mantle cell lymphoma at age 57 in 2005 and acute myelogenous leukemia at age 60 in 2008 in Orland Park, Illinois

• • •

I THINK THE MOST important help was the comfort of knowing that God was in control, and I also was certain that I was going to be cured.

Charose, nurse
Diagnosis of Hodgkin disease at age 17 in 1972 and breast cancer at age 51 in 2006 in Omaha, Nebraska

• • •

ALL THE PEOPLE in the world who prayed for me. There was a lot of prayer—in Catholic churches, at the Wailing Wall in Israel, and in numerous other churches and synagogues.

Sheri, actress
Diagnosis of Hodgkin disease at age 29 in 1993 in Columbia, Maryland

THE LORD GOT ME through this journey, especially after the treatment had ended. I did a lot of praying, and I felt like God was right beside me. I had what I thought were cancer scares, and He was always there. I finally learned to trust in the Lord and [know that] everything would be okay. He will take care of me.

Joyce, educational assistant at an elementary school
Diagnosis of breast cancer at age 41 in 1995 in Knoxville, Tennessee

• • •

"It really shocked me when people told me that they were praying for me!"

MY JEWISH FAITH GETS me through all of life, and it did not desert me during cancer. I did not have a synagogue or rabbi within a thousand miles, so I was on my own. Since I have lived most of my adult life outside of the traditional Jewish community, I was used to turning inside to my faith—to the faith I keep within. I just knew that I would not be handed any more than I could handle and that prayer would see me through the good and the bad. It worked, and it continues to work to this day.

Ruthanne, bookkeeper
Diagnosis of breast cancer at age 51 in 1995 in Thorne Bay, Alaska

• • •

I MOVED INTO a deeper place in my own being. I learned how "to be" rather than "to do."

Pat, retired
Diagnosis of colon and bladder cancer at age 74 in 2005 in Como (Western Australia)

• • •

GOD HAS GIVEN ME a new lease on life.

Roxanne, disabled
Diagnosis of mantle cell lymphoma at age 48 in 2003 in Palm Beach Gardens, Florida

KNOWING THAT NOTHING TAKES God by surprise and that He would carry me through this time gave me hope and probably helped me the most.

Patti, financial administrator
Diagnosis of ovarian cancer at age 51 in 2005 in Colorado Springs, Colorado

• • •

AS A CATHOLIC, I'D love to say yes, but my cancer journey wasn't so much spiritual as it was emotional.

Mary, administrative assistant
Diagnosis of breast cancer at age 42 in 2003 in Simi Valley, California

• • •

MY CANCER EXPERIENCE HAS drawn me closer to God and has shown me what truly is important in life. I feel calmer and more positive about life. I know that through adversity comes strength and knowledge. I am enjoying the little things that, before the diagnosis, I would have missed.

Cynthia, administrative assistant
Diagnosis of breast cancer at age 55 in 2003 in Highland Lakes, New Jersey

• • •

SPIRITUALITY WAS THE REAL core of what helped me cope with cancer. It provided hope. Reading the Bible gave me insights into God as my rock and my support.

Jan, retired hospice chaplain
Diagnosis of breast cancer at age 55 in 2006 in Wichita, Kansas

• • •

IT REALLY SHOCKED ME when people (that I didn't really know that well) told me that they were praying for me! The first time someone told me that, I think I cried! It was so touching. But obviously, all the prayers helped me in my fight against cancer.

Marla, executive assistant
Diagnosis of breast cancer at age 35 in 1994 in Jasper, Indiana

I PRAYED, and I sat in the graveyard talking in my mind to the spirits and asking them to show me the way out of the nightmare I was faced with.

Andrew, self-employed
Diagnosis of non-Hodgkin lymphoma at age 45 in 2005 in Greater Manchester, Cheshire (United Kingdom)

• • •

I KNOW THAT GOD will bring me through this.

Melody, medical secretary
Diagnosis of breast cancer at age 39 in 2004 and lung cancer at age 42 in 2007 in Jessup, Maryland

• • •

I WAS ALONE the day the call came in and I first knew just how sick I had become. It was bigger than I knew I could handle alone. I asked God to allow my journey to be a witness for Him. I claimed Phil. 4:13: "I can do all things through him who gives me strength" (NIV). I called my husband, and then we called our sons. It became a family journey. We told our church, and they became our Prayer Warriors. At my worst point, they rallied together to host a prayer vigil in the hospital while I struggled to survive in the ICU. There is so much power in prayer for I am a miracle, and God chose me to be here. Our family, friends, and our community became involved in supporting my family in my absence. All told, it was fifteen months equaling 281 days in the hospital. As I was being cared for by the doctors and staff, I ministered to them and got involved in their lives to give back what I could.

Susan, homemaker
Diagnosis of acute myelogenous leukemia at age 50 in 2003 in Medina, Ohio

• • •

I KNEW GOD. I have a lot of faith. I do know that one day I will be leaving this world. I just felt like that it was not the time.

Lovey, homemaker
Diagnosis of uterine cancer at age 52 in 2000 in Cadiz, Kentucky

AT FIRST, I BLAMED God. I wondered, "Why me? What did I do to deserve this?" Then I realized that pity thinking was getting me nowhere. I started praying for healing, and I began eating healthier. I began to count my blessings—and still do! I went to a Healing of the Sick. My dad was beside me during the mass (he was going through [recovery for] alcoholism). I'm proud to say that he has not touched a drop of alcohol since and has seven years of sobriety under his belt.

Danielle, financial service specialist
Diagnosis of melanoma (skin cancer) at age 30 in 2000 in Ramstein (Germany)

When I first received my diagnosis, I found that my spiritual faith actually made things *harder* rather than easier. I thought, "If God loved me so much, why had He allowed something so devastating in my life?" As I hurled my questions heavenward, in time God showed me the answers—or at least gave me the peace to live with the unanswered queries. My spiritual faith deepened as I was forced to pray, trust, and soul-search in new ways. Eventually, God even took the whole experience and made something good come from it. Today, I work for my oncologist as a patient advocate, offering emotional and spiritual encouragement to his cancer patients and their caregivers.

LYNN EIB received a diagnosis of stage III colon cancer at age 36 in 1990. She is the author of several books on cancer and spirituality, including *When God & Cancer Meet: True Stories of Hope & Healing*.

GOD IS GOOD. TRUSTING in Him, I am in remission for the second time.

Marie, retired
Diagnosis of ovarian cancer at age 59 in 2004 in Lebanon, Ohio

NOT REALLY, THOUGH I have to admit that I did pray, with the hope that my prayers were heard.

Bryna, management development consultant
Diagnosis of tongue cancer at age 35 in 1985 in Brockton, Massachusetts

• • •

SURVIVING CANCER MEANS a whole new life. I was a troubled youth and young woman, so I think God stepped in and forced me to wake up the hard way. I look at my life before [cancer] and my life now, and I am so thankful to have my beautiful daughter and the chance to prove to myself that life is worth living when you have something wonderful to live for.

Cheryl, billings account clerk
Diagnosis of Ewing's sarcoma (bone cancer) at age 21 in 1987 in Malden, Massachusetts

• • •

GOD, JESUS, AND ALL the angels and saints have armed my family and me to beat this cancer. Prayers from everyone help. I also feel that my personal prayer time helps. I am now at peace living with cancer. My cancer is under control—not gone, but inactive. God gave me the tools, and I am using them to live a healthy life with cancer.

Kathryn, homemaker
Diagnosis of multiple myeloma at age 39 in 2001 and basal cell carcinoma (skin cancer) at age 45 in 2007 in St. Charles, Missouri

• • •

I FELT AN ENORMOUS spiritual presence that I had been unaware of before. The more I allowed myself to acknowledge that this was God's grace in my life, the more I felt an overwhelming aura of peace and self-assurance. I wish I could explain it better than that. It was and continues to be absolutely remarkable.

Jerry, computer software instructor
Diagnosis of acute myelogenous leukemia at age 43 in 2003 in Anoka, Minnesota

MY AUNT GAVE ME Bibles, tapes, and healing prayers. She took me to fellowship services and prayer groups and keeps me spiritually connected.

Yvonne, paralegal
Diagnosis of colon cancer at age 48 in 2004 in San Antonio, Texas

• • •

PRAYING IS A WONDERFUL thing. I do believe in the power of prayer, or I really don't think I would be here now.

April, disabled
Diagnosis of breast cancer at age 34 in 1999 in Wichita, Kansas

• • •

> "…I realized that pity thinking was getting me nowhere. I started praying for healing…"

SPIRITUAL GROWTH APART FROM "religion" has been the greatest blessing I have experienced from [having] cancer, as well as other difficult challenges of life. I have also come to have a greater thankfulness for and enjoyment of "the simple life." Nature is now my familiar friend, rather than a challenge to be fought against.

Barbara, homemaker
Diagnosis of breast cancer at age 38 in 1986 in Conway, Arkansas

• • •

I AM CATHOLIC and found comfort in going to Sunday Mass and sharing my progress with my pastor. I was able to thank God for some simple things, like the fact that it was springtime and great weather for walking to work after my radiation treatments. I prayed an Our Father or a Hail Mary during every radiation treatment and offered the prayer for someone else or someone else's soul. My best friend had breast cancer and suggested this as a great way to pass the brief minutes lying on the table.

Barbara, nurse
Diagnosis of breast cancer at age 58 in 1995 in Stoneham, Massachusetts

SPIRITUALITY BROUGHT ME CLOSER to the positive energy of the Universe. I learned to rely on the healing power of my own inner positive energy and that which surrounded me. I am able to connect with the angels of healing and actually heal myself physically. I have had several experiences wherein I summoned the angels of healing, and they healed that which needed to be healed or removed what should not have been there.

Debbie, hospice nurse
Diagnosis of breast cancer at age 52 in 2004 in Phoenix, Arizona

• • •

I HAVE ALWAYS LOOKED to the heavens every day to say, "Thank you."

Kathleen, retail manager
Diagnosis of breast cancer at age 48 in 2007 in Washington Township, New Jersey

• • •

MY GIRLFRIEND TOOK ME to church with her one Sunday. The preacher started his sermon. After a few minutes he stopped and said, "I am being told to stop this sermon and help someone understand." He turned to me and said, "The Lord has told me to let you know that many things are happening, and you have no understanding of why [they are happening]. In times of need, trouble, or the turmoil of not knowing, all you have to do is ask for my help, and I will be there for you." Then he continued his sermon.

Fran, postmaster
Diagnosis of breast cancer at age 42 in 1999 in LaVergne, Tennessee

• • •

"I know God heard these prayers."

MY BROTHERS-IN-LAW, who own their own business, would stop each day at noon and pray for me. This still brings tears to my eyes. I know God heard these prayers.

Michele, facilities manager
Diagnosis of colon cancer at age 42 in 2006 in Charles Town, West Virginia

I DO WISH that a survivor had approached me early in my treatment and informed me that I could live with cancer and that things do turn around. I would like to become a voice for anyone going through this ordeal.

Cindy, staffing specialist
Diagnosis of cervical cancer at age 32 in 1989 and colorectal cancer at age 48 in 2005 in Maryville, North Dakota

• • •

I PRAY DAY AND NIGHT asking God to help me and to give me a cure.

Amelia, unemployed
Diagnosis of acute myelogenous leukemia at age 29 in 2007 in Long Beach, California

• • •

THE SCHOOL WHERE MY daughter teaches would have prayers for me every morning.

Mariann, receptionist
Diagnosis of bladder cancer at age 50 in 2002 in West Haven, Connecticut

• • •

I AM A CHAPLAIN, and I am a Catholic. Religion and spirituality are my lifelines. I have a spiritual director who helps me see God's hand in the threads of my life. I was refreshed by the Sacraments. Hearing the Gospels through the ears of cancer is like a new translation.

Judy, chaplain
Diagnosis of colorectal cancer at age 48 in 2003 in Cudahy, Wisconsin

• • •

MY BIBLE STUDY GROUP was awesome. Cancer and fighting cancer elevated my dependence not only on others, but on God and His guidance.

Karen, real estate broker
Diagnosis of breast cancer at age 38 in 2001 in Loganville, Georgia

Creative endeavor, together with spiritual thinking about
the goodness of life, and gratitude for the love of our
Creator expressed to me in innumerable ways enabled me
to survive.

SUSAN VREELAND retired in 2000 after a 30-year career teaching high school
English in San Diego, California. Four years earlier, she had received a lymphoma
diagnosis at the age of 50. Susan's writing talents have led her to become a
New York Times bestselling novelist. She is the author five works of fiction on art-
related themes, including *Girl in Hyacinth Blue* and *Luncheon of the Boating Party*.

I AM NOT a religious person, but I am a spiritual one. When I found out I was ill,
I renewed my interest in the Buddhist philosophy, finding it very calming and
reassuring. I do not fear death or what may come afterwards.

Judy, retired accounting clerk
Diagnosis of lung cancer at age 64 in 2004 in Norwalk, California

• • •

I WAS NEVER a religious person, but I must say, I actually felt very good when I went
to synagogue. I felt connected, like I was doing yet another thing to help myself.

Laura, unemployed psychiatric social worker
Diagnosis of breast cancer at age 43 in 2006 in Avon, Connecticut

• • •

WHEN I FIRST RECEIVED the diagnosis, I allowed fear to grip me for three days.
But because of my faith in God, after three days of torment I turned to Him. He
was my total source. I read every scripture I could find on healing and I listened to
healing tapes; that is how I built up my faith. I continue to work and help others,
which also gives me some relief — it takes my mind off myself. I stayed upbeat
and told myself that "I could beat the little "c" because the great "C" was with me.

Marguerite, retired deacon
Diagnosis of breast cancer at age 60 in 1993 in Cheltenham, Maryland

WHEN I RECEIVED my cancer diagnosis, I was glad it was me instead of one of my family members. I didn't think I could handle watching my husband or children have cancer. I actually thanked God for making it be me. Shockingly, about two years into my cancer [experience], my youngest son also received a cancer diagnosis. When I was told, I went into the next room and said out loud, "God, you picked *me*. Don't do this to my son. I can't handle this…it's not fair. Help me, God." As I sat there, all of the sudden a sense of peace came over me—instantly. I took a deep breath and wiped my eyes. I went back into my son's hospital room and felt in complete control of myself. At that point, I realized that I could handle this. I did have the strength. I did have the support of God. My son is doing great and is in total remission.

Karen, medical assistant
Diagnosis of breast cancer at age 43 in 2001 in Cincinnati, Ohio

• • •

I REALIZED THAT I had been on a pathway to spiritual renewal and was not afraid to die.

John, retired
Diagnosis of prostate cancer at age 57 in 1995 and chronic lymphocytic leukemia at age 65 in 2003 in Jacksonville, Florida

• • •

I DON'T ATTEND CHURCH, but I do have a relationship with God. He has seen me through so many challenges in life, and He continues to lead me. I believe I have angels who watch over me and keep me safe.

Linda, purchasing agent
Diagnosis of breast cancer at age 47 in 2007 in Antioch, California

• • •

I GUESS IT WOULD be the healing power of prayer and positive vibes sent my way because I am not a church-going person. However, I do consider myself a spiritual person. I believe my spirituality helped me keep a positive mindset.

Barbara, retired art therapist
Diagnosis of pancreatic cancer at age 72 in 2006 in Golden, Colorado

> "I realized that I had been on a pathway to spiritual renewal and was not afraid to die."

OUR CHURCH DONATED the children's school tuition. Other churches gave us food and clothes. Churches on the East Coast mailed us gift cards for the kids from the prison ministry (my husband is in prison). We had garage sales and sold our furniture and personal items of value to make ends meet.

Alejandra, clerical worker
Diagnosis of uterine cancer at age 36 in 2005 in Torrance, California

• • •

QUIET REFLECTION HELPED ME find some peace so that I could sleep.

Jennifer, federal officer with U.S. Customs and Border Patrol
Diagnosis of cervical cancer at age 36 in 2007 in Montreal, Quebec (Canada)

• • •

MY PASTOR'S WIFE ORGANIZED thirty days of attention, and the ladies signed up for one of the thirty days. They brought flowers, visited, made meals, and cleaned my house one day.

Judi, nurse
Diagnosis of breast cancer at age 40 in 2000 in Pen Argyl, Pennsylvania

• • •

I WISH I HAD known that a church full of caring people was right down the road. We did not have a church home at that time, even though there were two churches who pitched in to provide a few meals and other things. But there is a church—we are now on staff at that church—which is filled with people who are looking for hurting people to help.

Carlyn, administrative assistant
Diagnosis of Hodgkin disease at age 30 in 2004 in Willow Spring, North Carolina

MY FAITH GOT STRONGER; the relationship between me and God became very tight. I kept thinking, "I have a baby girl who needs a healthy mom." I called everyone I knew and asked for prayers. I reevaluated my life and what is most important. I also thought about my mom who has always been there for me, no matter what. She's walked by my side in the best and worst times of my life, and I needed to be there for my daughter just the same way. My husband has been in Iraq three times, and I've been blessed to have him back every time. So I needed to fight, too, to be home with him as well.

Candy, teacher
Diagnosis of thyroid cancer at age 31 in 2007 in El Paso, Texas

• • •

PRAYER HELPED ME the most. I believe it is the one thing that healed me. I was never a strong believer, but now I have so much feeling for anyone who says prayer is the answer.

John, retired
Diagnosis of esophageal cancer at age 76 in 2006 in Jamestown, North Carolina

• • •

> "...I renewed my interest in the Buddhist philosophy, finding it very calming and reassuring. I do not fear death or what may come afterwards."

MY FAITH IN GOD and my husband got me through. When I received the diagnosis, I was a little afraid at first. Not of dying but of telling my twelve-year-old daughter. But after that, I was sort of at peace because I just felt it wasn't my time to go and God was going to get me through. I kept [a] positive [attitude], went to church, and wore a lot of silly hats during chemo.

Lisa, unemployed
Diagnosis of lung cancer at age 42 in 2007 in Colebrook, New Hampshire

THE FIRST THING I did was pray. The second step I took was to ask for guidance and healing prayers from everyone I knew.

Pam, retired dental hygienist
Diagnosis of breast cancer at age 57 in 2005 in Lakeland, Florida

• • •

JUST KNOWING THAT SO many people were praying for us helped me. When my brain tumor was diagnosed in 1998, my husband and I were working at the same place. Some of my husband's coworkers organized a group to meet in the chapel one day where they held a prayer service for us. Everyone joined hands, and they were all praying for us and asking God to heal me and help our family. That was so uplifting! Our prayers were answered!

Angela, registered nurse
Diagnosis of brain cancer at age 32 in 1998 and cervical cancer at age 37 in 2003 in Fulton, Mississippi

References

Kliewer, S. Allowing spirituality into the healing process. 2004. *Journal of Family Practice* 53(3):616–624.

Larson, D.B, J.P. Swyers, and M.E. McCullough. *Scientific research on spirituality and health: a consensus report.* Rockville, MD: National Institute for Healthcare Research; 1997, quoted in Kliewer 2004, 616.

Michael, J. 2005. *Flying crooked: a story of accepting cancer.* Vancouver, B.C., Canada; Berkeley, CA: Greystone Books (Distributed in the U.S. by Publishers Group West).

Zinnbauer B.J., K.I. Pargament, and B. Cole, et al. 1998. Religion and spirituality: unfuzzying the fuzzy. *Journal for the Scientific Study of Religion* 36:549–564, quoted in Kliewer 2004, 616.

CHAPTER 11

• • •

What I Wish I Had Known at Diagnosis

Cancer is a phenomenal teacher. Weeks, months, or even years after a cancer diagnosis, survivors look back in awe at what they have learned in the process. For the uninitiated and unwilling student, the lessons are difficult. I know, from my own personal and professional experience, the elements of a typical "cancer education." There is so much to learn about the diagnosis, treatment options, potential side effects, and so on. However, I was curious about how survivors would respond to this topic: what they wished they had known—right from the start. I figured these veterans could impart some valuable information to the new cancer patients and their loved ones. And I was right. This chapter is devoted to that important issue, and I hope that health care providers and those who offer cancer support services and education will pay close attention to the responses.

Knowing what you need to know before you go through an experience is practically impossible. In medicine we have a saying: "The mind doesn't know what the eyes haven't seen." Still, much can be learned from others' experiences that may pave the way to an easier road for you or a loved one who is going through the cancer journey.

In medical school, one of the first things future doctors learn is a new way of thinking and talking about health and disease. There is a hierarchy of knowledge that goes from very general to quite specific. For example, in grade school, one learns about the human body and its major parts. Most children know what muscles are and have a basic understanding of how they work. Teens and young adults usually can be more specific and name certain muscles, such as the quadriceps in the thigh. In medical school, students must learn many more details, for example, that the four muscles that make up the quadriceps work together to extend the knee. If they don't work in a coordinated manner, they'll throw the kneecap (patella) out of alignment, resulting in *patellofemoral tracking syndrome*, a common cause of knee pain. Furthermore, the culprit is usually not all four quadriceps muscles, but rather the vastus lateralis, which is usually more powerful and fully developed than the vastus medalis. Even more specifically, this problem usually occurs only in the last few degrees of range of motion of knee extension.

Only over time and with a significant amount of education can one achieve an in-depth understanding of any health problem. Most people know something about cancer before diagnosis, but in order to make good treatment decisions and to navigate this difficult and complicated experience, they usually need to become much more educated about their diagnosis and treatment options, as well as potential side effects from the therapy. Not only do they need to become more educated, but they must do it incredibly quickly, with the pressure of literally having their lives on the line.

This pressure can be overwhelming; but certainly there is help. Doctors, nurses, social workers, and other health care providers are terrific sources of information. Nonprofit organizations that are dedicated to providing cancer education and outreach are wonderful resources as well. Of course, many people turn to the Internet and, with discretion, this approach can also help fast-track learning about a particular type of cancer and the treatment options.

A recurrent theme in survivors' survey responses was that, before undergoing cancer treatment, they wished they had known more about its potential side effects. This is not a book about cancer treatment and its related side effects. However, setbacks are a normal part of going through a serious illness. Not to experience a setback would be the exception—not the norm. Although some setbacks can be quite devastating, the vast majority of problems can be dealt with or even completely overcome. Many health setbacks, during and after cancer treatment, will have no effect on the patient's long-term prognosis. Having this perspective from the beginning helps people recognize and appropriately deal with setbacks without becoming too discouraged (though they are almost always discouraging to some degree).

In her book, *There's Always Help; There's Always Hope*, Eve Wood, MD, nicely summarized the healing process. She wrote, "First and foremost, I want to reiterate that the process of growth and healing is not a straight line. None of us moves from dysfunction to fulfillment without a lot of setbacks, pauses, and mistakes. The path to health is a bumpy road" (Wood 2004, 194–195).

Knowing that it's normal to experience some setbacks during this process is useful to know from the start. There are many other pearls of wisdom that survivors shared for this book. I hope they will help you and your loved ones on this journey.

• • •

I WISH I HAD KNOWN that I was going to be physically well throughout my surgery, chemotherapy, and radiation. I was pretty worried about how I was going to manage my busy and complicated life through many months of treatment. On the other hand, had I known, I might not have done so much to prepare myself—taking almost everything off of my plate so that I could completely devote my energy toward recovery. Also, I wish I had known how cute my bald head was! I never realized that I have a nicely shaped head! And when my hair grew back it was curly, and I always wanted curly hair! It has straightened out in the year since, but I now keep it short. I love having short hair!

Mary, attorney
Diagnosis of breast cancer at age 54 in 2005 in Brookline, Massachusetts

• • •

LIFE IS SO MUCH sweeter after treatment!

Karen, real estate broker
Diagnosis of breast cancer at age 38 in 2001 in Loganville, Georgia

• • •

WHEN I FIRST FOUND out I had cancer, I was still in shock about the news. I did not find out the stage of my cancer until a month after surgery.

Rosi, student accounts office assistant
Diagnosis of colon cancer at age 52 in 2007 in Austin, Texas

> "Life is so much sweeter after treatment."

I WISH I HAD KNOWN that there were different chat groups available with whom to discuss my journey. Now, I am online and volunteer with several groups to be a contact for others who are going through treatment.

Greg, disabled
Diagnosis of mantle cell lymphoma at age 57 in 2005 and acute myelogenous leukemia at age 60 in 2008 in Orland Park, Illinois

• • •

THAT IT IS an ongoing process. The cancer experience never truly goes away. It is so huge and devastating that it actually changes you. It is always in the back of your mind. You have to learn how to coexist with it and not let it get you down.

Eileen, teacher
Diagnosis of breast cancer at age 43 in 2006 in Hilton, New York

• • •

I WISH I HAD KNOWN about all of the services that are available to help cancer patients. For example, the American Cancer Society's Look Good...Feel Better® program, the Patient Navigator program, support groups, and clinical trials.

Beth, health educator
Diagnosis of liver cancer at age 32 in 1990 in Fort Hood, Texas

• • •

I WISH I HAD KNOWN that chemo treatments were cumulative in the body and that recovery from each successive treatment would be more difficult.

David, journeyman sheet metal worker
Diagnosis of breast cancer at age 63 in 2005 in Missoula, Montana

• • •

THE RADIATION TREATMENTS could have been easier had I known about radiation burns. I could have self-treated the burns.

John, retired
Diagnosis of esophageal cancer at age 76 in 2006 in Jamestown, North Carolina

I WISH MY DOCTOR had told me about the constipation. Gross, I know, but significant. The pain from constipation was far worse than the pain from surgery (and they cut through my abdominal wall—who knew being backed up could be so painful?). I wish my doctor had told me that follow-up treatment would not be determined until after the final pathology [report]. I was told my cancer was diagnosed early. My scans were excellent. I would have a radical, abdominal hysterectomy, and that was it. Finding out I needed radiation was hard. Finding out that not only did I need external radiation therapy, but brachytherapy as well was also somewhat difficult. I also learned that when doctors say this should be the last test, it rarely is. That when they say this is the last treatment session, it rarely is. That medicine is a philosophy before it is a science (that part is not always easy to accept). That your work structure—not your friends or colleagues, but your management structure—will change. [Employers] will treat you differently, just because you have cancer. Perhaps I would have told them less, had I known how they would react. That's doubtful, as I am pretty open, but you never know.

Jennifer, federal officer with U.S. Customs and Border Patrol
Diagnosis of cervical cancer at age 36 in 2007 in Montreal, Quebec (Canada)

• • •

I WISH I HAD KNOWN about breast MRIs, so my cancer could have been diagnosed earlier.

Pam, retired dental hygienist
Diagnosis of breast cancer at age 57 in 2005 in Lakeland, Florida

I challenge my patients to think of healing not so much as an endpoint, but rather as a lifelong journey. To recognize and continually strive toward those activities, people, and thoughts that are most nourishing to them. This helps survivors to be better equipped to handle the bumps along the road.

KELLY PAUL, MD, is a physiatrist, with a special interest in oncology rehabilitation at Indiana University.

> ## "I wish I had known about breast MRIs, so my cancer could have been diagnosed earlier."

I WISH MY DOCTOR had told me that I have to pamper my surgery arm for life. I was told about lymphedema but not [enough].

Tracey, radiation oncology information analyst
Diagnosis of breast cancer at age 37 in 2002 in Villa Park, Illinois

• • •

CANCER TREATMENT IS NOT as scary as all the rumors lead you to believe. If you live through the treatments, one day at a time (sometimes one moment at a time), you really can get through it. I wish I knew that people adapt to what they need to adapt to when faced with dire circumstances and that I could find internal strength that I never knew was there.

Elena, arts administrator
Diagnosis of inflammatory breast cancer at age 44 in 1999 in Silver Spring, Maryland

• • •

IT'S IMPORTANT TO OPEN up about cares and worries and to accept offers of help.

Don, retired
Diagnosis of prostate cancer at age 74 in 2003 in Ocean Pines, Maryland

• • •

I WISH I HAD been told how critically important are the skills of the doctors we don't even choose for ourselves...like the radiologists who perform the needle biopsies and the pathologists who read the slides. Their skill drives the decisions for diagnosis and therapy, yet we may never even meet them or know to check out their credentials and experience.

Sandra, assistant professor of nursing
Diagnosis of breast cancer at age 54 in 2002 in Atlanta, Georgia

THE BEST ADVICE I give to anyone is this: Find something in your life to focus on other than your cancer...it can be a hobby, or work, or a relationship—pretty much anything other than your cancer. You deal with the medical aspects as necessary, but your mind needs something other than the cancer to focus on.

Ronald, business owner and entrepreneur
Diagnosis of testicular cancer at age 20 in 1975 in Dover, New Hampshire

• • •

DO OTHER SURVIVORS TALK about buying new, pretty underwear to go see their doctors? I ended up going to doctors so often and getting undressed and dressed so often I decided I needed better-looking underwear.

Carrie, information management specialist
Diagnosis of breast cancer at age 44 in 2002 in New York City, New York

• • •

GET SECOND OPINIONS, PARTICIPATE in your treatment; do not "go with the flow" of treatment. Question everything. Because of complications, I ended up having over and above the normal number of surgical procedures. I didn't know about the possible complications of breast reconstruction surgery after a mastectomy. With my reconstruction, everything that could go wrong did. Had I known what some of the end results would be, I would never have had it done. I could have lived just fine without it.

Michele, administrative assistant
Diagnosis of breast cancer at age 45 in 1999 in Detroit, Michigan

• • •

I WISHED MY DOCTOR had suggested freezing my eggs before the radiation (that destroyed my ovaries) from the first cancer's treatments, so I could have retained the option of having more children.

Angie, volunteer and cancer advocate
Diagnosis of vulvar cancer at age 31 in 1998 and breast cancer at age 36 in 2003 in Anderson, South Carolina

"Find something in your life to focus on..."

MY BACKGROUND, IRONICALLY, is in the field of cancer biology. For awhile, I thought that being familiar with the biological underpinnings of the disease would help me coast through treatment. I wish I had known back then that knowing the science would not shield me from the emotional aspects surrounding cancer.

Federico, cancer chemical biologist
Diagnosis of testicular cancer at age 32 in 2006 in Brookline, Massachusetts

I didn't realize at first that there would be a rich and full life after cancer.

CAROLYN RUNOWICZ, MD, received a diagnosis of breast cancer at age 41 in 1992. She specializes in gynecologic cancers and women's health. Dr. Runowicz is the director of the Carole and Ray Neag Comprehensive Cancer Center at the University of Connecticut Health Center. She is also a past president of the American Cancer Society.

I DIDN'T TELL my family about my diagnosis—they still don't know. Only some of my friends knew. I wish I'd known that this, too, shall pass. I felt that I was to blame, like I was "damaged goods." I felt so incredibly alone because I never was the type of person to ask for help—it was always my friends asking me to help them. This [experience] taught me how to ask for help and support. My friends being there for me, without my having to ask them, was super. I would tell them I was going alone to Sloan-Kettering* for a visit, and they'd show up there, unasked.

Jaime, graduate student
Diagnosis of cervical cancer at age 24 in 2005 in Blackwood, New Jersey

• • •

JOIN A SUPPORT GROUP. That has been a big help to me. Not only to talk to others, but to get ideas about how they handle things.

Cathy, retail district manager
Diagnosis of pancreatic cancer at age 45 in 2005 in Columbus, Ohio

---

*Memorial Sloan-Kettering Cancer Center.

I WISH MY DOCTOR had laid out [discussed with me] the option of mastectomy versus lumpectomy. At the time, I was very happy not to lose my breast. In hindsight, had I chosen mastectomy, I might have felt more secure about my prognosis.

Joyce, legal secretary
Diagnosis of breast cancer at age 44 in 2006 in South Amboy, New Jersey

• • •

I HAD BREAST CANCER, and my initial reaction was to have a mastectomy. My husband fell apart at the prospect of a mastectomy. So when I saw his reaction, I chose to undergo a lumpectomy. One thing I did not know was that patients who have chosen lumpectomy might need to go in for a re-excision because the margins are not "clear." I was one of those patients. Not only that, but the margins were still not clear after my second surgery. So, in the end, my third surgery was a mastectomy. Had I known more about my particular case, I would have chosen to undergo a mastectomy immediately after diagnosis, along with the breast reconstruction at that time. It would have saved me many trips under the surgeon's knife.

Ann, homemaker
Diagnosis of breast cancer at age 47 in 2003 in Mechanicsburg, Pennsylvania

• • •

WHEN I COULDN'T FIND a support group that was appropriate for my cancer, I wish I had known to start my own support group earlier.

Ric, public relations director
Diagnosis of thyroid cancer at age 50 in 1995 in Londonderry, New Hampshire

> "When I couldn't find a support group that was appropriate for my cancer, I wish I had known to start my own support group earlier."

I WISH I HAD KNOWN from the start that I had to be my own advocate. I lost a couple of weeks before I realized that my original doctor was dragging his feet and was not qualified to handle my case. Thankfully, I found a wonderful doctor at Indiana University Medical Center who immediately saw the seriousness of my situation and was capable of performing the intricate surgery I needed to begin beating this cancer! Because my cancer was very advanced and very aggressive, I would not be here today if I had not been aggressive in seeking treatment.

Sherri, elementary school teacher
Diagnosis of endometrial (uterine) cancer at age 42 in 2004 in Bruceville, Indiana

• • •

> "...one mammogram can save two lives!"

I WISH I HAD better understood that it is an up-and-down process, with progress and some setbacks. I initially looked at the treatment plan as linear, but found that there can be changes along the way.

Midge, accountant
Diagnosis of non-Hodgkin lymphoma at age 52 in 2005 and breast cancer at age 54 in 2007 in Westford, Massachusetts

• • •

FIND A GOOD SUPPORT system, be it a friend, stranger, survivor, or support group—and use it. Don't rely on or expect a lot out of those you are close to. They hurt, too, and so often they don't know what to say or what to do. They are dealing with their own issues and fears and may not know the best way to react to yours. If they want to help by doing chores or just sitting and staring at you, respect the fact that that is how they are dealing with it and welcome it. Don't look too closely at statistics either. They can be misleading and do nothing but induce further fear. None of us flows on numbers alone. Some lose the battle, but many win. Just go to a Relay for Life®, and take a long look at the thousands fighting right along with you. Don't ever feel like you are fighting the battle alone. March on, brave warriors! Someday our fight will be won!

Kathie, nurse and social worker
Diagnosis of kidney cancer at age 53 in 2005 in Kingston, New York

I spent countless hours reading information and asking questions. It's really important to advocate for yourself and be sure that the treatment you are getting is the best treatment for you. I got a second opinion, which can be tough to do. We are inclined to not question our doctors and to trust them implicitly. That being said, the second opinion I got was the right one for me, so I would encourage people to seek more opinions. Ask the tough questions, get a second opinion, take good care of yourself, surround yourself with family and friends, and do whatever it takes to keep hope alive. I believe that unity is strength, knowledge is power, and attitude is everything—and that is true for every person affected by cancer.

LANCE ARMSTRONG had testicular cancer that had spread to his brain, lung, and abdomen. One year after his 1996 diagnosis, he founded the Lance Armstrong Foundation, which is dedicated to helping cancer survivors.

IWISH I HAD KNOWN that I wasn't going to die within moments or months or even years of the diagnosis.

Jennifer, psychotherapist
Diagnosis of breast cancer at age 39 in 2004 in Pennington, New Jersey

• • •

IT WOULD HAVE HELPED me to know that there was a good, but different, life after all the treatment—that I would probably never feel so much heartbreak as I did, but that it would ease in time.

Pearl, nurse
Diagnosis of breast cancer at age 32 in 2004 in Glasgow (Scotland)

> "I wish I had known that I wasn't going to die within moments or months or even years of the diagnosis."

THAT IT IS POSSIBLE to survive after the devastation of a cancer diagnosis.

Mark, retired nuclear pharmacist
Diagnosis of chronic lymphocytic leukemia at age 59 in 2001 in Bay Shore, New York

• • •

I HAVE NO CHILDREN, but was offered information about cryogenics since my treatment would make me sterile. I was twenty-five at the time and had no idea when I might be thinking of children, so I did not go that route. I wish I had taken more time to consider it. It is the one regret that I now have.

Todd, oncology social worker
Diagnosis of chronic myelogenous leukemia at age 25 in 1997 and kidney cancer in 2005 at age 33 in Warwick, Rhode Island

• • •

I HAVE A GREAT family doctor who is a close friend as well. He told me, "Matt, you will have to learn to be responsible for all of your records and information that we medical people provide you with; don't trust us to do everything right or coordinate perfectly." I took that information to heart, and it has made a huge difference. In short, I've managed my own case to the best of my ability.

Matt, carpenter
Diagnosis of chronic lymphocytic leukemia at age 51 in 2003 in Bath, New York

I WISH I HAD KNOWN that chemo didn't have to be such an ordeal. I wish I had known that I could survive it—although that learning process itself was an incredible gift to me, so I guess I'm glad I had to learn it. I wish I'd known that having breast cancer—and surviving it—would bring blessings and transformation, not just anxiety and hard times.

Cathi, clinical social worker
Diagnosis of breast cancer at age 52 in 2003 in Waban, Massachusetts

ONE THING I WISH I had known is that my emotions would go haywire with the chemo. I found myself often crying at commercials.

Shelly, program coordinator for adults with disabilities
Diagnosis of breast cancer at age 32 in 2004 in Concord, New Hampshire

• • •

THE BIGGEST SURPRISE to me was how challenging the emotional/psychological side of this turned out to be. I have been able to talk about prostate cancer and the fact that I had it very calmly, intelligently, almost dispassionately. Yet, when I would finish one of those discussions, I would just want to go in a closet, pull the door shut, and sit down to cry.

Bill, administrator
Diagnosis of prostate cancer at age 62 in 2007 in Jefferson, Wisconsin

• • •

I WISH I HAD KNOWN that I carried a mutant gene (HNPCC); then I would have had a prophylactic hysterectomy at the same time as my colectomy.

Kirsten, distribution assistant
Diagnosis of colon cancer at age 49 in 2006 and endometrial (uterine) cancer at age 50 in 2007 in Buford, Georgia

• • •

THAT IT WOULD HAVE been less traumatic down the road had I felt comfortable talking about my fears and feelings with my husband, rather than pretending to be okay all the time.

Lindy, hospice volunteer
Diagnosis of breast cancer at age 35 in 1984 and radiation-induced sarcoma at age 55 in 2004 in Lexington, Massachusetts

"It would have been less traumatic down the road had I felt comfortable talking about my fears and feelings..."

I NOW KNOW that anyone can do it if they have to. I did not think I could stand having my blood drawn; it was too scary and might hurt. I did not think I could find a way through the medical system; it was too intimidating.

Matt, carpenter
Diagnosis of chronic lymphocytic leukemia at age 51 in 2003 in Bath, New York

In 1988, when I was thirty-nine years old, I had my spleen removed because of a high-grade, diffuse lymphoma. After the surgery, I underwent treatment with high-dose chemotherapy for three months. My prognosis was very poor—from a few months to less than two years. Actually, I am a twenty-year survivor! I learned that being a survivor could be a chance to go ahead, to be resilient. What cancer gave me was an incredible opportunity to stay away from futility and take care of the most important people and things in my life.

CLAUDE-ALAIN PLANCHON, MD, is an oncologist in the field of nuclear medicine and leader of the French branch of Vital Options® International, an organization dedicated to cancer survivors.

WHEN I FOUND OUT my mammogram was abnormal, I called my twin and asked her if she was getting her mammograms, because her risk would be higher if I had breast cancer. She was not getting mammograms. She went home and found a lump, got a mammogram, and found out she had invasive breast cancer (stage I). I learned that one mammogram can save two lives!

Deb, nurse practitioner
Diagnosis of melanoma (skin cancer) at age 21 in 1974 and breast cancer at age 52 in 2006 in Evansville, Indiana

THAT HAVING AN NG [nasogastric] tube pulled out sucks! That radiation makes you really, really tired. That I was going to lose my memory because of chemo.

Evelyn, executive assistant
Diagnosis of colon cancer at age 33 in 2004 in Boston, Massachusetts

• • •

I WISH SOMEONE had shared with me all the success stories. More and more people are living with cancer than ever before.

Andrea, hospital administrator
Diagnosis of Ewing's sarcoma (a form of bone cancer) at age 15 in 1992 in Norfolk, Massachusetts

• • •

THAT I WOULD STILL be here four years on! The initial diagnosis is terrifying.

Elizabeth, retired administrator
Diagnosis of breast cancer at age 58 in 2003 in Plymouth, Devon (England)

• • •

THAT CANCER IS NOT a death sentence. It is treatable.

Debra, administrative assistant
Diagnosis of ovarian cancer at age 51 in 2007 in Chicago, Illinois

• • •

> "I wish the doctor had explained 'thyroid storm' to me, so I wouldn't have been so incredibly scared by it when it happened."

THAT SOMETIMES DOCTORS DON'T really go into detail on possible side effects, and they downplay the seriousness of some of the long-term effects. But honestly, in hindsight I think that my choices were the right ones.

Pat, office manager
Diagnosis of breast cancer at age 53 in 2001 in Canton, Michigan

I WISH I HAD KNOWN which functions are controlled by the thyroid. The only way I found out what it controls was by getting every symptom, one at a time. I wish the doctor had explained "thyroid storm" to me, so I wouldn't have been so incredibly scared by it when it happened. I had no idea what was happening to me; I thought I was going to die.

Nicki, homemaker
Diagnosis of thyroid cancer at age 20 in 2005 in Union, Missouri

• • •

WHAT MY DOCTORS WOULD have chosen for treatments if it was them [if they had cancer] or a loved one.

Kelley, massage therapist
Diagnosis of breast cancer at age 36 in 2006 in Rochdale, Massachusetts

Every time I see a new patient with cancer, I share with them that cancer is a treatable and increasingly a curable disease. Along with medical treatments, every patient needs a prescription for hope, which is free, powerful, and has few side effects.

KEN MILLER, MD, is an oncologist and the director of the Yale Cancer Center Survivorship Program. He is the editor of the book *Choices in Breast Cancer Treatment*.

MY BREAST CANCER was initially misdiagnosed. Had I not followed up with another doctor after finding the lump in my breast, I probably would not be alive today. I wish I had asked more questions, had not taken what the doctors told me as gospel concerning my surgery and treatment, as well as reconstruction. Not doing that cost me dearly years later.

Eileen, technology specialist
Diagnosis of breast cancer at age 34 in 1984 and acute myelogenous leukemia at age 49 in 1999 and basal cell carcinoma (skin cancer) at age 55 in 2005 in Framingham, Massachusetts

I ONLY KNEW ONE person locally who had breast cancer—a man at our church. When my cancer was first diagnosed, we talked about what chemo would be like, and that was beneficial. I was invited to join Bosom Buddies but did not because I was actually embarrassed at the thought of someone reassuring me when they might have more advanced cancer than mine! It would have been better for me to talk with them and learn in advance what to expect with chemo and radiation. Other than book learning, I experienced it on my own.

Linda, genealogy associate at a historical library
Diagnosis of breast cancer at age 59 in 2006 in Sulphur, Louisiana

• • •

THAT I COULD DIE, and that the treatments were experimental. This was the 1960s. It took a long time for doctors to diagnose Hodgkin disease and eleven years to cure it. I also wish they had told me that the treatments would leave me sterile.

> **"Cancer is not a death sentence. It is treatable."**

Randy, respiratory therapist
Diagnosis of Hodgkin disease at age 6 in 1965 in Ewa Beach, Hawaii

• • •

I WISH I HAD had the initial information from the doctor in writing (stage/treatment), because most of the original records have been lost, and we have only been able to piece some of it together. A lot of things were not known at the time. I remember I focused on the 95 percent cure rates at the time and obviously have survived thirty-five years, even with multiple issues from treatment. I do believe patients were not told as much then as they are now. Even my parents didn't seem to have much information, and since I was a teenager, I wasn't given as much information. Perhaps I was given more info than I remember; that was a long time ago.

Charose, nurse
Diagnosis of Hodgkin disease at age 17 in 1972 and breast cancer at age 51 in 2006 in Omaha, Nebraska

HOW TO ASK FOR help. I wish that I had given weekly updates to everyone to let them know what I was going through—how I felt and what I needed. One can never have enough support!

Sheri, actress
Diagnosis of Hodgkin disease at age 29 in 1993 in Columbia, Maryland

• • •

I WISH I HAD gotten counseling from professionals who work with cancer patients. It would have been easier and less stressful for me. I handled it okay, but it would have been better to have had counseling. I had two close friends, but I did not tell them everything I was feeling. They would have listened; I chose not to reveal my feelings. I am a private person, but it would have helped me to talk to them. I could have talked to my husband about it, but he is not good at dealing with situations like this. He keeps his feelings hidden, too.

Joyce, educational assistant at an elementary school
Diagnosis of breast cancer at 41 in 1995 in Knoxville, Tennessee

• • •

HOW IMPORTANT FAMILY IS.

Laurie, medical assistant
Diagnosis of breast cancer at age 43 in 2006 in Sacramento, California

• • •

I WISH THEY HAD told me it [the cancer] could recur and that cigarette smoking was a big factor.

LaDonne, retired
Diagnosis of kidney cancer at age 40 in 1978 in Mundelein, Illinois

• • •

I WISH I HAD KNOWN how important it is to have a doctor who has experience with your type of cancer and its treatment.

Vera, personal assistant
Diagnosis of thyroid cancer at age 51 in 2002 in Milwaukee, Wisconsin

WHEN I FOUND that they didn't find clear margins after my first surgery, I fell apart. An hour later, I got a phone call from a survivor who worked at the hospital where I was getting treatment, and she talked to me about her mastectomy. I realized that losing a breast wasn't the end of the world!

Mary, administrative assistant
Diagnosis of breast cancer at age 42 in 2003 in Simi Valley, California

• • •

I LEARNED NOT TO listen to survival statistics. I felt that if one person had survived my type of cancer, I could do it too.

Janet, elementary school teacher
Diagnosis of colon cancer at age 42 in 1993 in Philadelphia, Pennsylvania

• • •

> "Educating yourself on your disease and your options allows you to be your own best advocate."

SIX MONTHS BEFORE the diagnosis, I knew I was bruising easily, and I thought I was just clumsy. Now I know the bruises, so slow to disappear, were the early warning signs. Also, my joints were aching so much, and I was taking naps. I worked two part-time jobs and was in denial until I got a very large bruise that I just could not ignore.

Susan, homemaker
Diagnosis of acute myelogenous leukemia at age 50 in 2003 in Medina, Ohio

• • •

I WISH I HAD KNOWN that I would grieve the loss of my breast. It had been part of my identity and my self-image, besides my body image. It was my breast, but to my doctor it was just another breast.

Jan, retired hospice chaplain
Diagnosis of breast cancer at age 55 in 2006 in Wichita, Kansas

THAT I WAS *NOT* going to die within the next five years or so. I had a mastectomy and did not have reconstruction, because I thought I was dying at the time!

Marla, executive assistant
Diagnosis of breast cancer at age 35 in 1994 in Jasper, Indiana

• • •

> "I wish I had known that I would be a survivor and had not wasted so much time in self-pity."

THAT IN THE VERY beginning, educating yourself on your disease and your options allows you to be your own best advocate.

Nancy, administrative assistant
Diagnosis of breast cancer at age 54 in 2006 in Fowlerville, Michigan

• • •

I WISH I HAD KNOWN that I would be a survivor and had not wasted so much time in self-pity. Why me? Why not me? Why anyone? We'll never know...

Danielle, financial service specialist
Diagnosis of melanoma (skin cancer) at age 30 in 2000 in Ramstein (Germany)

• • •

IT WOULD HAVE HELPED to know that I would lose some friends and that it shouldn't bother me because all people are not supportive. I needed to move on to the new friends I made and to appreciate the ones that stuck around to be there for me and my family. I did have a bit of a broken heart when I realized some friends would drop our friendship. I could have been more prepared for that and, therefore, experience no disappointing surprises. Dealing with cancer was enough without the drama of worrying about friends and family members who could not deal with my cancer. Seven years later, I am doing great and do not expect anything, but I'm pleased to get help, love, and caring when it is offered.

Kathryn, homemaker
Diagnosis of multiple myeloma at age 39 in 2001 and basal cell carcinoma (skin cancer) at age 45 in 2007 in St. Charles, Missouri

THAT IT IS OKAY to be scared. It is normal to have fear, but by talking with others you feel so much better.

Dorothy, receptionist
Diagnosis of breast cancer at age 44 in 2005 in Chesapeake, Virginia

• • •

I WISH I HAD reached out to the American Cancer Society for help, guidance, and information. I should have taken others' offers of help—not pushed people away. I felt this was my disease, my problem, and only I could fix it. I definitely shut people out.

Allie, Director, Distinguished Events; American Cancer Society
Diagnosis of thyroid cancer at age 46 in 2003 in Fair Haven, New Jersey

On a practical note, ask for copies of all your medical reports and films and start a folder to keep track of things, just like you would keep track of your insurance or any business matter. Bring your folder and films to all doctors' appointments, along with a notebook of your questions so you won't forget them.

SUSAN PORIES, MD, FACS, is a breast surgical oncologist at Mount Auburn Hospital in Cambridge, Massachusetts, and the Beth Israel Deaconess Medical Center in Boston, Massachusetts. She is the lead editor of the book *Soul of a Doctor,* which is a collection of stories about young doctors-in-training. Dr. Pories encourages doctors to write and is the faculty advisor for the Harvard Medical School student writing group.

"CANCER" ISN'T THE INVINCIBLE monster it once was. There is plenty of reason for optimism.

Jerry, computer software instructor
Diagnosis of acute myelogenous leukemia at age 43 in 2003 in Anoka, Minnesota

I DO WISH that a survivor had approached me early in my treatment to inform me that I could live with cancer and things do turn around. I would like to become a voice [of encouragement] for anyone going through this ordeal.

Cindy, staffing specialist
Diagnosis of cervical cancer at age 32 in 1989 and colorectal cancer at age 48 in 2005 in Maryville, North Dakota

There are so many things that I know now that I wish I had known when I was diagnosed, both about cancer and about myself. I know so much more about lymphoma, so much more about immune system–enhancing supplements and diet, so much more about new treatments, and so much more about myself and my ability to cope and, indeed, just how much I really do want to live.

JAMIE RENO is a *Newsweek* correspondent. He was diagnosed in 1996, at age 35, with stage IV, low-grade, follicular non-Hodgkin lymphoma. He went through a very difficult chemotherapy treatment in 1997 and then, when the cancer returned in 1999, participated in a clinical trial of a new radioimmunotherapy (RIT) cancer drug called Bexxar, which saved his life. He has been in remission ever since.

THAT IT COULD HAPPEN to me. I always thought it would be someone else—never me. I have no family history. I am young and healthy.

Jocelyn, social worker
Diagnosis of breast cancer at age 43 in 2006 in Macedon, New York

• • •

THE TERROR DOES SUBSIDE.

Laura, unemployed psychiatric social worker
Diagnosis of breast cancer at age 43 in 2006 in Avon, Connecticut

I WISH I HAD KNOWN how much control I had over my treatment options. I was stressed to the max, weighing options under incredible deadlines, and then I spoke with a social worker who calmed me down and taught me that I was in control.

Robin, college professor
Diagnosis of breast cancer at age 50 in 2006 in Costa Mesa, California

• • •

I WISH I HAD DECIDED to get a bilateral mastectomy, so I would not have to worry so much. I still worry, and I think I always will.

Cheryl, homemaker
Diagnosis of breast cancer at age 49 in 2006 in Garland, Texas

• • •

I WISH I HAD KNOWN that I had time! I could have taken as much time to decide my treatment as possible. My doctors did not tell me that, so I was in a very big hurry. Also, knowing that there is financial help out there if you know where to go to find it, but you have to ask everybody.

Jennifer, housekeeper
Diagnosis of breast cancer at age 40 in 2004 and skin cancer at age 41 in 2005 in Craig, Colorado

• • •

> "It is survivable. Chemo really does suck. Your hair will grow back...just not fast enough!"

ACTUALLY, IT OCCURRED to me that if I beat this, not much else is likely to take me out anytime soon. I could live to be one hundred years old after all. With breast cancer being the most frightening thing, it's somewhat reassuring to have already come a long way in that battle.

Deborah, physician
Diagnosis of breast cancer at age 47 in 2007 in Overland Park, Kansas

I WAS SEVEN MONTHS pregnant, working full-time and taking care of four other children when my cancer was diagnosed. Labor was induced [to deliver my baby] at thirty weeks, and I started chemo the next day. One year later, I am still having a hard time, but I am optimistic it can only get better. The only advice I have is, "Do not make it seem as though it is 'no big deal' because it is!"

Ann, physical education teacher
Diagnosis of non-Hodgkin lymphoma at age 41 in 2006 in Random Lake, Wisconsin

• • •

BREAST RECONSTRUCTION IS NOT what it is cracked up to be. To look normal, I should have had the other breast removed at the same time, but my nerves couldn't handle it then.

Polly, human resource administrator
Diagnosis of breast cancer at age 54 in 2005 in Port Gibson, Mississippi

• • •

IT IS SURVIVABLE. Chemo really does suck. Your hair will grow back...just not fast enough!

Linda, purchasing agent
Diagnosis of breast cancer at age 47 in 2007 in Antioch, California

• • •

YOU CAN GET THROUGH THIS. It is a marathon that needs to be anticipated and planned for. Keep on with your life, and don't make the illness your life.

Anne, psychologist
Diagnosis of breast cancer at age 50 in 2005 in Boston, Massachusetts

Reference
Wood, E. A. 2004. *There's always help; there's always hope.* Carlsbad, CA: Hay House.

CHAPTER 12

• • •

What Would Have Helped but Was Too Hard to Ask For

I have to be honest; there are some comments in this chapter that I found a bit heartbreaking. It can be incredibly difficult to ask for what we need or what would help us the most. I admit that I didn't always let people know what would have really helped—they were already doing so much, and I didn't want to burden them further.

If you are a friend or family member of someone going through cancer, this chapter offers some important insights, and I encourage you to read what survivors shared about this topic. Knowing what will help someone (who might be hesitant to tell you what he or she needs most) can allow you to really make a difference. Keep reading to learn what no one may ever tell you.

• • •

WHAT I DESIRED MOST, for which I found it hard to ask, was physical contact with people. Just the mere contact of someone touching my arm, shaking my hand, giving me a hug, I found to be very comforting. And occasionally, someone to cry with.

Bill, administrator
Diagnosis of prostate cancer at age 62 in 2007 in Jefferson, Wisconsin

• • •

I HAVE A DIFFICULT time asking for help in general, so I had to really work at asking for help and letting people know when I needed them to do things for me and when I just needed some time alone.

Sarah, paralegal
Diagnosis of breast cancer at age 28 in 2000 in Miami, Florida

MORE HUGS from my husband.

Kirsten, distribution assistant
Diagnosis of colon cancer at age 49 in 2006 and endometrial (uterine) cancer at age 50 in 2007 in Buford, Georgia

• • •

I WISHED I HAD had someone to clean my house, because I was too tired to do anything during radiation. I would never ask someone to clean my house!

Sally, research laboratory administrator
Diagnosis of breast cancer at age 40 in 1990 in Salem, Massachusetts

• • •

"Just the mere contact of someone touching my arm, shaking my hand, giving me a hug, I found to be very comforting."

OUTSIDE SUPPORT GROUPS. I wanted to just talk to someone who did not know me. Just to vent. I needed to just release some of my feelings, and I did not know where to turn.

Beth, health educator
Diagnosis of liver cancer at age 32 in 1990 in Fort Hood, Texas

• • •

THE THING I THINK my family needed most during that time was help with transportation. I needed frequent rides back and forth to the hospital, and my brothers needed rides back and forth to their baseball games, karate classes, and other activities. We never really felt comfortable asking people for help with driving me or my brothers, but there were a few people who offered to help with transportation, and it was really appreciated.

Andrea, hospital administrator
Diagnosis of Ewing's sarcoma (a form of bone cancer) at age 15 in 1992 in Norfolk, Massachusetts

PHYSICALLY, I WAS JUST overwhelmed and tired and would have loved some help with cleaning and chores like laundry. One friend sent her kids to cut my grass and take out garbage.

Luanne, registered nurse
Diagnosis of breast cancer at age 45 in 2007 in Morris, Illinois

"More hugs from my husband."

• • •

MORE SUPPORT for my husband from his family and friends.

Kathi, retired special education teacher
Diagnosis of breast cancer at age 49 in 2003 in Wrightstown, Wisconsin

• • •

I WISHED THAT I had had someone to talk to about my feelings. Back in 1983, I really couldn't share my inner feelings with anyone. We didn't talk much about the cancer. Cancer was a private matter at that time.

Pamela, bookkeeper
Diagnosis of Hodgkin disease at age 23 in 1983 and basal cell carcinoma (skin cancer) at age 41 in 2001 and breast cancer at age 46 in 2006 in Gardiner, Maine

• • •

A ONE-ON-ONE DISCUSSION with a survivor of the same or similar cancer would have been very helpful. I did repeatedly ask professionals for this type of support, but it took ten months to find someone.

Mike, management professional
Diagnosis of rectal cancer at age 38 in 2006 in Rochester, New York

• • •

HELP FROM OTHERS with day-to-day things. I'm not a person who likes to ask for help, so I would overdo it and regret it later.

Kelley, massage therapist
Diagnosis of breast cancer at age 36 in 2006 in Rochdale, Massachusetts

MORE HELP WITH HOUSEHOLD chores. Going from housewife and stay-at-home mother to bedridden cancer patient was a hard transition. I felt really guilty about my husband going to work all day and then having to come home and take care of the house, too.

Nicki, homemaker
Diagnosis of thyroid cancer at age 20 in 2005 in Union, Missouri

• • •

JUST ABOUT ANYTHING. I am a person who handles everything—from the bills, changing diapers, taking care of our entire house. It is hard to let go and let someone help me, let alone ask for it.

Rochelle, manicurist
Diagnosis of melanoma (skin cancer) at age 34 in 2007 in Las Vegas, Nevada

• • •

WHAT I DIDN'T LIKE was for people to tell me that they were sorry. That I hated. One person I knew didn't say anything when I first saw her after I received my diagnosis. All she did was come up to me and give me a big hug. That meant so much to me, and I will never forget what she did.

Joyce, educational assistant at an elementary school
Diagnosis of breast cancer at 41 in 1995 in Knoxville, Tennessee

• • •

FOR MORE OF MY FRIENDS that I had prior to diagnosis to just be there. They didn't have to have the perfect thing to say or do...just be there.

Laurie, medical assistant
Diagnosis of breast cancer at age 43 in 2006 in Sacramento, California

• • •

I DIDN'T HAVE a problem asking for anything. I was very proactive with my care.

Julie, real estate agent
Diagnosis of thyroid cancer at age 34 in 1996 and breast cancer at age 43 in 2005 in Torrance, California

TWO THINGS WERE HARD for me to ask for. One was the support I really needed from my husband—just the reassurance that everything was going to be okay. The second thing was help with housework. Fatigue drained my energy.

Vera, personal assistant
Diagnosis of thyroid cancer at age 51 in 2002 in Milwaukee, Wisconsin

• • •

I WISH I HAD had help with my self-image. When I was bloated from steroids, bald, and unibreasted, it would have been nice if someone (like my husband!) had convinced me that I was still pretty, that I was okay the way I was. It was hard for him, too.

Mary, administrative assistant
Diagnosis of breast cancer at age 42 in 2003 in Simi Valley, California

• • •

I AM A LITTLE stubborn, so asking for any kind of help was difficult for me. I would have liked to have a little more help with my mother after my recurrence, as her Alzheimer's disease had progressed.

Kathleen, teacher
Diagnosis of Hodgkin disease at age 40 in 1997 in Lisbon, Connecticut

• • •

I WOULD HAVE LOVED to have spoken to a long-term survivor of stage IV colon cancer. Now, I take calls from newly diagnosed colon cancer patients through the Bloch Cancer Hotline and the Colon Cancer Alliance, so that others can know it is possible to survive and become healthy.

Janet, elementary school teacher
Diagnosis of colon cancer at age 42 in 1993 in Philadelphia, Pennsylvania

• • •

INTIMACY WITH MY HUSBAND.

Jan, retired hospice chaplain
Diagnosis of breast cancer at age 55 in 2006 in Wichita, Kansas

IT WOULD HAVE HELPED to have had a closer relationship with my sister. She never even called me.

Glenda, disabled
Diagnosis of ovarian cancer at age 60 in 2004 in Chanute, Kansas

Asking for what you need and then being open to receiving it can be one of the unexpected challenges of the cancer experience. Many of us are much more comfortable helping others rather than being on the receiving end of someone's assistance.

One of the first steps is to let yourself find out what you really need. Be honest with yourself as you ask what it is that will help you be as strong and supported in your healing as possible. You may need someone to help with the laundry, to drive you to the clinic for treatment, to bring your child to a sports activity, or mow the lawn. You may wish for some financial help as the bills pile up. You may want someone to come watch a funny movie with you or simply sit with you in shared silence or listen as you speak from your heart. Or perhaps what you long for is to have some time alone, doing what you can do on your own, without anyone asking if they can help you.

Asking is a risk. It takes courage. You might not get what you ask for after you have made yourself vulnerable enough to say what you need. You may be disappointed. You may also be wonderfully surprised by who comes through in unexpected ways. But it is true that you won't get what you need unless you ask for it.

One of my patients said he was learning how to receive help with gratitude [instead of] guilt. He said it was one of the most challenging and important lessons he has had to learn. He realized that in being open to others' offers to help, he was allowing them a chance to feel helpful, not helpless, about his cancer diagnosis.

It is remarkable how, in receiving someone's care, you in turn are giving them an opportunity to feel stronger.

AMY GROSE, LICSW, is an oncology social worker with the Lance Armstrong Foundation Adult Survivorship Clinic and Perini Family Survivors' Center at Dana-Farber Cancer Institute in Boston, Massachusetts.

I FOUND IT HARD to ask for counseling after all of it was over (meaning after my chemo treatments and after my hair started to grow again). This might have helped with my acceptance of myself as I am now, after a mastectomy.

Marla, executive assistant
Diagnosis of breast cancer at age 35 in 1994 in Jasper, Indiana

• • •

HOW CAN YOU ASK someone to clean your house or to pay for some housecleaning help? People forget that life goes on as you lay on the bathroom floor or in bed dealing with the chemo drugs, etc.

Kathryn, homemaker
Diagnosis of multiple myeloma at age 39 in 2001 and basal cell carcinoma (skin cancer) at age 45 in 2007 in St. Charles, Missouri

SOMEONE TO CLEAN my house. Friends were very gracious about bringing meals, stopping by the pharmacy. But I don't think I vacuumed for six months. One friend offered once to clean—I was so grateful. And instead of flowers, a certificate for a massage would have been better.

Carmela, technical writer
Diagnosis of endometrial (uterine), bladder, and ovarian cancer at age 48 in 2005 in Clinton Township, Michigan

• • •

IT IS HARD for me to ask for help in any area—whether it be help at home, financial, emotional, anything.

April, disabled
Diagnosis of breast cancer at age 34 in 1999 in Wichita, Kansas

• • •

AN EAR TO LISTEN to, a shoulder to cry on. I didn't want to hear how sorry anyone was...I just needed family and friends to be there for me.

Danielle, financial service specialist
Diagnosis of melanoma (skin cancer) at age 30 in 2000 in Ramstein (Germany)

• • •

> "I wished I had had someone to clean my house, because I was too tired to do anything..."

I NEEDED MORE EMOTIONAL support. My family could not *always* be there, and sometimes it's hard even to ask them because you're always concerned about scaring them. I was never really prepared to encounter the enormous psychological battle that I faced. I'm sure that's different for everyone, but there were times that, despite everyone else's best attempts at consolation, I just turned into an emotional Twinkie. It was very scary to me to be so out of control.

Jerry, computer software instructor
Diagnosis of acute myelogenous leukemia at age 43 in 2003 in Anoka, Minnesota

I NEEDED MORE REASSURANCE about my body image and physical changes in my breasts, and this was very hard to share with my husband.

Barbara, nurse
Diagnosis of breast cancer at age 58 in 1995 in Stoneham, Massachusetts

· · ·

FINANCIAL HELP. We lost our house; we couldn't pay our bills.

Lisa, unemployed
Diagnosis of lung cancer at age 42 in 2007 in Colebrook, New Hampshire

· · ·

> "It is hard to let go and let someone help me, let alone ask for it."

MONEY. Because I was not working, and we had just moved into a new house, we were strapped—almost to the point of losing our house. Occasionally, someone would pay our electric bill or get some groceries or just give us money. But there were other weeks that we simply went without in order to pay the bills.

Carlyn, administrative assistant
Diagnosis of Hodgkin disease at age 30 in 2004 in Willow Spring, North Carolina

· · ·

HELP DOING CHORES that I was not able to do myself.

Marie, retired
Diagnosis of ovarian cancer at age 59 in 2004 in Lebanon, Ohio

· · ·

MONEY. I could not work anymore, and my partner was temporarily out of work. Can you imagine fighting to live and not knowing how to pay the rent?

Yvonne, paralegal
Diagnosis of colon cancer at age 48 in 2004 in San Antonio, Texas

AFTER IT WAS ALL OVER and I was through with the chemotherapy, [I wish] I had been able to talk to my husband and tell him what I needed from him, so that I could learn to accept my new body image and be able to renew our relationship (intimacy).

Debbie, hospice nurse
Diagnosis of breast cancer at age 52 in 2004 in Phoenix, Arizona

• • •

RIDES BACK AND FORTH to the doctor, tests, and treatments, so my husband did not have to take any more time from work.

Mariann, receptionist
Diagnosis of bladder cancer at age 50 in 2002 in West Haven, Connecticut

• • •

I FOUND IT REALLY hard to ask my husband to get up with me at night when I was pacing the floor because he had done so much. Or to call my girlfriend when the fears hit me during those episodes. They both had to get up in the mornings, and even though I couldn't sleep, I felt I shouldn't disrupt their sleep.

Fran, postmaster
Diagnosis of breast cancer at age 42 in 1999 in LaVergne, Tennessee

• • •

I FOUND IT VERY hard to ask for people to just come and visit.

Cheryl, homemaker
Diagnosis of breast cancer at age 49 in 2006 in Garland, Texas

• • •

PERMISSION TO FALL APART once or twice in those early days when I was so terrified. There is only my husband and me, and I could not do it with him here. After my diagnosis, he would not leave me out of his sight, so I cried only in the shower.

Judy, retired accounting clerk
Diagnosis of lung cancer at age 64 in 2004 in Norwalk, California

FOR PEOPLE TO SPEND time with me. Just sitting and holding my hand. Or watching a movie together. Or being by my side while I slept. It's easy to ask people to do specific, necessary tasks—please go shopping, please bring dinner, please do my laundry, please pick up the kids. I found it much harder (and still do) to ask people to just come and be with me. Human contact and connection are vitally important, as the cancer journey can be very lonely. Although friends were eager to perform chores, their lives were so busy, I felt uncomfortable asking them to forfeit two to three hours on a Sunday afternoon to just sit with me and keep me company and distract me.

> "Human contact and connection are vitally important, as the cancer journey can be very lonely."

Elena, arts administrator
Diagnosis of inflammatory breast cancer at age 44 in 1999 in Silver Spring, Maryland

• • •

I FOUND IT HARD to accept help and even harder to ask for it. I still find that difficult. I am a caretaker in every aspect of my life: wife, mother, nurse, and teacher. Never did I ever need to be cared for. It felt very humiliating to me. I had to learn (I'm still learning) that to accept help is to give a gift to the one helping. It feels really good to be the one who can help. It helps people to offer specific things, such as: "I am free tomorrow afternoon and would like to come over to clean your house" or "I am on my way to the grocery store; what do you need right now?" or "I just made soup and would like to bring it over." Those specific offers were easier for me than "I'm here, just ask." It's so hard to ask.

Sandra, assistant professor of nursing
Diagnosis of breast cancer at age 54 in 2002 in Atlanta, Georgia

• • •

TO BE LEFT ALONE.

Carrie, information management specialist
Diagnosis of breast cancer at age 44 in 2002 in New York City, New York

MOST TIMES, I WENT alone for my all-day treatment. It would have been nice to have company, but I found it hard to ask people. It was difficult because my close friends and other family members do not live nearby. My husband had to take care of getting the children off to school.

Midge, accountant
Diagnosis of non-Hodgkin lymphoma at age 52 in 2005 and breast cancer at age 54 in 2007 in Westford, Massachusetts

• • •

I WAS EMBARRASSED to ask for extra help with household chores, errands, and so forth. My husband did not help out much in that area and, although my in-laws offered many times, I didn't feel comfortable asking for their help.

Joyce, legal secretary
Diagnosis of breast cancer at age 44 in 2006 in South Amboy, New Jersey

Breast Cancer Foundation of the Ozarks provides short-term, nonmedical financial assistance to families dealing with breast cancer treatment. As a breast cancer survivor and a health care provider, I know that there are many resources within each community. When cancer is first diagnosed, everything seems overwhelming. At the time, you may not think about the things to which you have access. Area hospitals, local nonprofit organizations, friends, and families are wonderful contacts for direct access to helpful resources. Every way you can empower your healing process is important.

MARY BETH O'REILLY is a nurse and founder and chairperson of the Breast Cancer Foundation of the Ozarks in Missouri. She received a breast cancer diagnosis at age 51 in 1995.

I WISH I HAD ASKED for more help with grocery shopping, cleaning, clothes washing—all the household chores we take for granted.

Michele, administrative assistant
Diagnosis of breast cancer at age 45 in 1999 in Detroit, Michigan

• • •

ADMITTING TO OTHERS that I didn't feel well and that I needed more rest.

Angela, registered nurse
Diagnosis of brain cancer at age 32 in 1998 and cervical cancer in 2003 in Fulton, Mississippi

• • •

I WOULD HAVE GIVEN anything for someone to tell me they were scared, too, but I never got that. Everyone—and I do mean everyone—had the brave front with responses like, "You'll be fine," or "At least they caught it early," or "Oh, lots of people live just fine with one kidney," or "Well, at least you don't have to go through that horrible chemo." Damn it! All I wanted was someone to say, "I'm scared for you, too."

Kathie, nurse and social worker
Diagnosis of kidney cancer at age 53 in 2005 in Kingston, New York

• • •

A CONCRETE PLAN for therapy.

Mark, retired nuclear pharmacist
Diagnosis of chronic lymphocytic leukemia at age 59 in 2001 in Bay Shore, New York

• • •

I FOUND IT DIFFICULT to ask about my prognosis, but as the information slowly leaked out, I felt more in control, knowing the statistics.

Todd, oncology social worker
Diagnosis of chronic myelogenous leukemia at age 25 in 1997 and kidney cancer at age 33 in 2005 in Warwick, Rhode Island

PSYCHOLOGICAL HELP, I THINK. I had no idea I would feel so emotional, so heartbroken. But then again, nothing prepares you for breast cancer. So realistically, I could never have been prepared. Mums and teachers don't teach you about this one!

Pearl, nurse
Diagnosis of breast cancer at age 32 in 2004 in Glasgow (Scotland)

• • •

I THINK I ASKED for everything I could think of. It became one of those times when nothing was hard to ask for anymore. That, too, was a life lesson.

Cathi, clinical social worker
Diagnosis of breast cancer at age 52 in 2003 in Waban, Massachusetts

• • •

I WANTED MORE COMPANY. After awhile, people stopped calling because the shock and the newness wore off. There were times when I was sitting in the chemotherapy room for six hours by myself. (The nurses were wonderful!) There were also times when the dinners stopped coming, and the cards or phone calls stopped coming. That made me sad and lonely sometimes.

Shelly, program coordinator for adults with disabilities
Diagnosis of breast cancer at age 32 in 2004 in Concord, New Hampshire

• • •

MONEY. When I took advantage of the Family and Medical Leave Act, I could not work and began falling behind with my bills.

Jo Anne, nurse's aide
Diagnosis of breast cancer at age 51 in 2003 in Brownstown, Michigan

• • •

FOR MY HUSBAND to ensure that the children would leave me alone when I needed to take a shower or do something that required me to be alone.

Judi, nurse
Diagnosis of breast cancer at age 40 in 2000 in Pen Argyl, Pennsylvania

I COULD HAVE USED more help with household duties and children. I have a hard time asking for help and felt a little silly asking for help since I wasn't bedridden. (We could just eat more cold sandwiches for dinner.) I know people wouldn't have minded helping more, but for some reason, it was a little awkward asking for help.

> **Laura, stay-at-home mom**
> *Diagnosis of breast cancer at age 31 in 2006 in Hope Mills, North Carolina*

• • •

I COULD HAVE USED more mentoring from someone who had gone through the process.

> **Sheila, legal secretary**
> *Diagnosis of breast cancer at age 65 in 2006 in Walnut Creek, California*

• • •

IT WOULD HAVE HELPED to be able to call my husband (he's in prison), but that was impossible.

> **Alejandra, clerical worker**
> *Diagnosis of uterine cancer at age 36 in 2005 in Torrance, California*

• • •

"I needed more emotional support. I was never really prepared to encounter the enormous psychological battle that I faced."

I BECAME DEPRESSED after about four months. It would have been helpful to have a support group, with people who had gone through my same circumstances.

> **John, retired**
> *Diagnosis of esophageal cancer at age 76 in 2006 in Jamestown, North Carolina*

Treating cancer extends beyond just the physical aspects of the disease. Cancer's emotional impact may cause feelings of helplessness and hopelessness for the patient and family members. The financial burden is another problem and many people are faced with high costs and practical concerns, such as whether they can continue to work and who will take care of their family. In fact, a recent report by the Institute of Medicine recommends that as a standard part of their care, people with cancer should receive help with any psychological and social challenges they may be facing as a result of their diagnosis. Cancer patients should expect and receive systematic screening by their health care team, and be referred to needed psychosocial services, including the many free and low-cost services that are already available through professional and nonprofit organizations. No one with cancer need face his or her diagnosis alone, and supportive services help cancer patients overcome obstacles that have the potential to interfere with their treatment.

DIANE BLUM, MSW, is the executive director of CancerCare.

CHAPTER 13

• • •

How My Body and Intimacy Were Affected

During the 2006 National Breast Cancer Awareness Month, Geralyn Lucas, author of *Why I Wore Lipstick to My Mastectomy,* and I were on *ABC News NOW* on the same day. Though we weren't actually filmed together, we had the opportunity to meet and chat before the interviews. I told Geralyn one of the things that most impressed me from her memoir was her description of how she resumed intimacy with her husband just days after having a mastectomy. Here is the excerpt from her book:

> I put on some perfume. And I line my lips with lipstick. I can't even feel Tyler's hand when he puts it on the bright red diagonal scar across my chest. In fact, I have been walking into strangers with my reconstructed right boob because I cannot feel where it starts.
>
> But the great thing about sex is that it's like riding a bicycle. I know that Tyler still loves me—my laugh, our conversations—but will he still be turned on? Yes, yes, and definitely yes. I cannot believe that Tyler wants me so much. The way he is kissing me and touching me, I know that it's not my hair or my boob that ever made him fall in love with me. It was my mojo. It was always there, just waiting for me to meet it.
>
> After Tyler and I have sex again I feel so hot that I still can't get that Shania Twain song out of my head: *Man, I Feel Like a Woman!* (Lucas 2004, 93–94).

Later, this exact scene was reproduced by actress Sarah Chalke of *Scrubs* fame, who portrayed Geralyn, the then twenty-seven-year-old successful television producer, in the CBS movie version of her memoir. Though I know that many, perhaps most, women would not want to resume sexual relations this quickly after a mastectomy, I've often thought about how meaningful it must have been to Geralyn to have her husband immediately welcome her back into his embrace.

At the time we met, Geralyn's memoir had recently been published in a French version. She had a copy with her and showed me the cover. While the American version shows Geralyn in a flashy pink tank top with red lipstick, the French version has her discretely nude from the waist up. Her arms are crossed over her chest, partially hiding her breasts (one now reconstructed). Geralyn is a gorgeous woman, largely because of her personality, but also her physical appearance. Though she is small in stature, her presence envelops you and her energy is contagious. Whenever I think of Geralyn, I think of her unbridled energy that is so attractive.

For this chapter, I asked survey participants to respond to two questions:
1. *Did cancer/cancer treatment have an impact on your sexuality? If yes, how?*
2. *Did cancer/cancer treatment affect the way you feel about your body? If yes, please explain.*

As with all of the questions on the survey, survivors could choose to respond or not. A few people left one or both of these questions blank; however, many people answered both questions. It's interesting to see glimpses of the survey participants' personalities in these responses. As you read them, you'll find a mix of emotions and human characteristics—humor, pain, resilience, sadness, anxiety and, of course, love. You'll also find what Geralyn would call "mojo." Some people's mojo really came through in their responses.

Many survivors struggle with the issues of body image and when/how/-whether to resume physical intimacy. For those who are struggling now, it's worthwhile to note that time really does help when dealing with these issues. Barbara, whose breast cancer was diagnosed in 1986 when she was thirty-eight, perhaps best summed up this sentiment when she wrote, "I find as I get older that I am much more able to appreciate the 'story' that my body tells and am less and less concerned with the physical appearance."

Everyone who's been through cancer has a story, and the changes to each person's body are part of that tale. Read on to learn what survivors wanted to share with you from their story.

• • •

OUR MARRIAGE HAS GROWN even closer. After my first cancer treatment was over, my husband told me that he never knew before that I really needed him. I was always so self-reliant and "together." While I was in chemotherapy and receiving radiation, I needed his help and support daily. It was a real gift to him to feel needed.

Sandra, assistant professor of nursing
Diagnosis of breast cancer at age 54 in 2002 in Atlanta, Georgia

• • •

AT FIRST, CANCER IMPACTED my sexuality, but that was part of the emotional healing.

Angie, volunteer and cancer advocate
Diagnosis of vulvar cancer at age 31 in 1998 and breast cancer at age 36 in 2003 in Anderson, South Carolina

• • •

WITH TESTICULAR CANCER, it took me at least six to eight weeks before I could feel comfortable performing. Since then, it has not been an issue.

Federico, cancer chemical biologist
Diagnosis of testicular cancer at age 32 in 2006 in Brookline, Massachusetts

• • •

I WAS EMBARRASSED about my scars at first, but my husband helped me work through that, and now it is like they are not even there. The bald head was an issue in the beginning, too, but now I seem to forget about it. My husband tells me it looks sexy.

Cathy, retail district manager
Diagnosis of pancreatic cancer at age 45 in 2005 in Columbus, Ohio

"Our marriage has grown even closer. After my first cancer treatment was over, my husband told me that he never knew before that I really needed him."

> "I was embarrassed about my scars at first, but my husband helped me work through that and now it is like they are not even there."

I HATE TO CHANGE my clothes in the locker room at the gym.

Ann, homemaker
Diagnosis of breast cancer at age 47 in 2003 in Mechanicsburg, Pennsylvania

• • •

ABSOLUTELY, MY CANCER and treatment have had an effect on my sexuality. The most immediate impact comes from periods of pain and not feeling well enough to give a damn about that aspect of life. Then, you have fears and concerns over your appeal to your partner. Whether from the scars or weight changes or being bald or emotional issues, there is a lot to deal with that impacts your self-esteem, and you feel there is no way it could not have the same effects on your partner. The changes are real. It takes a lot to get past "poor me" and communicate with yourself on an intelligent level. Then, it takes even more effort to communicate with your partner. Closeness is critical in such trying times. It's good to find ways to communicate when it's time to be held and reassured as a person or when it's time to be intimate and how to make that happen in a comfortable, satisfying way for both of you.

Beth, massage therapist
Diagnosis of breast cancer at age 39 in 2006 in Tempe, Arizona

• • •

THE CHEMO PUT ME into [early] menopause, which has created a series of sexual ups and downs.

Joyce, legal secretary
Diagnosis of breast cancer at age 44 in 2006 in South Amboy, New Jersey

IN THE BEGINNING, I thought people would care about my baldness, scars, etc. I had been dating a guy for nine months and when I received my cancer diagnosis, he dropped me like a hot potato. I called him after about a year and said, "You didn't even call to see if I was dead or alive." He replied, "I'm a coward." There were a few of those out there but, for the most part, men didn't care if I was bald or scarred. So once I realized it was not an issue for anyone I cared about, that was a good thing. It was [a source of] worry for me for a very short time. Now, I feel great about myself and have a wonderful boyfriend.

Myra, service representative, internal technical support
Diagnosis of breast cancer at age 52 in 2003 in Sharon, Massachusetts

• • •

DIVORCING MY HUSBAND HELPED me heal the most after I finished cancer treatment. Now [that I am] divorced with one breast, sex is not an issue. The issue is when to tell a potential sexual partner about my mastectomy.

Linda, patient advocate
Diagnosis of breast cancer at age 47 in 1998 in Selden, New York

• • •

IT IS STILL VERY hard for me to see myself as anything but "damaged". [The cancer] has really impacted my sense of femininity. I see my body as something to contend with, something not to be trusted. This makes intimacy hard. It's as if my body has betrayed me.

Jaime, graduate student
Diagnosis of cervical cancer at age 24 in 2005 in Blackwood, New Jersey

• • •

I COULD HAVE SAT around and felt sorry for myself because my belly looks like a road map and now I'm a little lopsided because of the surgical procedures. But instead, I got my belly button pierced at the age of forty-two. Why not? I don't have any feeling in my belly. My hubby thought it was sexy, and my kids thought it was cool. My mother thought I had lost it.

Kimatha, medical laboratory technician
Diagnosis of kidney cancer at age 42 in 2001 in Edinburgh, Indiana

I THOUGHT, "IT MIGHT be the last time, so let's try."

Kenneth, career transition teacher to Navy retirees
Diagnosis of kidney cancer at age 64 in 1999 in San Diego, California

• • •

BLOOD PRESSURE MEDS and fatigue have had a large effect on me.

Kyle, pastor
Diagnosis of kidney cancer at age 60 in 2004 in Johnstown, Pennsylvania

• • •

DURING TREATMENT, IT SUFFERED because I was too sick and tired to want to be intimate. But once I was through chemo, it returned to normal...maybe better [than normal] because we don't take it or each other for granted.

Sherri, elementary school teacher
Diagnosis of endometrial (uterine) cancer at age 42 in 2004 in Bruceville, Indiana

• • •

DURING MY TREATMENT, I had no energy or desire. I expended the little I had on work and children. My husband was very supportive, and we got back on track once the treatments were over.

Midge, accountant
Diagnosis of non-Hodgkin lymphoma at age 52 in 2005 and breast cancer at age 54 in 2007 in Westford, Massachusetts

• • •

I LOST THIRTY POUNDS from the chemo and have not put a pound back on. I have a poor self-image at this point, and that hasn't really changed, even with the weight loss. I feel deformed to a degree but it is okay—we never had much of a sex life before, and it is even less now.

Jennifer, psychotherapist
Diagnosis of breast cancer at age 39 in 2004 in Pennington, New Jersey

HUGE IMPACT. I LOST my libido halfway through chemo and haven't really regained it. I just feel physically disinterested in sex, although before breast cancer, we had a good sex life. I feel sad that I am missing out on some great years of my life sexually—like I've lost the fun, sexy, and vivacious me I once was. I feel a bit like a freak with my strange-looking, fake breast. I feel as though no one other than my husband would ever find me attractive sexually.

Pearl, nurse
Diagnosis of breast cancer at age 32 in 2004 in Glasgow (Scotland)

Cancer and its treatment inevitably affect body image and sexuality. Whether a couple is eventually brought closer, an individual learns to accept a different body, or damage to sexual freedom and joy seem permanent, every cancer patient (and partner) must deal with change. As always, honest communication, mutual respect, and genuine love make it more likely to achieve a positive adaptation. Sometimes, unfortunately, even in the best of relationships, physical intimacy never fully recovers. In already-troubled relationships, it is even more difficult to adjust and accept new physical realities. Often, the saving grace is a renewed appreciation for life that almost every cancer survivor experiences. Yes, sex is important, but being alive to love, to laugh, to grow into a richer, deeper, more thoughtful life is more important. Maturity and perspective always help.

HESTER HILL SCHNIPPER is a clinical social worker and chief of Oncology Social Work at the Beth Israel Deaconess Medical Center in Boston, Massachusetts. She is also a two-time breast cancer survivor and author of the book *After Breast Cancer: A Common-Sense Guide to Life After Treatment.*

> ## "I feel sad that I am missing out on some great years of my life sexually..."

I AM NOT HAPPY about the way my swollen lymph nodes give me a gut that makes me appear very overweight when, in fact, I am only slightly overweight. There are unsightly red blotches on my hands and arms caused by the steroids I'm taking. But above all, I feel that my body has let me down by getting CLL, and I am now constantly on the alert for complications and ailments that may be brought on by the disease. My testosterone has dropped dramatically since I have had CLL, but I am reluctant to pump it up with injections. Whereas we used to make love at least twice a week, it is now once every seven to ten days.

Colin, writer and author
Diagnosis of chronic lymphocytic leukemia at age 62 in 1998 in Roma (Italy)

• • •

AT FIRST IT DID [affect my sexuality] because the way my CML was diagnosed was that I presented in the emergency room with priapism (a sustained erection). I required a shunt for that, and it was unknown whether I would permanently lose functionality. For a while following that procedure, I was unable to obtain an erection, but that was really the least of my worries at the time. I was very relieved when I learned it was not permanent.

Todd, oncology social worker
Diagnosis of chronic myelogenous leukemia at age 25 in 1997 and kidney cancer in 2005 at age 33 in Warwick, Rhode Island

• • •

I USED TO BE pretty laid back and not too worried about makeup, clothes, and hair, but now I feel that since I have a new breast that cost more than my two cars, I should try to look a little better. Plus, I have a thing about not wanting people to feel sorry for me. So if I look good, they won't tend to feel sorry for me.

Peggy, pathologist's assistant
Diagnosis of breast cancer at age 47 in 2003 in St. Augustine, Florida

DURING THE YEAR or so after the bone marrow transplant, it was not so great, but it's better now.

Matt, carpenter
Diagnosis of chronic lymphocytic leukemia at age 51 in 2003 in Bath, New York

• • •

I WENT THROUGH MENOPAUSE, and my libido has dipped; I have vaginal dryness. That's probably more related to menopause than to the medications, but I guess they contribute, too. That's really no fun. I think I love my body more now, because it's mine and I'm still here. My breast is a little lumpy, but it's still here, too. I am in better shape than I was before, I like my body more, and I have learned how precious it is.

> # "I love my body more now, because it's mine and I'm still here."

Cathi, clinical social worker
Diagnosis of breast cancer at age 52 in 2003 in Waban, Massachusetts

• • •

MY HUSBAND had a difficult time since he's the type who could "fix" anything and found there was nothing for him to do here. I felt protective of him and tried to spare him what I was actually going through. He seemed to "need" me more. Looking back, I believe that was because he thought I might die. We were separated in 1999, then divorced, but we have remained friends. I believe the two of us were probably in denial during that time. Four years ago, I began seeing a man I had known for many years who lives in Tennessee. He has gone through this second round of cancer with me, albeit sometimes from a distance, and he has made me feel just as sexy with no breasts (I also had a simple mastectomy on the right side) as I felt with two. I'm definitely sad that I no longer have breasts, but I'm also realistic. I can live without my breasts, but I could not have lived with the cancer that had grown in them. For years, my sister has said that "life's a trade," and that has become my mantra.

Lindy, hospice volunteer
Diagnosis of breast cancer at age 35 in 1984 and radiation-induced sarcoma at age 55 in 2004 in Lexington, Massachusetts

WHILE IT IS UNFORTUNATE, it is true that society puts a great deal of focus on women's breasts. Consequently, when a woman has a diagnosis of breast cancer and loses one or both of her breasts, it forces her to look at her body in a different way. I had a reconstruction with an implant, so with clothes on my breasts look "normal" and you cannot tell that I had a breast removed. However, the long scar from my underarm to the middle of my chest tells otherwise. I am self-conscious about the way my reconstructed breast looks when I am naked or in a bathing suit, but I am thankful that I have made it seven years cancer free, so I try to keep things in perspective. When I was in treatment, I went into chemo-induced menopause. It was difficult to deal with the effects from that, such as vaginal dryness, but we found ways to make things work easier and different ways to work around any obstacles and please each other. My husband was very understanding and made a point to do things to make me feel attractive and sexy, so that helped immensely. Physically, I struggled with the way my scar and my reconstructed breast looked, and I still do sometimes. But my husband isn't bothered by any of it, so that helps a great deal.

Sarah, paralegal
Diagnosis of breast cancer at age 28 in 2000 in Miami, Florida

• • •

MY HUSBAND'S POSITIVE OUTLOOK. We were in it together, no matter what. He married me for my heart and for love—not my body.

Bernadette, cardiovascular technician
Diagnosis of breast cancer at age 48 in 2001 in Oxnard, California

• • •

UNFORTUNATELY, I WASN'T SEXUALLY active right before, and I haven't had the chance to be after. I do have a special person [in my life], but I haven't got to the point of allowing him to see what I look like with a lopsided breast. It's scary to think about when it will happen. One small thing that always was an issue before was my hair. I kept the same hairstyle for thirty years. But after chemo and losing my hair, I discovered that it grows! So now I experiment and have fun...it's a small thing, but also a big mind change.

Linda, retired
Diagnosis of breast cancer at age 54 in 2003 in Placentia, California

HELL NO! LOL! I am aware of my big scar...but I am not ashamed of it. If a man can't handle seeing it and understanding the reasons why it's there, then he will never be able to have a relationship with me.

Evelyn, executive assistant
Diagnosis of colon cancer at age 33 in 2004 in Boston, Massachusetts.

> ## "We were in it together, no matter what."

• • •

MY INTEREST IN SEX has never waned; however, my erections have not been as strong, reliable, or long-lasting as before, which has been embarrassing to me and caused me not to initiate sex very often. Further, for several months I had an ileostomy bag and dressings over several surgical incisions across my stomach. As a result, my wife and I have only had sexual intercourse a few times during my hospitalization and my entire nineteen months of chemotherapy, a fact that hasn't particularly bothered me and has not seemed to bother her either. It's just an effect that "came with the territory." But now that my treatments have ended, my ileostomy bag and dressings have been removed, and I've regained my health and vitality, our mutual enjoyment of sex is returning and becoming more frequent again.

Mike, retired real estate developer and cattle rancher
Diagnosis of colon cancer at age 66 in 2006 in Red Lodge, Montana

• • •

I HAD A FEEDING tube for about seven months, so I had no interest in sex.

Julie, account executive in advertising/marketing
Diagnosis of laryngeal cancer at age 46 in 2002 in New York City, New York

• • •

I AM ONE SCAR—from left to right and right to left. I don't like to look at that, as it reminds me of the three surgical procedures. My right side is still swollen (it always will be), so I look funny when I wear a belt. But hey, at least I am here.

Beth, health educator
Diagnosis of liver cancer at age 32 in 1990 in Fort Hood, Texas

I HAVE SURGERY SCARS, but I consider them battle scars.

Eileen, teacher
Diagnosis of breast cancer at age 43 in 2006 in Hilton, New York

• • •

I'M NOT ABLE to have children at this point, so that definitely impacts my feelings about relationships. I believe that most men are interested in having a family and, since that is not an option for me, I feel it's not fair of me to get too involved in a relationship. I realize adoption is an option, but I also realize that four cancer recurrences over fifteen years may prevent me from seeing children reach adulthood, and so I don't think it's fair to adopt a child and not be able to see him or her grow up. In our society, I think you're expected to get married and have kids. Because I don't see this as an option for me, I do feel a little like an "outcast" from that perspective.

Andrea, hospital administrator
Diagnosis of Ewing's sarcoma (a form of bone cancer) at age 15 in 1992 in Norfolk, Massachusetts

• • •

WHAT WAS AMAZING was that at this exact time of my life, my husband to whom I have been married for twenty-two years, came to me and told me he was having an affair. My life was turned upside down. He left for awhile. My time alone was therapeutic; I journaled all that I was feeling. I had to put the situation with my husband on the back burner and take care of my health. I stayed as focused as possible on my health. The affair he had seemed minute.

Laura, housecleaner
Diagnosis of esophageal cancer at age 45 in 2002 in Schenectady, New York

• • •

I HAVEN'T HAD SEX for about fifteen years, and it doesn't bother me in the slightest.

Elizabeth, retired administrator
Diagnosis of breast cancer at age 58 in 2003 in Plymouth, Devon (England)

I TRIED TO LOOK good every day...bought cute wigs and wore more makeup than usual.

Debra, administrative assistant
Diagnosis of ovarian cancer at age 51 in 2007 in Chicago, Illinois

• • •

MY HUSBAND HELPED ME the most. He loved me, and has told me and showed me that he loves me, whether I'm bald or I have a misshapen breast or no breasts. No matter what, he loves me and desires me as a woman, as his wife. He went with me to every appointment, every test, every surgical procedure, every treatment—and he still does. He listened to my every fear and kept me grounded. He helped me sort out treatment options and was my sounding board as I made hard decisions. As much as possible, he truly shared the cancer experience with me, and I was never alone.

Kathi, retired special education teacher
Diagnosis of breast cancer at age 49 in 2003 in Wrightstown, Wisconsin

• • •

I DON'T TRUST my body. I am afraid of what it will do next. I've just gone through my third cancer diagnosis, I know it will develop again. I just don't know when or where. I have dozens of scars, but they don't bother me. They remind me of my strength.

Pamela, bookkeeper
Diagnosis of Hodgkin disease age 23 in 1983 and basal cell carcinoma (skin cancer) at age 41 in 2001 and breast cancer at age 46 in 2006 in Gardiner, Maine

• • •

WE WERE TOLD that I was sterile because of treatment. If we had known that wasn't true, we would have used protection and probably wouldn't have our second son now.

Nicki, homemaker
Diagnosis of thyroid cancer at age 20 in 2005 in Union, Missouri

> ## "I have dozens of scars, but they don't bother me. They remind me of my strength."

ONE OF MY NURSES urged me to go to Merle Norman Cosmetics for a complete makeover—to help me feel attractive. I was fortunate that there was a studio not far from my house. The owner was very compassionate and spent a great deal of time helping me learn which makeup would help my skin (which was very dry and flaky from all of the radiation) and how to look good without people knowing I was wearing makeup. I still go to Merle Norman today, and they have added wigs [to their product line] for folks losing their hair from the effects of chemo. The company actively works with the Reach to Recovery® program. It is a place where I always feel welcomed and accepted.

Eileen, technology specialist
Diagnosis of breast cancer at age 34 in 1984 and acute myelogenous leukemia at age 49 in 1999 and basal cell carcinoma (skin cancer) at age 55 in 2005 in Framingham, Massachusetts

• • •

I AM STERILE for one thing. Also, I believe my sex drive has diminished sooner than most people my age...but it's not gone!

Randy, respiratory therapist
Diagnosis of Hodgkin disease at age 6 in 1965 in Ewa Beach, Hawaii

• • •

I AM STILL HEALING from surgery, but I can tell you I will love the person I am, inside and out. I have let my weight come between my husband and my sex life, but it won't anymore. I am thankful to be here and thankful to have a husband who loves me for me. All of me! I will love my body more. I want to treat it better as it's giving me another chance at life. I want to give it the same chance in return.

Rochelle, manicurist
Diagnosis of melanoma (skin cancer) at age 34 in 2007 in Las Vegas, Nevada

I THINK BREAST RECONSTRUCTION helped me personally with my own sexual identity.

Charose, nurse
Diagnosis of Hodgkin disease at age 17 in 1972 and breast cancer at age 51 in 2006 in Omaha, Nebraska.

Address the issues that undermine your confidence. If you suffer from hair loss or eyebrow loss, for example, find out how to remedy these temporary problems. Counteracting the physical side effects of treatment will vastly improve your mindset and overall well-being.

RAMY GAFNI is a celebrity makeup artist and the creator of RAMY Beauty Therapy cosmetics. He is the author of *Ramy Gafni's Beauty Therapy: The Ultimate Guide to Looking and Feeling Great While Living with Cancer.*

I HAD A LOT of fun with my breast prosthesis, removing it and showing it to those interested. Children were particularly fascinated with it. My prosthesis started many conversations, which probably would have never occurred without "the boob."

Ruthanne, bookkeeper
Diagnosis of breast cancer at age 51 in 1995 in Thorne Bay, Alaska

• • •

BECAUSE I HAD SURGERY on my leg to remove a bone tumor, I have a big scar on my leg and my ankle is also unaligned so that I cannot wear sandals. This means that I am unable to achieve the "woman look" I want, but I've learned to adapt and make the best of a bad situation.

Cheryl, billings account clerk
Diagnosis of Ewing's sarcoma (bone cancer) at age 21 in 1987 in Malden, Massachusetts

I HAD BEEN A WIDOW for five years when I was diagnosed. But even though I am seventy-seven now, I still miss sex and my fantastic man.

Pat, retired
Diagnosis of colon and bladder cancer at age 74 in 2005 in Como (Western Australia)

• • •

I MARRIED MY BOYFRIEND.

Sheri, actress
Diagnosis of Hodgkin disease at age 29 in 1993 in Columbia, Maryland

• • •

> "I will love my body more. I want to treat it better as it's giving me another chance at life."

OF COURSE, THE CHEMO treatments are very intense, but intimacy all falls back into place.

Roxanne, disabled
Diagnosis of mantle cell lymphoma at age 48 in 2003 in Palm Beach Gardens, Florida

• • •

I GREATLY DISLIKED HAVING a port. It rubbed against my children's heads when they hugged me and against my bra straps. When I undressed, it was a definite reminder that I was sick and in treatment.

Janet, elementary school teacher
Diagnosis of colon cancer at age 42 in 1993 in Philadelphia, Pennsylvania

• • •

WHEN I LOST MY HAIR and had to wear a wig, I found a new hairstyle that I like, and I will probably use that style when my hair grows back. For the moment, I never have a "bad hair day."

Nancy, administrative assistant
Diagnosis of breast cancer at age 54 in 2006 in Fowlerville, Michigan

I NO LONGER AM CONSUMED about gaining a few pounds. Any weight is better than the eighty-six pounds my treatment took me to.

Danielle, financial service specialist
Diagnosis of melanoma (skin cancer) at age 30 in 2000 in Ramstein (Germany)

• • •

AFTER SURGERY on my tongue, I was badly scarred on my neck, left arm, and both upper legs (skin grafts). So, for a very long time, I was self-conscious about how I looked. However, it has been five years since that surgery and I no longer am concerned about my scars.

Bryna, management development consultant
Diagnosis of tongue cancer at age 35 in 1985 in Brockton, Massachusetts

• • •

I WAS SHOCKED to find myself crying the first time I shopped for new bras after surgery. Now I feel comfortable with my body again. It really just took time to get used to the change.

Barbara, nurse
Diagnosis of breast cancer at age 58 in 1995 in Stoneham, Massachusetts

• • •

I RECEIVED MY BREAST cancer diagnosis after fifteen months of marriage. I never asked, "Why me?" I only asked "Why now?" I wish I had known how it would affect my marriage. I wish I had known what a struggle it was going to be. We took separate paths to get through the grieving process and lost touch with "us." Now the road back is a struggle.

Debbie, hospice nurse
Diagnosis of breast cancer at age 52 in 2004 in Phoenix, Arizona

• • •

MY HUSBAND STILL THINKS I'm sexy, so that's all that really matters, right?

Laura, unemployed psychiatric social worker
Diagnosis of breast cancer at age 43 in 2006 in Avon, Connecticut

I know now that the cancer experience can take a huge toll on a relationship, especially a new relationship. I am alive today in large part because of the unabating love and support of my then fiancée, Cecilia. Without her daily visits, home cooked meals brought to my bedside, and around-the-clock attention to my care whether I was in or out of the hospital, I would never have survived treatment.

We were married shortly after my successful blood stem cell transplant for acute leukemia but, unfortunately, the cancer experience changed the nature of our relationship. The realization of my tenuous mortality caused me to fear that I might never achieve my remaining life goals. So, as painful as it is for me to admit, I became even more focused, intense, and driven than I had been before my illness. I would often lose my temper over even the smallest things. This caused her to become more distant.

If I had known that my reaction to cancer would play such a significant, albeit not exclusive, role in the dissolution of my marriage, I would have tried to lighten my approach to life rather than darken it. Unfortunately, as the saying goes: "Life can be understood backwards, but it must be lived forwards." So, I take forward with me the gratitude for being alive, the thanks that she was there for me when I most needed her, and the lessons that I have learned about myself because of her departure from our marriage. I choose to focus on the priceless gift of life I have been given rather than the equally priceless gift of love that I have lost. Nothing in life is free. I have paid that price, but gained equally priceless new perspectives in the process. The end result is that cancer has made me a better, wiser, more compassionate and humble man.

ALAN HOBSON is a Mount Everest climber, summiteer, and leukemia survivor. He received a diagnosis of leukemia at age 42 in 2000 in Calgary, Alberta (Canada). Alan is the co-author of the book *Climb Back from Cancer*, which he wrote with his now ex-wife.

AFTER MY MASTECTOMY, it was difficult to feel feminine again. But my husband was so great through all of it, and he still is. Now, I'm forty-four years old, and we are trying to have a baby. It has made us closer than ever.

Karen, real estate broker
Diagnosis of breast cancer at age 38 in 2001 in Loganville, Georgia

• • •

I BELIEVE THE SCAR I carry from where my right lung was partially removed is a testament to the triumph of medicine and my stubborn insistence on living. I don't feel a bit worse off for the cancer.

Judy, retired accounting clerk
Diagnosis of lung cancer at age 64 in 2004 in Norwalk, California

• • •

I DIDN'T REALIZE how badly my self-esteem would be shaken. One-breasted, bald, with no eyelashes or eyebrows, and a twenty-pound weight gain from chemo made it difficult for me to look in the mirror. My fiancé called me every day (we lived four hours apart), even if I only spoke ten words after chemo. He's stood by my side and still tells me I'm beautiful. Today, he is my husband. He loved me unconditionally, which helped so much.

Linda, purchasing agent
Diagnosis of breast cancer at age 47 in 2007 in Antioch, California

> "I have learned to deal with the fact that I might be unhappy with the way I look, but at least I'm alive."

THE EFFECTS OF BREAST cancer and treatment on body image are awful. We're not back to where we need to be in our sexual relationship because of so many factors—fatigue, sadness, pain, fear. This is going to require some continued attention. For the first time after my bilateral mastectomy, I was in a public locker room and took off my shirt. Two young girls nearby shrieked and ran to their mom; of course, she was terribly embarrassed. I'd forgotten how horrible I looked. When I rejoined my husband, all I could say was how very, very grateful I was that no matter what he was thinking when he looked at me, I never saw anything on his face like [the shock] I saw in those children. We're moving forward from there.

Deborah, physician
Diagnosis of breast cancer at age 47 in 2007 in Overland Park, Kansas

• • •

I CAN'T TAN ANYMORE, so obviously I don't feel as pretty at times because I felt my best when I was tanned. I have learned to deal with the fact that I might be unhappy with the way I look, but at least I'm alive. If I meet someone who really cares whether I'm tanned, then he is probably not worth knowing at all.

Jennifer, publicity coordinator
Diagnosis of melanoma (skin cancer) at age 21 in 2004 in San Diego, California

• • •

I FEEL MORE COMFORTABLE in my body now. I have very pale skin and was always ridiculed growing up because I was so white. Now, if anyone were to make fun of me, I would explain what happened to me and why I don't care about being so white. "Pale is the new tan."

Mary Anne, word processor
Diagnosis of melanoma (skin cancer) at age 26 in 2007 in Dixon, California

MY NECK AND JAW are scarred from radiation and several incisions. I also had one third of my tongue removed. My speech [ability] is poor, and my voice is hoarse as well. So definitely, this has an impact on my sexuality. Actually, there is the good and bad with this. I am two hundred fifty pounds lighter than I used to be, so I feel a lot better about my body in that respect.

Kathy, babysitter
Diagnosis of tongue cancer at age 38 in 1997 in Niles, Illinois

• • •

I COULD HAVE USED frank discussions about resuming sexual relations after the hysterectomy. I still could. But I am totally psyched not to have my period anymore.

Jennifer, federal officer with U.S. Customs and Border Patrol
Diagnosis of cervical cancer at age 36 in 2007 in Montreal, Quebec (Canada)

• • •

IT'S AMAZING HOW UNSEXY having a bald head can make you feel. My husband did his best to make me feel sexy, but I did not. He was constantly telling me how beautiful I looked and how much he loved me. It was hard to let it sink in. It was hard for me to look in the mirror at times. The scar where I had a port bothers me mentally. I am slowly trying to look at it as a trophy, but I have a long way to go down that road!

Carlyn, administrative assistant
Diagnosis of Hodgkin disease at age 30 in 2004 in Willow Spring, North Carolina

• • •

I HAD ALWAYS STRUGGLED with self-image. Even though I'm tall and thin, I always felt my breasts were too small, so having scars and misshapen breasts was difficult. I really struggled with feeling sorry for my husband about having to make love to a deformed, bald woman. But he was very loving, and we talked about it and prayed about it. Gradually, I've come to really believe and see my scars as beautiful reminders that I am still here. That's pretty sexy!

Laura, stay-at-home mom
Diagnosis of breast cancer at age 31 in 2006 in Hope Mills, North Carolina

> **"I've come to…see my scars as beautiful reminders that I am still here."**

I JUST HAD MY radiation treatments, so no sex for a couple of weeks. My husband is very understanding. We'll see how my body reacts.

Candy, teacher
Diagnosis of thyroid cancer at age 31 in 2007 in El Paso, Texas

• • •

I WAS SOMEWHAT OVERWEIGHT, and radiation caused me to lose fifty pounds. Now, I am back to my best weight—the same as when I got married fifty years ago.

Sigrid, registered nurse
Diagnosis of endometrial (uterine) cancer at age 72 in 2006 in Oceanside, California

A little secret my husband and I share is that we actually enjoyed my time with breast cancer treatment because it was the first time in our adult lives (especially since becoming parents) that we stopped long enough to talk to each other and spend a little down time together. We talked and talked during the chemo sessions and enjoyed each other tremendously.

HALA MODDELMOG is a breast cancer survivor and the president and CEO of Susan G. Komen for the Cure.

Reference
Lucas G. 2004. *Why I wore lipstick to my mastectomy*. New York: St. Martin's Press.

5 Things

People Should Tell a Partner Who Has Cancer

1. **I love you and we'll get through this together.** Women (and men) need a lot of reassurance from their partners during this time. Tell your partner every day that you love her and that you are there for her.

2. **Your body is beautiful, no matter what.** Cancer takes a toll on how survivors feel about their bodies. Women tend to be particularly hard on themselves about their physical appearance—even before a cancer diagnosis. After surgery and other treatments, they worry about being unattractive. Reassure the woman (or man) you love over and over. It goes a long way.

3. **I find you sexually attractive.** It's not enough just to tell your partner you find her attractive. It's important to reinforce that you desire her and want to continue to be physically intimate. It's difficult for couples to maintain intimacy when one feels uncomfortable for any reason. Let your partner know that this is an important part of your relationship and that you still find her sexually attractive and desirable. If you are a woman whose male partner is going through cancer, you may be the one who encourages intimacy. Perhaps this wasn't the case in the past, but things can change and so can people. Try it out and see what happens.

4. **I'll help you in any way that I can—now and in the future.** Some people can't handle the news that their partner has been given a cancer diagnosis, especially if the relationship was not solid to begin with. Many women, in particular, fear being left, either now or in the future. If you are the kind of guy who's going to stay, tell her so— even if you think she knows it already.

5. **You are still the same person I fell in love with.** A cancer diagnosis can be overwhelming, and sometimes people feel as though the disease defines them. It's important to put cancer in perspective as a medical condition and an experience that a survivor may have. Tell your partner all the reasons why you fell in love with her, and remind her that she is still that same smart, funny, kind (or whatever) person.

Questions about Intimacy and Infertility to Ask Your Doctor

For Women

✓ Will cancer treatment leave me with a temporary or permanent loss of sensation? If so, what can I expect from this?

✓ Will I experience painful intercourse (due to reduced vaginal lubrication or changes in the genital tissue)? If so, what can I do about this?

✓ Will I undergo premature menopause? If so, how can I treat the symptoms of this?

For Men

✓ Will I have less feeling in my genitals? If so, how will this affect me?

✓ Will I be left impotent or have difficulty maintaining an erection or ejaculating? If so, what can I do about this?

For Men and Women of Childbearing Age

✓ How will my cancer or the treatment affect my fertility?

✓ Can I freeze my sperm or eggs?

✓ What are my options for having children after treatment?

For Everyone

✓ When can I safely resume sexual activity?

✓ Will I experience less sexual desire (decreased libido)?

✓ Will I experience less physical pleasure with intimacy and sexual intercourse?

✓ Are there any special precautions that I should take?

✓ Are any of the medications (or other treatments) I am currently taking affecting me emotionally or physically with regard to intimacy?

✓ Are my issues with intimacy going to be permanent?

✓ Can you offer me suggestions (e.g., creams, devices, medications, etc.) on how to improve my ability to be physically intimate?

✓ Can you refer me to a professional who specializes in the type of intimacy issues that I am dealing with?

Reprinted with permission from After Cancer Treatment: Heal Faster, Better, Stronger *(Johns Hopkins University Press, 2006) by Julie K. Silver, MD.*

Improving Emotional Intimacy

- Set aside time to have a conversation about issues you have been avoiding or that are emotionally charged. During this "date," be encouraging to your partner and listen to him or her at least as much as you talk. Sharing your feelings is a great way to build emotional intimacy.

- Do something together that doesn't involve a lot of verbal communication. Go to a movie or a concert.

- Take time to enjoy nature together. Have a picnic, take an outdoor hike, or go for a walk or bike ride.

- Join something together such as a cooking or foreign language class.

- Go out for a non-alcoholic drink at your favorite coffee shop.

- Plan a romantic dinner at a local restaurant.

- Read to each other.

- Do a crossword puzzle together or play a board game.

Reprinted with permission from After Cancer Treatment: Heal Faster, Better, Stronger *(Johns Hopkins University Press, 2006) by Julie K. Silver, MD.*

CHAPTER 14

• • •

What Helped Me Heal

After a speech I gave at a breast cancer conference, a woman came up to me and said, "It's been six weeks since I finished radiation, and I'm not yet back to my normal energy level. My husband thinks everything is fine, but I'm upset about this." She said she felt as though she was getting more support from a close girlfriend than from her husband whom she thought just didn't "get it."

I'm sharing this story for two important reasons. First, it can take months, even years, to heal as optimally as possible after cancer treatment. Six weeks is not enough time for your body to heal when it has been exposed to toxic therapies. Second, loved ones are so incredibly invested in a survivor's well-being that husbands or wives, for example, may seem like they are not "getting it" when actually, they just want the person they love to be okay. Compounded with this intense desire to see a loved one improve quickly is the fact that it's often not easy for others to see how difficult it really is for their loved one to recover from cancer and its treatments. Survivors may look healthy to friends and family but, in reality, may be struggling with lingering after-effects.

While I was writing this book, my youngest daughter wanted to do something to help someone far away. So our family signed up to become "angels" who would support a soldier who was deployed away from home. We were assigned a man named Charles who had just left for Afghanistan. We didn't know anything about him, and, of course, he didn't know us. However, through correspondence (mostly letters and e-mails), we found out that he's been in the military his entire career, worked in the Pentagon during the September 11, 2001, attack (though he wasn't in the building when it was hit), and likes to run. Just before Charles was deployed, he received diagnoses of two different types of cancer. I asked him how, in a single calendar year, he was able to heal from two different cancers and then go to help rebuild Afghanistan—a remote and potentially very dangerous country with few resources. He explained to me, "I had diagnoses of both prostate cancer and skin cancer during my annual military physical examination. After six months of treatment, I accepted a position in Afghanistan, working in the headquarters for a year. With the consent of my doctors, I decided I could commit to a year and get stronger in Afghanistan just as well as I could at home. I strengthened my body by running daily and doing sit-ups, push-ups, and chin-ups. With God's help, I am getting better every day." Certainly, Afghanistan does not seem like the perfect healing environment; however, people can recover in many situations that are not ideal.

In other books, I have written a lot about healing and what it takes to recover from cancer or another serious injury or illness. Obviously, in those books, I focused exclusively on healing and recovery, but space doesn't permit adequately covering those subjects here. Therefore, I've created this summary, which includes a few important things about healing that people need to know:

1. *Aim for optimal healing.* Many people don't heal as well as they can. Before you accept a "new normal," try to heal as optimally as possible. In short, don't accept more pain, disability, and fatigue than you have to.

2. *Take time to heal.* You need to carve out time in your day to focus on healing. Most cancer survivors will place "having better health" at the very top of the list of things they want to achieve. Yet, when one looks at their daily "to do" list (after the acute cancer treatments are finished), the things that facilitate healing are not on it. Daily activities, chores, work, and so on make up the majority of the list, with healing activities ranking very low or not included. In order to heal optimally—both physically and emotionally—you need to bump the things that will help you heal to the top of your "to do" list, and keep them there.

3. *Make a plan.* It helps to have a plan to heal as well as possible. If you know what you want to achieve and you have goals that are aimed to get you there, it's easier to improve your health—even if you are living with cancer as a chronic condition. Having a plan means that you can see your progress as you go from one goal to the next. This helps both physically and emotionally.

If your goal is to heal as well as possible and you take the time to heal and have a plan, then it's likely that you can improve your physical and emotional health. However, healing can take months or years—even in someone who is very dedicated to recovering as well as possible. This is frustrating for many cancer survivors who want to heal quickly and well. Healing is a process that can be *facilitated* but not *rushed*. I think of this as tempo gusto, a musical term that means "at the right speed."

As a medical doctor who specializes in rehabilitation medicine, I think and write about healing on a daily basis. However, I thoroughly enjoyed reading what the survey participants had to say on this subject. They wrote some wonderful things about healing. See if you agree.

• • •

MY DOCTOR TOLD ME that it would be a minimum of two years before my life would start to turn around. I just didn't believe her. Since she was truthful, I know I can trust her.

> **Pam, retired dental hygienist**
> *Diagnosis of breast cancer at age 57 in 2005 in Lakeland, Florida*

> ## "I believe God had a plan for me..."

• • •

I WISH THE VARIETY of resources we have now had been available when I received my diagnosis. The Internet did not exist and, therefore, the ability to access information and to connect with others was limited. For all purposes, I was alone except for my wife and parents, though they were not very involved . One doctor told me it would be unlikely for me to survive and even said he specifically knew of only one patient with my pathology who had lived. Within hours after receiving this information, I never again even considered the possibility (in the doctor's mind, "probability") that I would not survive! I was silent about my cancer for more than thirty years—it has been only within the last couple of years that I have begun to share my story and, hence, to heal myself.

> **Ronald, business owner and entrepreneur**
> *Diagnosis of testicular cancer at age 20 in 1975 in Dover, New Hampshire*

I ATTENDED A CONFERENCE for cancer patients and their support person. I read Bernie Siegel's books. I listened to tapes. I began attending a church where the messages about living were positive and healing was emphasized. I also attended a Casting for Recovery® weekend. It was awesome!

Judi, nurse
Diagnosis of breast cancer at age 40 in 2000 in Pen Argyl, Pennsylvania

• • •

I ATTENDED ALL SEMINARS I could from the center where I did my treatment.

Elizabeth, self-employed
Diagnosis of breast cancer at age 52 in 2006 in Sanford, Florida

The view. The view from center ice at an audience that gave me so much every night of my career. I may have even been taking it for granted. When I received a diagnosis of testicular cancer on March 17, 1997, I thought my skating life was over. My inspiration was getting back to the place I loved the most—the ice. I thought of little else while going through chemotherapy. I was one step closer after the surgery required to remove what was left of the tumor. And on October 29, 1997, I was standing center ice in front of a large audience in Los Angeles, declaring my victory over cancer. Without the support of everyone across the United States who helped me love my job, I don't know how I could have dealt with my illness. I think every cancer patient has that "carrot" to get back to life, and it is different for everyone.

SCOTT HAMILTON is an Olympic gold medal ice skater who received a diagnosis of testicular cancer in 1997.

IN 2000, I WAS blessed with a five-week-old Chihuahua. I named him Taco, and he has brought me such comfort and joy! Having to get up and let him outside, making sure he had water and food, and taking care of him required most of my attention. Being his caregiver kept me going.

Michele, administrative assistant
Diagnosis of breast cancer at age 45 in 1999 in Detroit, Michigan

• • •

SITTING IN THE FRESH air and never tiring of watching the world around me [helped me heal]. It was soothing to my soul to watch the world continue around me. I took walks as soon as I could. I also had to undergo some significant physical therapy to get my body working again. As I made certain benchmarks of progress, I was greatly encouraged.

Robert, fire chaplain
Diagnosis of melanoma (skin cancer) at age 57 in 2003 in La Habra, California

• • •

GOING THROUGH PHYSICAL THERAPY helped me regain some of my strength. My physical therapist sent me home with exercises to do that would help me. I was doing exercises at home and taking brisk walks, which also helped. Doing more for myself— this made me feel better.

Rosi, student accounts office assistant
Diagnosis of colon cancer at age 52 in 2007 in Austin, Texas

> "The most reassuring realization... is that *I am not alone.*"

• • •

MY FAITH AND SHARING my story with other cancer survivors has helped me heal. My faith in God was the major factor in my coping. I believe God had a plan for me, and it had to involve cancer for me to get there. Seventeen years later (a long cry from six months!), here I am, working with cancer patients.

Beth, health educator
Diagnosis of liver cancer at age 32 in 1990 in Fort Hood, Texas

> ## "My faith and sharing my story with other cancer survivors has helped me heal."

YOU CANNOT BE IMPATIENT with yourself. Chemo is almost like trying to self-destruct. Let the internal forces play. Relax. You will emerge again.

Suza, self-employed
Diagnosis of mantle cell lymphoma at age 41 in 2005 in Johannesburg, Gauteng (South Africa)

• • •

WHILE I REALIZE it's not over and I will have to remain diligent about my health, I feel like I am "done" and will not have cancer again.

Lynne, Web coordinator
Diagnosis of breast cancer at age 43 in 2006 in Rome, New York

• • •

I DON'T THINK I was ever emotionally damaged by my cancer diagnosis, my treatment, or my prognosis, so healing was not a problem or an issue for me. It was (and still is) simply a process I'm going through—it's another stage in my life. I'm doing the best I can, and I am very content and happy with my state of mind.

Mike, retired real estate developer and cattle rancher
Diagnosis of colon cancer at age 66 in 2006 in Red Lodge, Montana

• • •

I DON'T THINK I have fully healed, but helping out in the online Forum* has helped tremendously in getting me on track. It is crucial to meet and share experiences with other survivors. The most reassuring realization—the one that has helped me most in healing emotionally—is that I am not alone. There are many others like me, and there's no reason to go through this journey by myself.

Federico, cancer chemical biologist
Diagnosis of testicular cancer at age 32 in 2006 in Brookline, Massachusetts

*TC-Cancer.com

I USED TO TELL myself—when I was experiencing side effects of the treatment—that if the chemo was kicking my butt, it must have been even harder on the cancer. I saw the side effects as confirmation that chemo was killing the cancer.

Elizabeth, American Cancer Society volunteer coordinator
Diagnosis of breast cancer at age 44 in 2002 in Des Moines, Iowa

The days that followed my diagnosis were filled with so many questions and deep breaths. The funny thing is that the world went right back to its normal routine. Grasping my own mortality was the next step. I knew I was far too young to leave this world. I had too many responsibilities, too many people counting on me. Every time I allowed myself to think that I was finally safe, I would hear someone mention a friend or family member who had died of the disease. In time, I learned how lucky I was to have caught the melanoma early. To me, the process took too long. I believe I only started to breathe again once I was confident I had done everything possible at that point to protect myself. If the melanoma came back after that, it wasn't because of something I had neglected.

SHONDA SHILLING is the wife of major league baseball player Curt Shilling. Shonda received a diagnosis of melanoma (skin cancer) in 2001.

I WAS SO STUNNED in the beginning that I really needed time to get used to the idea that this was really happening and that I had to get through it. There were no other choices.

Cathi, clinical social worker
Diagnosis of breast cancer at age 52 in 2003 in Waban, Massachusetts

IN ALL HONESTY, it hit me hard. The shock, coupled with the pregnancy hormones. It was really rough. I had a support system, but was unable to "grab" onto them. In my pain, I took on theirs. I never wished it on myself, let alone my family and friends. I felt bad that they, too, had to go through this. I have to say, time has helped me.

Nancy, office manager
Diagnosis of bladder cancer at age 25 in 1997 in Levittown, New York

• • •

I LOVE MY VISITS to the cancer hospital, M. D. Anderson. Everyone there is upbeat. Patients encourage one another. I get into great conversations every time I visit—especially when a bunch of patients are all sitting around, partially dressed with tubes up their arms, waiting for the next CT scan.

Edward, professor
Diagnosis of basal cell carcinoma (skin cancer) at age 42 in 1985 and mantle cell lymphoma at age 56 in 1999 in Chapel Hill, North Carolina

• • •

MY FAMILY WAS NEARBY, but because my prognosis was grim, we moved to the country. It was one of the best and most rewarding things we could have done. We have had continual family support and community and friends who have rallied nonstop. I have learned to focus on the moment at hand and make as many memories as possible with my family and friends. My daughters have grown up riding horseback under a full moon, getting lost in a cornfield, smelling flowers on the side of the road, camping, walking, and having many memorable adventures.

Suzanne, wife and mother
Diagnosis of colon cancer at age 31 in 1998 in Canton, Texas

• • •

I HAD LYMPH NODES removed beside my breast, and let me tell you, never underestimate the power of a sports bra!

Rochelle, manicurist
Diagnosis of melanoma (skin cancer) at age 34 in 2007 in Las Vegas, Nevada

I WOULD NOT PRESUME to tell someone else how to get through cancer. I was so damn lucky. What can I say, "Get lucky, dude?" My children are grown or mostly on their own. My wife has a great job, with plenty of money. We have the best insurance. My brother is a 6/6 match [for a bone marrow transplant].

Matt, carpenter
Diagnosis of chronic lymphocytic leukemia at age 51 in 2003 in Bath, New York

• • •

I HAVE FOUND that the human spirit is much more resilient than I had imagined. I have found that friends appear, unasked and undemanding, just when they are needed most—the love of friends is incredibly reaffirming.

Bill, administrator
Diagnosis of prostate cancer at age 62 in 2007 in Jefferson, Wisconsin

• • •

THE DOCTOR at the beginning said I had a 50/50 chance of survival. There are no words to describe how helpless I felt. I was introduced to the radiation specialist and the chemo specialist—the surgeon who put in my port. I lost my hair and my identity. I found myself in deep prayer and searching the scriptures for words of comfort. I wish I could have had time to prepare more. They were in a hurry to get started, but I truly thought I had cancer in my brain and I was so scared and overwhelmed, and my whole body just trembled. I kept telling the doctor that I would be glad when I could stop my legs from shaking.

Mary, business assistant
Diagnosis of synovial sarcoma of the right forearm at age 44 in 2006 in McPherson, Kansas

> "I have found that friends appear, unasked and undemanding, just when they are needed most—the love of friends is incredibly reaffirming."

BE HONEST WITH EVERYONE, and don't try to be a superhero.

Shelly, program coordinator for adults with disabilities
Diagnosis of breast cancer at age 32 in 2004 in Concord, New Hampshire

> The turning point in my true healing was when I read a quote that changed my way of thinking for good: "Hope and hopelessness are both a choice, so why not choose Hope?"
>
> **HEATHER WARRICK (AKA CANCER PRINCESS)** received a breast cancer diagnosis at age 24 in 1994. Her cancer recurred nine times, and she now lives with cancer as a chronic condition. Heather is the manager of Health Programs for the American Cancer Society.

WHEN I FIRST RECEIVED my diagnosis, antidepressants helped me the most. I still am not healed. After receiving another cancer diagnosis, I was very angry and depressed. My doctor increased my antidepressants, and my friends and family are coming through again.

Kirsten, distribution assistant
Diagnosis of colon cancer at age 49 in 2006 and endometrial (uterine) cancer at age 50 in 2007 in Buford, Georgia

• • •

SLEEP, SLEEP, SLEEP.

Sally, research laboratory administrator
Diagnosis of breast cancer at age 40 in 1990 in Salem, Massachusetts

• • •

I FEEL CONFIDENT that my treatments have worked and will keep cancer at bay. I get check-ups consistently, every six months, and will be doing so for the rest of my life. This feels fine to me.

Laura, housecleaner
Diagnosis of esophageal cancer at age 45 in 2002 in Schenectady, New York

I HAD COMPLEMENTARY THERAPIES (i.e., acupuncture, aromatherapy, massage). My husband paid for my friend and me to go to a health spa for five days.

Elizabeth, retired administrator
Diagnosis of breast cancer at age 58 in 2003 in Plymouth, Devon (England)

• • •

I NEVER FRETTED OVER recurrence. Initially, the thought of it would cross my mind, but from the first moment I realized I had cancer, I never expected it would kill me. I always felt I would survive it. If it does come again, I will deal with it... just like I did the first time.

Pat, office manager
Diagnosis of breast cancer at age 53 in 2001 in Canton, Michigan

• • •

I AM STILL HEALING, but I eventually had to seek help and get prescription drugs. Depression from the cancer, coupled with postpartum depression, left me no choice. Recently, though, I have been making leaps and bounds in [dealing with] the anxiety that comes along with a cancer diagnosis. I just made a conscious decision to take back my life and quit worrying about every little twitch and pain. It was getting to a point where every time I had a stomach ache or sore throat, I would think it was some type of cancer attacking me again. I am now over that and am focusing on the here and now instead of the "What if."

Nicki, homemaker
Diagnosis of thyroid cancer at age 20 in 2005 in Union, Missouri

Cancer is a journey. This isn't a cold that you just get over. There are certain kinds of cancer that may be cured, but oftentimes that is not the case. Thus, it becomes a part of your life. I never forget that I had it.

NANCY BRINKER received a diagnosis of breast cancer at age 37 in 1985. She had founded the Susan G. Komen for the Cure in 1981 in memory of her sister and best friend.

> "No one really explains the post-surgical depression… I used the Internet to put me in touch with other cancer survivors whom I could talk to."

THE DIAGNOSIS REALLY DIDN'T hit me until after surgery. No one really explains the post-surgical depression that (I have since discovered) so many women have experienced. I used the Internet to put me in touch with other cancer survivors whom I could talk to. Some I called just to cry to, which they openly welcomed. Participation in my local support group has been a savior. These women are my family, and I enjoy our weekly meetings. I will be perfectly honest; I did start taking Zoloft to help with the anxiety and depression that I just couldn't kick myself.

Kelley, massage therapist
Diagnosis of breast cancer at age 36 in 2006 in Rochdale, Massachusetts

• • •

WITH THE DIAGNOSIS OF AML [acute myelogenous leukemia], knowing I had beaten the breast cancer gave me the impetus to fight again.

Eileen, technology specialist
Diagnosis of breast cancer at age 34 in 1984, acute myelogenous leukemia at age 49 in 1999, and basal cell carcinoma (skin cancer) at age 55 in 2005 in Framingham, Massachusetts

• • •

FROM THE AGE of eight to fourteen, I spent much time at Oak Knoll Naval Hospital in Oakland, California. This was during the 1960s while the Vietnam war was going on. The human sacrifice I witnessed registered more with me than the internal cancer I was experiencing. I had internal mental and physical defects from my illness, but the external physical harm I saw in the returning Vietnam veterans diminished my thought of how sick I really was.

Randy, respiratory therapist
Diagnosis of Hodgkin disease at age 6 in 1965 in Ewa Beach, Hawaii

GETTING BACK on my sailboat and taking a three-week cruise with my husband helped me heal. We visited friends who had been unable to get to me during my treatment. We did a lot of fishing, sightseeing, and even a little hunting. It was good to get back into the real world.

Ruthanne, bookkeeper
Diagnosis of breast cancer at age 51 in 1995 in Thorne Bay, Alaska

Cancer has made me appreciate every single day of life since I received my diagnosis at the age of 24. Cancer made me want to give back something, to make cancer survivorship easier for those less privileged who do not have access to quality care. Mostly, cancer gave me a specific focus for a lifelong desire to work with organizations committed to social change. What helped me heal was an indescribable succession of circumstances, which included getting up every morning to be a parent to our son; having the peer support of fellow survivors, as well as wonderful professional psychosocial support; the love of a devoted husband, friends, and family; working for a cause I am deeply committed to; a sense of humor; taking our dog for long walks; and chocolate!

ELLEN STOVALL is the president and CEO of the National Coalition for Cancer Survivorship. She had three cancer diagnoses: Hodgkin disease at age 24 in 1971, recurrence of Hodgkin disease at age 36 in 1983, and breast cancer at age 61 in 2007. When she is not working as a cancer advocate, you can find her taking long walks with her golden retriever.

GETTING BACK TO SOME sense of normalcy...no doctors visits, no tests. This was emotionally difficult because it had become a way of life. Counseling helped, and setting new goals was very healing.

Sheri, actress
Diagnosis of Hodgkin disease at age 29 in 1993 in Columbia, Maryland

• • •

WHEN YOU RECEIVE a cancer diagnosis, make up your mind to go on living your life.

Eileen, retired registered nurse
Diagnosis of endometrial (uterine) cancer and basal cell carcinoma (skin cancer) at age 64 in 2006 in Charlotte, North Carolina

• • •

> "When you receive a cancer diagnosis, make up your mind to go on living your life."

I WAS FORTUNATE TO have had early-stage cancer both times, so I felt confident of a physical cure, which helped the emotional healing. Sometimes I think one can never be totally "healed" emotionally. In regard to emotion, the breast cancer was harder. I knew I would have real issues without having breasts, and breast reconstruction truly helped my recovery. With my most recent (breast cancer) diagnosis, I focused on getting plenty of sleep, eating as nutritiously as possible (even more organic), and getting as much exercise as possible, given the stage of recovery. One thing that especially helped with the recovery after breast surgery/reconstruction was physical therapy, with an excellent team that was experienced specifically with that. It made a dramatic difference with my pain and flexibility.

Charose, nurse
Diagnosis of Hodgkin disease at age 17 in 1972 and breast cancer at age 51 in 2006 in Omaha, Nebraska

I HAD A VERY hard time healing emotionally after cancer treatment. I felt I didn't do well with it. For one thing, I'm a Type A personality. Another thing is that I kept a lot bottled up inside, and I resented what my husband, my family, and my husband's family did not do or try to do for me. Also, I feared a [cancer] recurrence in the worst way. Prayer helped me, and cancer survivors helped me. I was also in a support group that really helped. I now realize that I should have had counseling on how to deal with [my fears]. Dumb me—I didn't think about doing that, and the doctors never suggested or told me about services that were available for those who needed them.

Joyce, educational assistant at an elementary school
Diagnosis of breast cancer at 41 in 1995 in Knoxville, Tennessee

• • •

I DON'T KNOW if one ever heals from the emotional scars of cancer. I've engaged in discussions with other survivors and developed a positive outlook on my future. But I don't know if that sword over my head will ever go away.

Mike, management professional
Diagnosis of rectal cancer at age 38 in 2006 in Rochester, New York

> "Counseling helped, and setting new goals was very healing."

• • •

I TALKED TO a social worker who specialized in dealing with patients who had been through treatment for cancer.

Laurie, medical assistant
Diagnosis of breast cancer at age 43 in 2006 in Sacramento, California

• • •

I HAVE A FRIEND who is a ten-year survivor of ovarian cancer. She has been my "cheerleader" throughout everything, offering advice and encouragement.

Patti, financial administrator
Diagnosis of ovarian cancer at age 51 in 2005 in Colorado Springs, Colorado

I WAS DEPRESSED WHEN I was diagnosed—now I'm not. Emotionally, I'm in a much better place.

Mary, administrative assistant
Diagnosis of breast cancer at age 42 in 2003 in Simi Valley, California

• • •

MY SYNAGOGUE HELD a healing service that met once a month, for those who were in need of healing themselves or were praying for others. It was a wonderful, supportive group that allowed me to focus on myself in an honest, open, and safe environment.

Janet, elementary school teacher
Diagnosis of colon cancer at age 42 in 1993 in Philadelphia, Pennsylvania

• • •

I PERSONALLY PRAYED to be healed and to get through it with endurance and dignity and to keep the cancer from ever coming back.

Marla, executive assistant
Diagnosis of breast cancer at age 35 in 1994 in Jasper, Indiana

• • •

AFTER COMING out of the ICU, I had to learn to walk, talk, feed myself, and so on, because every bodily function had shut down. My brain stayed engaged, and I did pull through. Physical therapy helped me then and again a year later when things were not good. I had to work to get strong.

Susan, homemaker
Diagnosis of acute myelogenous leukemia at age 50 in 2003 in Medina, Ohio

• • •

I THINK MY HEALING was greatly improved by keeping a positive attitude, continuing my life as normally as possible, and not giving in to the disease.

Cynthia, administrative assistant
Diagnosis of breast cancer at age 55 in 2003 in Highland Lakes, New Jersey

I AM NOW GOING to a counselor to work through grief and anger.

Jan, retired hospice chaplain
Diagnosis of breast cancer at age 55 in 2006 in Wichita, Kansas

My will to live and having a positive attitude.

SHARON OSBOURNE explains what helped her heal after she was given a poor prognosis. Sharon is the wife of musician Ozzy Osbourne and is best known for her role in the reality MTV series *The Osbournes*. Sharon has three grown children—two daughters and a son—as well as a house full of animals. She received a colon cancer diagnosis at the age of 49 in 2002.

AT ONE POINT I almost gave up. I couldn't take it anymore—the needles, the tests, and chemo. It was too much. But eventually, I turned it around. Something inside told me to keep on going, to fight it, and I would win. Today, I'm a parent to my daughter, my most precious gift of all, and my life is somewhat back to normal. To enjoy life with her made it so worth it. And I thank God every day for saving me and forcing me to go on.

Cheryl, billings account clerk
Diagnosis of Ewing's sarcoma (a form of bone cancer) at age 21 in 1987 in Malden, Massachusetts

• • •

WHAT HELPED ME the most was getting back to a semblance of real life—work, activities, and family gatherings!

Bryna, management development consultant
Diagnosis of tongue cancer at age 35 in 1985 in Brockton, Massachusetts

• • •

I SLEPT A LOT. I believe rest helps the body heal faster.

Yvonne, paralegal
Diagnosis of colon cancer at age 48 in 2004 in San Antonio, Texas

> "I personally prayed to be healed and to get through it with endurance and dignity and to keep the cancer from ever coming back."

I HAD STAGE IIIA breast cancer. But, you know what? Statistics are what they are. You can read anything into them that you want to see. I'm constantly looking for "survivor" stories and survivor statistics. I look for the positives in life, not the negatives.

Jerri, state employee
Diagnosis of breast cancer at age 48 in 2006 and endometrial (uterine) cancer at age 50 in 2008 in Standish, Michigan

• • •

AS TRITE AS THIS may sound, I took great comfort from a poster that was hanging in my room. It said something to the effect that "courage" isn't always about succeeding, but more about allowing yourself to come back ready to fight another day.

Jerry, computer software instructor
Diagnosis of acute myelogenous leukemia at age 43 in 2003 in Anoka, Minnesota

• • •

THE SHOCK OF CANCER is enough to send anyone into a panic, but I chose not to cry. I chose to put my trust in my doctors, my family, and myself.

Kathleen, retail manager
Diagnosis of breast cancer at age 48 in 2007 in Washington Township, New Jersey

• • •

IT HELPED ME to consider from the onset that I am involved in a fight. I am not a fighter by nature, but I quickly developed the attitude that cancer is my enemy and I must defend myself.

Barbara, nurse
Diagnosis of breast cancer at age 58 in 1995 in Stoneham, Massachusetts

THE LONGER I GO, the less I worry.

Fran, postmaster
Diagnosis of breast cancer at age 42 in 1999 in LaVergne, Tennessee

• • •

SOMETIMES A SMELL or a bald lady in a crowd will make it come back...like a flashback to a bad car wreck. It's weird, but just another way of making us realize how little control we have in life.

Karen, real estate broker
Diagnosis of breast cancer at age 38 in 2001 in Loganville, Georgia

• • •

CANCER STINKS. It is unfair; it is cruel. But if I sit around being mad at cancer, I will be stuck and not move on. Yes, I live in "Cancer World," and I will always live there, but my life is good and blessed in so many ways.

Judy, chaplain
Diagnosis of colorectal cancer at age 48 in 2003 in Cudahy, Wisconsin

• • •

I AM VERY AWARE of having high anxiety, specifically when it comes to my health. I work with a counselor and will be seeking advice from a psychiatrist for changing my medication to reduce my anxiety and depression. I pray. I make an effort to learn about how others cope. I go to the doctor to get reassurance when something doesn't seem right.

Judi, nurse
Diagnosis of breast cancer at age 40 in 2000 in Pen Argyl, Pennsylvania

• • •

I WAS SO SCARED. When I look back, I can't believe how scared I was and how that made me feel. I wish there was something to take that feeling away...there is and there will be—a cure!

Cheryl, homemaker
Diagnosis of breast cancer at age 49 in 2006 in Garland, Texas

In recent years, much more attention has been given to psychosocial issues that impact life after a cancer diagnosis. People can feel hopeful because quality of life during and after cancer treatment is highly valued. Improvements in methods to prevent, minimize, or alleviate many side effects of treatment, both short-term and long-term, have made the treatment experience easier in many instances.

ELYSE CAPLAN is the education director for Living Beyond Breast Cancer (LBBC) and oversees large-scale conferences and teleconferences; the LBBC Survivors' Helpline; written and online publications; networking programs for young women, women with metastatic breast cancer and women of color; and workshops and trainings for health care professionals. She received a breast cancer diagnosis at age 34 in 1991.

THERE IS A LARGE dragon boat community of breast cancer survivors, which has given me inspiration, information, and a laugh or two along the way.

Robin, college professor
Diagnosis of breast cancer at age 50 in 2006 in Costa Mesa, California

• • •

IT HELPS TO LEARN a new hobby. I took a class on beading.

Brenda, government clerk
Diagnosis of breast cancer at age 58 in 2006 in Madison, Tennessee

• • •

KNOWING THAT I HAVE an awesome support group in my life. I am not scared about the possibility of getting [cancer] again, now that I've been through the treatment process once already.

Mary Anne, word processor
Diagnosis of melanoma (skin cancer) at age 26 in 2007 in Dixon, California

I'M STILL HEALING.

Laura, unemployed psychiatric social worker
Diagnosis of breast cancer at age 43 in 2006 in Avon, Connecticut

• • •

I ATTENDED SPORTING EVENTS (which I love).

Karen, medical assistant
Diagnosis of breast cancer at age 43 in 2001 in Cincinnati, Ohio

• • •

IT'S ONLY BEEN TWO months since my last chemo. I still get weepy, but I am getting stronger with every passing day. I got married two days ago, and I know I will be around for many years to come. I choose to be positive and keep planning our future. I want to see my children and grandchildren grow up.

Linda, purchasing agent
Diagnosis of breast cancer at age 47 in 2007 in Antioch, California

> "I choose to be positive and keep planning our future. I want to see my children and grandchildren grow up."

Cancer survivors are living with the ill effects of the complications and toxicities of cancer treatment. Rehabilitation services can ameliorate some of these after-effects to improve function and quality of life.

MABEL CABAN, MD, is a physiatrist (a doctor who specializes in physical medicine and rehabilitation) and an assistant professor at The University of Texas Medical Branch in Galveston. Dr. Caban focuses her research and clinical work in oncology rehabilitation.

Believing I'd survive was the best healing medicine I had! I realized that my body was in need of some radical attention that would not make me feel all that good, but I never believed that this disease would take me out! I have a very loving and special family; their belief that I would be around for a long time healed me and kept my fears at bay.

TERRY MUSIC was 46 years old when her breast cancer was diagnosed. She is the chief mission delivery officer of the American Cancer Society.

It is no longer acceptable to leave cancer patients debilitated, demoralized, depressed, and unable to work or enjoy life after cancer treatment when the side effects of cancer treatment could have been anticipated, prevented, treated, or palliated. With the excellent oncology care that has produced dramatic increases in survival, cancer rehabilitation and cancer survivorship programs are emerging as the completion of the process of returning cancer survivors to a meaningful quality of life after cancer treatment.

NANCY A. HUTCHISON, MD, CLT, is the medical director for lymphedema and cancer rehabilitation at the Sister Kenny Rehabilitation Institute at the Virginia Piper Cancer Institute in Minneapolis, Minnesota.

CHAPTER 15

• • •

How Cancer Changed My Life

I once asked my father-in-law, who is now nearly eighty years old, how his life was changed by his diagnosis of thyroid cancer approximately thirty years ago (when treatments for this condition were not nearly as advanced as they are today). He told me that it wasn't really a big deal and didn't change his life at all. I found that hard to believe. In fact, as frightening as a cancer diagnosis is today, it was even worse three decades ago. I've thought about his rather cavalier response and have come to the conclusion that on the one hand, this Korean War veteran and former semi-professional baseball player was raised with the "tough guy" values so common in his generation of men. To complain or acknowledge fear just wasn't done. On the other hand, it's probably true that he really isn't concerned about having had thyroid cancer as a younger man. Time, especially a lot of it, really does help survivors to heal emotionally.

Cancer definitely changed me and the course of my life. At first, it was all-consuming and I thought about it constantly. During that time, I worked hard at helping myself to heal. When I was strong enough, I channeled my energy into helping other survivors to recover physically. After my cancer diagnosis, I joined the medical staff at Dana-Farber Cancer Institute in Boston, Massachusetts, where I treat cancer survivors with rehabilitation needs. I write a lot about survivorship issues and devote considerable time to speaking to cancer survivors at meetings and conventions.

Despite the fact that I am spending an increasing amount of each workday focusing on cancer survivorship issues, as the years go by, I am thinking and talking about cancer less and less in my personal life. Whereas not a day goes by that I don't think about cancer at some point, it's not part of what I typically talk about with friends and family. I have other things on my mind and, thankfully, my own cancer is becoming increasingly less important to me. Still, there is no doubt that cancer changed the course of my life.

Not surprisingly, most of the people who responded to the surveys also reported that cancer had changed their lives. Some survivors wrote that having cancer turned out to be a good thing—even a blessing. Many survivors, who didn't necessarily consider cancer a blessing, still used it as an opportunity to change their lives for the better. They described what Shakespeare wrote, "Sweet are the uses of adversity" (*As You Like It*, 2.1.14).

Quite a few of the survey participants expressed how much they like to talk to other cancer survivors and to help those who have just learned of their diagnosis. Ruthanne, who had breast cancer in her early fifties, wrote from Alaska, "Because of my association with the American Cancer Society and Relay for Life®, I have met so many special people. I love speaking about my battle and about cancer in general, trying to help others come to grips with their own diagnosis or the diagnosis of a loved one. Cancer has given my life a new purpose, for which I will always be grateful." Indeed, Ruthanne and all of the other survey participants agreed to share their stories because they wanted to reach out to you and your loved ones—to bring hope and inspiration as you go through your own experience.

• • •

EVERY DAY IS PRECIOUS to me. I feel that my life is actually better now than when I was younger. I am married to a great person, we are financially okay, and his family is loving and supportive. I am grateful for every day that I have.

Sheila, legal secretary
Diagnosis of breast cancer at age 65 in 2006 in Walnut Creek, California

• • •

WORDS CANNOT DESCRIBE how I feel. When I first received my cancer diagnosis, it seemed that my world would become a much different place. Now I am beginning to feel like my old self again.

John, retired
Diagnosis of esophageal cancer at age 76 in 2006 in Jamestown, North Carolina

THERE ARE SO MANY blessings that, at times, they seem to outweigh the negatives. First, I never felt more fully embraced and loved by family and friends. It was the most heartwarming experience to have a reason to tell people on a daily basis how much they meant to me, and to hear the same from them. For the first time in my life, I learned to put my own needs first. I gave myself permission to take care of myself. Instead of saying "later" to things, I said "yes."

Mary, attorney
Diagnosis of breast cancer at age 54 in 2005 in Brookline, Massachusetts

• • •

I HAVE MADE SOME very big changes in my life. I have been a volunteer for the American Cancer Society's Reach to Recovery® program. I have been a survivor for many years! I am also in graduate school part-time, studying counselor education. I plan to be a guidance counselor in an elementary school. Cancer has changed my life for the better, because it has given me clarity in my life.

Lisa, administrative assistant
Diagnosis of breast cancer at age 38 in 2000 in Owings Mills, Maryland

• • •

CANCER WILL CHANGE YOUR life. How it changes it is completely up to you. You can isolate yourself and feel every insecurity and fear that come with cancer. Or you can reach out, surround yourself with positive people, and let your faith guide you.

> **"I gave myself permission to take care of myself."**

Susan, housewife
Diagnosis of colorectal cancer at age 43 in 2006 in Mobile, Alabama

• • •

CANCER DID NOT CHANGE my life for the better. I changed my life for the better as a result of having cancer!

Judi, nurse
Diagnosis of breast cancer at age 40 in 2000 in Pen Argyl, Pennsylvania

> "Cancer has changed my life for the better, because it has given me clarity..."

I'M CALMER AND MORE flexible. I enjoy writing poetry and continuing many pre-cancer activities.

Don, retired
Diagnosis of prostate cancer at age 74 in 2003 in Ocean Pines, Maryland

• • •

CANCER IS SCARY, and you have the right to be scared. Don't go through it alone. Be with family, friends, even a support group. This is a test of your strength, so keep fighting! You have the right to be mad and moody.

Cathy, retail district manager
Diagnosis of pancreatic cancer at age 45 in 2005 in Columbus, Ohio

• • •

MY DAUGHTER, RACHEL, was ten years old when I learned I had cancer, and she never showed me a sad or scared face. She supported me and inspired me always to face the world with a positive and happy attitude. She provided the basis for my inner strength. She taught me that cancer does not have to define me. I was still her mom and still the same person. She's told me that I looked so bad, she thought I was going to die. Five years after my cancer diagnosis, Rachel asked to be excused from a biology lab on cancer cells. She just couldn't face looking through a microscope and seeing those nasty cells that caused so much pain and suffering for me. We have found it very helpful to do fundraising and programs together. I walked in the Avon and [Susan G.] Komen and American Cancer Society walks. Rachel did all sorts of activities with me. She saw me as a strong person, and I enjoyed her company. We also organized an annual family fundraiser, which we still hold every year, and donate all the proceeds to cancer research. Last year, we had two hundred fifty 9th graders attend a Think Pink Dance—we collected $5,600!

Carrie, information management specialist
Diagnosis of breast cancer at age 44 in 2002 in New York City, New York

I AM STRONGER for those who have cancer—they come to me to talk, and I listen. I am not there to give advice, but listening is the one thing I have found to be helpful.

Rose, government contractor
Diagnosis of stomach cancer at age 60 in 2002 in Centreville, Virginia

• • •

MY DIAGNOSIS HAS MADE me more motivated at work, and I feel a greater sense of purpose with my research. I mostly work on pediatric cancers, and every now and then I go on rounds with my boss. Seeing the kids in the cancer ward and interacting with them makes me gung-ho about beating the disease and fighting it in the lab.

Federico, cancer chemical biologist
Diagnosis of testicular cancer at age 32 in 2006 in Brookline, Massachusetts

• • •

FEW PEOPLE WOULD HAVE KNOWN I was going through treatment. I worked very hard to look normal, but I felt terrible. Now, when I see a crabby person, I realize I have no idea what he or she is going through. I have much more patience and empathy for others. At the same time, I have found an inner strength that many don't have. Pain means nothing to me anymore. It just means I am alive.

Ann, homemaker
Diagnosis of breast cancer at age 47 in 2003 in Mechanicsburg, Pennsylvania

• • •

CANCER IS BY NO MEANS fun or a path that I would either choose or wish on another person. It is inconvenient, distracting, disturbing, and scary. However, I can truly say, "Yes, cancer has changed my life for the better." I continue to grow as a person, expanding my knowledge, my compassion, my ability to love, and my ability to accept life as it comes. I have deeper, more meaningful relationships. I address things that are important, rather than letting them fester; and I dismiss things that bug me, but are not of any import. I find new reasons to be happy, new ways to enjoy life, new things to appreciate all of the time.

Beth, massage therapist
Diagnosis of breast cancer at age 39 in 2006 in Tempe, Arizona

I HAD BEEN LIVING my life like it was prologue to something else, something more. Then, one day in the waiting room, it hit me: "This is my life, right here, right now. This is it." It taught me to pursue my dreams, because life is way too short and you never know what can happen. It taught me to live in the moment, something I have a very hard time doing.

Jaime, graduate student
Diagnosis of cervical cancer at age 24 in 2005 in Blackwood, New Jersey

Getting a perspective on hearing that you have cancer takes some time. When my cancer was diagnosed more than twenty years ago, there were no support groups of people who had done this before, so I had to find my own way. What I finally learned is that cancer is a dual journey: one of the head that involves information and choosing treatment, and one of the heart and soul that is much more complicated because it has to do with the person who will emerge from the cancer experience. I have come to know that the treatment part is about being cured, and the heart part is about being healed. And if you can accomplish both, you have uncovered the mystery of life itself.

KATHY LATOUR received a breast cancer diagnosis at age 37 in 1986. She has dedicated her career to helping cancer survivors and is currently the editor-at-large for CURE Media Group, publishers of *CURE* and *Heal* magazines.

I GO TO THE DOCTOR sooner, rather than self diagnose.

Mark, retired nuclear pharmacist
Diagnosis of chronic lymphocytic leukemia at age 59 in 2001 in Bay Shore, New York

CANCER HAS GIVEN ME a gift of time. Since my diagnosis twelve years ago, I've never been in remission; six years ago, my prognosis was "terminal." I will lose my battle with cancer one day, but not today. Today, I am alive and living well.

Ric, public relations director
Diagnosis of thyroid cancer at age 50 in 1995 in Londonderry, New Hampshire

• • •

I DEAL WITH THE SICK for a living. [My cancer] experience has made me grow in that respect. I was always compassionate, but now I know how to be beneficial to others in this situation. I know what I needed, and so I try to give it back with all my soul. I try to listen and give empathy and support. I don't try to hide my feelings, and I do my best to let others know they can tell me how scared they are. It's okay to be scared...it's okay not to be strong 24 hours a day... it's okay to cry and ask others to cry with you...it's okay to be terrified of the outcomes of your periodic tests. For pity's sake, throw up on me—I wash; it's okay!

Kathie, nurse and social worker
Diagnosis of kidney cancer at age 53 in 2005 in Kingston, New York

• • •

BEING DIAGNOSED WITH TERMINAL cancer gave me a newfound freedom. I have done things I would never have done before, including appearing on *The Today Show*, talking to strangers about very personal experiences, walking the halls of Congress, learning to scuba dive and skydive. We've planned my funeral. Now we focus on living.

Suzanne, wife and mother
Diagnosis of colon cancer at age 31 in 1998 in Canton, Texas

> "Cancer will change your life. How it changes it is completely up to you. You can isolate yourself...Or you can reach out...and let your faith guide you."

NOT A DAY GOES BY that I don't think about my condition and wonder (and worry) about what the future may hold. I wish my doctor had spent more time discussing my specific prognostic factors and what they indicate about how my disease will progress and how I may react to chemotherapy when it's time for treatment. Thankfully, I have not yet had to have treatment. Although I am beginning to experience some symptoms of the disease, I am generally doing very well.

Kelly, financial services executive
Diagnosis of chronic lymphocytic leukemia at age 50 in 2003 and basal cell carcinoma (skin cancer) at age 53 in 2007 in Arlington, Virginia

• • •

IT DOES PUT THINGS in perspective. But, all things considered, I would not do it again.

Matt, carpenter
Diagnosis of chronic lymphocytic leukemia at age 51 in 2003 in Bath, New York

• • •

> ## "I have much more patience and empathy for others."

MY FRIEND BARBARA, whom I have known since high school, is an eight-year survivor of breast cancer, and she was there for me. She gave me two great books to read on survivorship. I will never forget how she signed one of them: "I know you can do this." Sometimes, I fell asleep reading the book.

Eileen, nurse
Diagnosis of colon cancer and melanoma (skin cancer) at age 50 in 2004 in Maple Glen, Pennsylvania

• • •

MANY BLESSINGS HAVE FOUND me this past year. But the best are these: (1) I am now much closer with my wife and children than ever before, (2) My friendships have grown stronger, and (3) I've found my meaning of life, which is simply to live every second.

Mike, management professional
Diagnosis of rectal cancer at age 38 in 2006 in Rochester, New York

THERE ARE MANY BLESSINGS. Every single day, I continue to feel the preciousness of every minute, of being here, of being alive. I am filled with gratitude. At moments, I can feel an incredible happiness well up inside of me. I am aware of how little is promised to any of us, how important it is to be and do and have whatever it is you want to be and do and have—now. There is little to gain by waiting to gain courage, to dare, to reach. This perspective has helped me keep the small stuff small and allow the really important things to surface. I am aware of how loved I am, and that is precious to me, too. I worry when something is amiss in my body; I worry that the cancer is back. I worry when I have to go for mammograms. I always had a slightly hypochondrical inclination, but now that I know that things really can go wrong, I'm more frightened when I have symptoms. Yet I am aware of how much I love my life, and I have been happier than I ever was before my diagnosis. If I had a guarantee that my cancer would not return, then I would be really glad that this whole experience happened for me.

Cathi, clinical social worker
Diagnosis of breast cancer at age 52 in 2003 in Waban, Massachusetts

• • •

SEVERAL FRIENDS HAVE TOLD me that, as time passes, I will come to view this experience as a "gift." Initially, this was a difficult concept to accept, but now I can see they were not wrong. One "gift" has been the recognition of what is truly important to me...and what is trivial and peripheral. There is little to no time left to waste. Since the surgery, I have found myself telling friends that I feel as though I have stepped through a doorway into a "new world." Not only can I look to the future again, but I realize that I am a different person now...a cancer survivor. With that survival comes the obligation to offer support, love, and understanding to those who are still undergoing their fight and those who have yet to face this nasty disease.

Bill, administrator
Diagnosis of prostate cancer at age 62 in 2007 in Jefferson, Wisconsin

> "I am aware of how little is promised to any of us... There is little to gain by waiting to gain courage..."

I DON'T BELIEVE I was ever emotionally damaged by having cancer. From the beginning, I was grateful to be alive and grateful that it had not happened to either of my sisters, since both had young children. My biggest fear was that they could get breast cancer, too, but I'm glad to say that they have not.

Lindy, hospice volunteer
Diagnosis of breast cancer at age 35 in 1984 and radiation-induced sarcoma at age 55 in 2004 in Lexington, Massachusetts

• • •

A BLESSING AND POSITIVE thing that came from my cancer experience was being able to spend my daughter's first year at home with her. Initially, I was going to take only three months for maternity leave and then go back to work. My cancer diagnosis came at the end of my leave, so I ended up spending a full year with my daughter. It certainly wasn't the circumstance I would have hoped for, but it was special nonetheless. Seeing her beautiful smiling face every morning helped me get through each day and look forward to the next.

Sarah, paralegal
Diagnosis of breast cancer at age 28 in 2000 in Miami, Florida

• • •

I DON'T HAVE ROAD rage anymore.

Kirsten, distribution assistant
Diagnosis of colon cancer at age 49 in 2006 and endometrial (uterine) cancer at age 50 in 2007 in Buford, Georgia

• • •

CANCER SUCKS. I hate having it, and I wish it would go away. I am still single with no kids, and now I have cancer. Yay? No way! Cancer has changed my life, but not for the better. I have accepted cancer as a part of me, and I am a happy person still. My life is not better, but it's not completely bad either. In fact, the only bad thing in my life right now is the cancer.

Evelyn, executive assistant
Diagnosis of colon cancer at age 33 in 2004 in Boston, Massachusetts

I WALK WITH a limp, and people are always asking me why (I tell them I fell roller skating to avoid the awkward conversation that would follow if they knew the truth). I have three big bald spots from where I had radiation on my head, so I have to wear my hair a certain way to cover those up. I have a huge scar down my back where my lung was removed and another scar on my chest from my port-a-cath. These are not the things I focus on every day, and I don't let them affect my quality of life, but they do impact my appearance in a way I wish they did not. I get really anxious before I go for my routine scans because I always dread that they will find another tumor. Most days, however, I move along with my life and don't give cancer a lot of thought. It's when I think about my future that cancer comes to mind. Having children doesn't seem like an option for me, so it's difficult to think about getting into a romantic relationship. I save money, but I don't go so far as to put it into tax-free retirement vehicles, because I don't think that living into retirement is a likely option for me. I feel like I can't really change jobs because I have good insurance now and an employer that I think would understand if I had another recurrence. And I can't move because all of my doctors are here. So, cancer limits me in several ways, but I have learned to reconcile these issues and not let them affect me on a daily basis.

Andrea, hospital administrator
Diagnosis of Ewing's sarcoma (a form of bone cancer) at age 15 in 1992 in Norfolk, Massachusetts

Having cancer had a tremendously positive impact on my life. I went from living life passively to living life actively. I realized that I had to attack life if I wanted to achieve anything. I lost a leg to cancer, but I gained a respect for life itself.

MARC WOODS received a diagnosis of osteosarcoma (bone cancer) of his leg at the age of 17. After a left lower extremity amputation, he went on to compete with Britain's Paralympic swim team, winning a total of twelve medals from five consecutive games, including four gold medals.

TODAY, I FIND IT hard even to remember most of that time, which is so strange because in the beginning, it consumed me. Every waking moment dealt with cancer in one way or another. Sometimes I feel like it happened to another person…and then I realize, it did. I will never again be that person who felt a lump in her breast one night and knew intuitively, "I have breast cancer."

Pat, office manager
Diagnosis of breast cancer at age 53 in 2001 in Canton, Michigan

• • •

> "I feel as though I have stepped through a doorway into a 'new world.'"

WITHOUT THIS EXPERIENCE, I would not have gone back into nursing (I had previously quit because of my fear of needles). Now, I know not to pass judgment on someone because of a seemingly harmless diagnosis. I got really sick and tired of people saying, "Oh, it's only thyroid cancer." Yes it is only thyroid cancer and it's probably not going to kill me, but it will control almost every aspect of my life for the rest of my life when my [thyroid] levels are not under control. I will go from dose to dose of medication forever.

Nicki, homemaker
Diagnosis of thyroid cancer at age 20 in 2005 in Union, Missouri

• • •

WITH EACH DIAGNOSIS, I was determined not to let cancer win. With the breast cancer, I had two young sons whom I was determined to watch grow up. I received the diagnosis of AML [acute myelogenous leukemia] just shy of my fiftieth birthday, and I was determined to make it. I wouldn't even contemplate giving up, no matter how lousy I felt.

Eileen, technology specialist
Diagnosis of breast cancer at age 34 in 1984 and acute myelogenous leukemia at age 49 in 1999 and basal cell carcinoma (skin cancer) at age 55 in 2005 in Framingham, Massachusetts

I HAVE BEEN a vegetarian for twenty-six years; I moved from Phoenix to the Haight-Ashbury district of San Francisco in 1980 and left in 1996. At age fifty, my favorite music is still punk rock. I have a profound appreciation of life. It's not always in the context of cancer, but I have been and always will be a "free spirit." Life is precious; I am anti-violence, anti-war, anti anything that compromises life or the quality of life in our world.

> ## "I will never again be that person who felt a lump in her breast one night..."

Randy, respiratory therapist
Diagnosis of Hodgkin disease at age 6 in 1965 in Ewa Beach, Hawaii

• • •

MY LIFE HAS CHANGED for the better. I've made a career change—from actuarial analyst to massage therapist. I'm so glad I made the move. I love what I'm doing now.

Kelley, massage therapist
Diagnosis of breast cancer at age 36 in 2006 in Rochdale, Massachusetts

• • •

IF I EXPERIENCE a new pain that lasts for a couple of weeks and doesn't go away, I get jittery about it and have it checked out. Every once in awhile, I get what I call "my cancer phobia," and I worry about things. I really don't think much about my cancer anymore, just when a new pain occurs without explanation and doesn't go away. I really worried after diagnosis and for a few years after. But as time went on, I became more secure. To minimize my worry, I talk to my best friend who also had cancer, and I talk to the Lord in prayer. After treatment is finished, one feels very insecure because you have been surrounded almost 24/7 by doctors or nurses who made you feel very secure. But then you are released and you're supposed to be like every other human body, but you're floundering around in the water without a life raft. At least, that's how I felt.

Joyce, educational assistant at an elementary school
Diagnosis of breast cancer at 41 in 1995 in Knoxville, Tennessee

I am always amazed by the incredible resilience of many people who have cancer. It is truly a privilege to share their journey and provide guidance when I can. There are other times when I am discouraged by the unfairness of the disease and, especially, the side effects of our treatments. These often wreak havoc with life plans—the absence of children, the inability to work and achieve other life goals—and the specter of recurrent cancer. We are working hard to prevent cancer and to reduce the burden and toxicity of treatments so that survivors in the future may have an easier time.

PATRICIA GANZ, MD, is a medical oncologist and professor at the University of California at Los Angeles (UCLA) School of Public Health and the David Geffen School of Medicine in Los Angeles. She is a founding member of the National Coalition for Cancer Survivorship (NCCS) and the director of the UCLA-LIVESTRONG Survivorship Center of Excellence at UCLA's Jonsson Comprehensive Cancer Center.

I DON'T KNOW if my children fully understood all of it, but they have done so much for me, physically and emotionally. They made me realize that my life is the most important [thing] to them. They need me and I need them. I was severely depressed before being diagnosed, and feel it even more so now. I now realize I do have a purpose in life, a very important one. I am a daughter, wife, mother, friend and, most important, a survivor!

Rochelle, manicurist
Diagnosis of melanoma (skin cancer) at age 34 in 2007 in Las Vegas, Nevada

• • •

I FIND MYSELF SMILING a lot more at people I meet in a store. I have more patience with things. I love to see things grow, and I love to get a hug from my kids and grandkids.

LaDonne, retired
Diagnosis of kidney cancer at age 40 in 1978 in Mundelein, Illinois

THREE THINGS: (1) I learned about it. I researched treatment facilities and located and talked with others who had prostate cancer and the type of treatment they sought. I did this with the belief that it would be beneficial to have as much factual information as possible. For me, uncertainty is the mother of anxiety, so I sought any action that would reduce uncertainty. (2) I laughed about it. For example, I told a friend he was going to plan a fishing trip as my "Make-A-Wish®" trip. He did so and has discharged me from the program at this point! (3) I broke the process into steps, focusing on one step at a time and no more. For example, I learned about treatment options by talking to people who had experienced various treatment approaches, researching treatment facilities, and so on.

Tim, clinical psychologist
Diagnosis of prostate cancer at age 65 in 2007 in Memphis, Tennessee

• • •

DURING CHEMOTHERAPY, I LISTENED to music that moved me on the little iPod Shuffle that an old friend brought me. I took walks by the river with my husband, looking at birds and taking photographs. He bought me a good pair of binoculars and a camera with good zoom lens. I went to a bookstore and bought a few books of poetry.

> ## "I find myself smiling a lot more at people I meet..."

Doris, library assistant
Diagnosis of breast cancer at age 60 in 2005 in Carmichael, California

• • •

I MADE THE DECISION not to try to work, as it was too draining with the type of chemotherapy regimen I was on. I rented movies through the mail and slept when I felt tired. I granted myself "amnesty" from doing things that were too taxing. I was in a fight for my life, so I devoted all my energies to that. I read books like *Angela's Ashes*, which actually made me grateful to have cancer instead of being a poor kid in pre-WWII Ireland. And if I wanted a trinket of some sort, I bought it.

Alycia, disabled
Diagnosis of breast cancer at age 44 in 2005 in East Berlin, Connecticut

"Every day I try to do something for someone else..."

I BECAME CLOSE FRIENDS with many other cancer patients, some who helped me through my ordeal and others who I have since helped through theirs. I know that I have inspired others who are going through what I went through, and I am grateful to be able to provide that and give others some hope when their cancer has just been diagnosed and they are feeling very low. I have become a stronger person, and my husband and I formed a very special bond through my cancer experience.

Janet, elementary school teacher
Diagnosis of colon cancer at age 42 in 1993 in Philadelphia, Pennsylvania

• • •

EVERY DAY I TRY to do something for someone else—either an e-mail or a card or a chat to encourage. I spend time with my small grandchildren, listening to them and praising their efforts.

Pat, retired
Diagnosis of colon and bladder cancer at age 74 in 2005 in Como (Western Australia)

• • •

WHEN I MEET PEOPLE who have been through what I have been through, we share our experiences and develop a bond. We belong to the same club—the survivors! I am a volunteer legislative ambassador with the American Cancer Society Cancer Action Network™ and participated in the Celebration on the Hill™ in Washington, D.C. It was a fabulous event; it was emotional and heartwarming to be among other survivors who are carrying the message to our legislators to support the fight to eliminate cancer! I also am co-chair of the publicity committee for my local community's Relay for Life®. Just this past year, we raised more than $400,000 for the American Cancer Society. So, has my life changed? You bet! I continue to lend my support to fight the battle against cancer!

Bryna, management development consultant
Diagnosis of tongue cancer at age 35 in 1985 in Brockton, Massachusetts

I HAVE HAD SO many blessings. I feel I am a different person, for the better now. I like myself now. I am a nicer, more compassionate person with everyone. I have God in my life and value everyday as a gift. I feel so much wiser and accept life as it comes; I enjoy life now. I feel as I am part of this world and in tune with everything in it.

Yvonne, paralegal
Diagnosis of colon cancer at age 48 in 2004 in San Antonio, Texas

• • •

CANCER IS A VERY individual experience. Each and every survivor (and we are all survivors from the day of diagnosis) will have a unique walk down the cancer path. However, we will all meet challenges and successes and failures that have been met and dealt with before us and will be met and dealt with again after us. It behooves us, therefore, not only to avail ourselves of the knowledge of those who have gone before us, but to endeavor to leave behind whatever we can that will benefit those who walk the path after us.

Barbara, homemaker
Diagnosis of breast cancer at age 38 in 1986 in Conway, Arkansas

• • •

WHEN I LET GO of my ego, I realized that I was letting go of the need to be perfect. I was no longer angry about my reflection in the mirror. I was able to look at my reconstructed breast and not have my heart sink to my stomach. When I let go of my need to be perfect, my ego, I was then able to experience the Universe as a loving place where I am free to be imperfect!

Debbie, hospice nurse
Diagnosis of breast cancer at age 52 in 2004 in Phoenix, Arizona

• • •

I HELP with the Cancer Survivors Network® and work on several survivor programs. Some days it is difficult to "do cancer," but it truly is an honor.

Karen, real estate broker
Diagnosis of breast cancer at age 38 in 2001 in Loganville, Georgia

I WAS ALWAYS a "control freak," and this made me learn more patience with people and to look at life for how precious it is.

James, retired police officer
Diagnosis of lymphoma at age 66 in 2007 in Sheridan, Wyoming

It means a great deal to me to be a survivor. I don't think most people realize how much it changes your life. It changed me for the better. Through this experience, I met some incredible people, and I appreciate my life more than ever before. I also appreciate other people more. It seems odd to say this, but being diagnosed with cancer was the best thing that ever happened to me—both physically and spiritually. If I could live my life over again, I wouldn't want to miss out on this life-changing experience.

SHARON OSBOURNE started The Sharon Osbourne Colon Cancer Program at Cedars-Sinai Medical Center in Los Angeles, California. Sharon received treatment there after her diagnosis of colon cancer in 2002.

I GRIEVE FOR WHAT I have lost through this experience. From my head to my toes, my body has been assaulted by the surgery, chemo, and radiation treatments (not from the cancer itself!). I no longer feel very feminine (no breasts; very short, thinning hair; short nails, no eye makeup). I am unable to lift heavy objects, especially with my left arm (where the lymph nodes were removed) so because of that, I do not feel as strong as I used to be. But I also hug myself and thank this body of mine for continuing to bounce back from treatment after treatment. It truly amazes me how my body can heal itself. So, on another level, I love my body. I also count all the scars as battle scars and am proud of them.

Elena, arts administrator
Diagnosis of inflammatory breast cancer at age 44 in 1999 in Silver Spring, Maryland

I AM MUCH BETTER to myself. I give myself permission to do totally silly things just because I feel like it. I turn my music loud and sing, even though I can't carry a tune. I got myself a sweet little dog from a rescue center. She brings such total joy to me. She reminds me how much fun it is to just be silly and free-spirited.

Brenda, government clerk
Diagnosis of breast cancer at age 58 in 2006 in Madison, Tennessee

• • •

DON'T IDEALIZE THE EXPERIENCE. Cancer is messy; cancer is painful. But it is part of life. Life is challenge. I describe the cancer experience as a train ride. Once you get on, you don't get off. I just keep going. I wish the train would stop, but it doesn't. So that is what I have in this life; that is what it is going to be for me. I'm going to enjoy my life.

Judy, chaplain
Diagnosis of colorectal cancer at age 48 in 2003 in Cudahy, Wisconsin

• • •

> "I give myself permission to do totally silly things just because I feel like it. I turn my music loud and sing, even though I can't carry a tune."

I HAVE BECOME a member of an entirely new community I knew nothing about before, namely, the community of cancer patients, cancer survivors, and caregivers. Previously, I would never have thought to concern myself with cancer or anyone involved with it, but I now stop and talk with everyone, especially other patients in the oncology waiting room at the clinic and those sitting next to me in the infusion center. I feel I am a part of something bigger than myself — it makes me proud, and it feels good.

Mike, retired real estate developer and cattle rancher
Diagnosis of colon cancer at age 66 in 2006 in Red Lodge, Montana

WE MOVED HOME to Ohio and were blessed to raise our daughter in a small town. I now work for the American Cancer Society with cancer patients, serving them with patient programs and survivorship programs.

Beth, health educator
Diagnosis of liver cancer at age 32 in 1990 in Fort Hood, Texas

• • •

TANNING BEDS are the devil. There is no "safe" tanning bed. I now know to never go to a tanning salon and have educated many of my friends about the dangers of tanning salons and how important it is to use sunblock at the beach. I pretty much set the example of what not to do, which thankfully made a lot of my friends think about their actions when it comes to the sun.

Jennifer, publicity coordinator
Diagnosis of melanoma (skin cancer) at age 21 in 2004 in San Diego, California

• • •

> "...this made me learn more patience with people and to look at life for how precious it is."

I THINK THE BEST thing was my mom and brother finally getting along. They hadn't talked for two years, and my diagnosis kind of brought them back together. That was better than anything anyone could have done to make my ordeal better for everyone.

Mary Anne, word processor
Diagnosis of melanoma (skin cancer) at age 26 in 2007 in Dixon, California

• • •

I LEARNED that it is better to tell people what they mean to us now, rather than to save it for a eulogy at a funeral service.

David, journeyman sheet metal worker
Diagnosis of breast cancer at age 63 in 2005 in Missoula, Montana

CANCER HAS FOCUSED ME.
Cancer has strengthened my relationships with my friends and family.
Cancer has brought me closer to God.
Cancer has made me a better, more compassionate physician.

Deborah, physician
Diagnosis of breast cancer at age 47 in 2007 in Overland Park, Kansas

I used to think that the biggest challenge I would face in my life would be climbing Everest, but that was until I was diagnosed with acute leukemia and given less than a year to live. My cancer experience was a huge wake-up call for me. It caused a fundamental shift in my perspective on many levels. Cancer scared the hell out of me and, to some degree, I guess I've been running from it ever since. I may be running from my past, but I am living fully in the present while climbing expectantly toward the future.

ALAN HOBSON is an adventurer who has climbed Mount Everest. Following his recovery from leukemia at the age of 42, he began to reach out to cancer survivors, encouraging them to exercise and to "climb back from cancer."

I DO WORRY MORE now, because you don't think that cancer can happen to you. I was only thirty-eight years old when I was diagnosed with a cancer that usually affects older men who smoke and drink. I did not smoke and would have an occasional cocktail. I try to let my doctors know if something concerns me, so that I do not go crazy with anxiety. I think fear of the unknown is worse than knowing what you are dealing with.

Kathy, babysitter
Diagnosis of tongue cancer at age 38 in 1997 in Niles, Illinois

I'M A DAMNED LUCKY lady. I know that any day, it could come back. But any day, a big bus could come along and run over me. Life is just like that. I wouldn't change it for anything because I'm a much happier person now than I was then—and I thought I was happy then!

Judy, retired accounting clerk
Diagnosis of lung cancer at age 64 in 2004 in Norwalk, California

As with many cancer survivors, having this disease made me understand what was really important. The small things I overlooked when I was well and fighting the rat race suddenly loomed very large. Now I value my husband more, watch my children more, hold my grandchildren more.

TERRY MUSIC was 46 years old when her breast cancer was diagnosed. She is the chief mission delivery officer of the American Cancer Society.

CHAPTER 16

• • •

What It Means to Be a Survivor

When I asked people what it meant to them to be a cancer survivor, I knew they would write some amazing things, and I was not disappointed. The survivors who participated in this book were so eloquent, this chapter needs only a brief introduction. I hope their powerful prose will resonate with you as this book comes to a close. Of the many excellent contributions in this chapter, none resonated more with me than the words shared by Tracey whose breast cancer was diagnosed in her thirties. She wrote, "I'm hope, grace, and mercy walking." I've thought of her statement a thousand times. Maybe you will, too.

• • •

A SMILE, ANOTHER DREAM that may come true (I still have a few of those). Another day I can love or even cry when I want to. A chance to tell my children the things they still need to learn and a chance for me to learn something new.

Kimatha, medical laboratory technician
Diagnosis of kidney cancer at age 42 in 2001 in Edinburgh, Indiana

• • •

I REFLECT that I am going to be sixty years old, and some survivors from my church's breast cancer support group are in their twenties. They have so much longer to deal with this disease, but they also will have more new technology to conquer their disease if it should return.

Pam, retired dental hygienist
Diagnosis of breast cancer at age 57 in 2005 in Lakeland, Florida

I FEEL I HAVE conquered the world, now that I am cancer free.

John, retired
Diagnosis of esophageal cancer at age 76 in 2006 in Jamestown, North Carolina

• • •

MY WIFE AND I prayed and, thankfully, my cancers were caught in time for me to have surgery. With the encouragement of my wife and the prayers of all, I am almost fully recovered. I continue to be allowed to work, run, and live another day...I too am a cancer survivor.

Charles, soldier in the United States Army
Diagnosis of prostate cancer and skin cancer at age 52 in 2007 in Colorado Springs, Colorado

• • •

I AM STILL HERE amongst the land of the living!

Celestine, property manager
Diagnosis of stomach cancer at age 45 in 2006 in Rosedale, Maryland

• • •

TO BE A SURVIVOR is to—
Celebrate every day that both feet hit the floor and you can take a step.
Celebrate every time we get together with friends, no matter what the reason.
Not assume that tomorrow will come; cherish this day for what it is.
Just smile; everything is so much better with a smile.

Mike, management professional
Diagnosis of rectal cancer at age 38 in 2006 in Rochester, New York

• • •

IT MEANS A LIFE ahead of me to guide my daughter in the right direction. To be there with her every step. To educate people so they know how to fight this cancer.

Candy, teacher
Diagnosis of thyroid cancer at age 31 in 2007 in El Paso, Texas

I TRIUMPHED OVER the scariest word in the English language.

Carlyn, administrative assistant
Diagnosis of Hodgkin disease at age 30 in 2004 in Willow Spring, North Carolina

• • •

I ACCEPT THE CHANGES and side effects, but recognize that I can improve beyond my former physical self.

Don, retired
Diagnosis of prostate cancer at age 74 in 2003 in Ocean Pines, Maryland

To me, survivorship is very much an attitude; it's a state of mind. How we interpret the experience of cancer and integrate it into our lives is fundamental to how we coexist with it. I have learned that hope is forever changing, and healing can come without curing.

SELMA SCHIMMEL is the founder of Vital Options® International and host of *The Group Room®*, a cancer talk radio show. A carrier of the BRCA1 mutation, she received a breast cancer diagnosis at age 28 in 1983 and a diagnosis of early-stage ovarian cancer in 2003, in Los Angeles, California.

I DON'T LIKE the term "survivor." I prefer "conqueror." To me, survival seems like something blew in and out like a storm, and somehow you made it through. No matter what, I want to be who I am and become a better person through my experiences. I want to take it almost as an opportunity to learn what I need to learn, to appreciate every little thing, to see the world from a different perspective. No matter what, I want to conquer a sense of hopelessness.

Judi, nurse
Diagnosis of breast cancer at age 40 in 2000 in Pen Argyl, Pennsylvania

IT MEANS EVERYTHING. It is who I am. I spent some fifty years searching for who I am, and now I can proudly say that I am a cancer survivor.

Linda, administrative assistant
Diagnosis of breast cancer at age 55 in 2006 in Superior, Colorado

• • •

PEACE.

> "I feel I have conquered the world, now that I am cancer free."

Kelly, certified nursing assistant
Diagnosis of cervical cancer at age 28 in 2003 in Holland, New York

• • •

THROUGHOUT LIFE I HAVE accepted what it brings: polio, cardiac bypass surgery, and cancer. I tell people I am a Triple Crown winner!

Phil, retired
Diagnosis of oral squamous cell carcinoma at age 78 in 2007 in Pawcatuck, Connecticut

• • •

BEING A CANCER SURVIVOR means I live with, absorb, and make as normal as possible the many side effects and ravages to my body, and I do so while celebrating the fact that I am alive at all! It is the mature recognition of how fragile life is and how valuable life is by respecting (without ignoring) all the messages your body and your life sends you. It means taking care of yourself well without shame or guilt, so that you are free to love others as long as you are able!

Dee, retired
Diagnosis of colon and kidney cancer at age 53 in 2000 in Wood Dale, Illinois

• • •

I WILL PERSIST, PERSEVERE, and live with passion!

Ronald, business owner and entrepreneur
Diagnosis of testicular cancer at age 20 in 1975 in Dover, New Hampshire

I FEEL WEIRD SAYING I am a cancer survivor. Asking what that is like is like asking what it means to be me. Do we ever have any idea about that? If you do, please help me get there; I am falling behind. All I can say is that I felt very fortunate before my diagnosis, and I feel very fortunate now. Each and every day, I think of how lucky I am.

Jennifer, federal officer with U.S. Customs and Border Patrol
Diagnosis of cervical cancer at age 36 in 2007 in Montreal, Quebec (Canada)

• • •

CANCER CANNOT TAKE from you what you refuse to give up. After two diagnoses of advanced cancers, I am cancer free! I have not lost my joy, my peace, or my laughter.

Angie, volunteer and cancer advocate
Diagnosis of vulvar cancer at age 31 in 1998 and breast cancer at age 36 in 2003 in Anderson, South Carolina

• • •

YOU BECOME A CANCER survivor the day your cancer is diagnosed. That's when the fight begins. Although the most obvious fight is physical, the mental fight is one that can wear people down. Having the right attitude, coupled with knowledge and its acquisition, helps in the journey. It made me realize that I am not invincible, but I can certainly put up a good fight while maintaining a decent quality of life.

Federico, cancer chemical biologist
Diagnosis of testicular cancer at age 32 in 2006 in Brookline, Massachusetts

I enjoy every day and every wrinkle!

CAROLYN RUNOWICZ, MD, received a diagnosis of breast cancer at the age of 41 in 1992. She specializes in gynecologic cancers and women's health. Dr. Runowicz is a past president of the American Cancer Society and remains a strong cancer advocate.

IT MEANS that I am a fighter, and I won.

Linda, patient advocate
Diagnosis of breast cancer at age 47 in 1998 in Selden, New York

• • •

SURVIVORSHIP MEANS that I can continue this life that I love and the ministry, which has been such a rich source of meaning in my life. It has also made me aware that healing, and not necessarily a cure, is now my goal.

Kyle, pastor
Diagnosis of kidney cancer at age 60 in 2004 in Johnstown, Pennsylvania

• • •

I'M PROUD TO BE a survivor, but I wish I had never been put in the position to play that role. Survivorship means you are alive to advocate for research, to help those who need help, and to gain a better perspective on what life is really about—loving and being loved, giving and sharing.

Kathie, nurse and social worker
Diagnosis of kidney cancer at age 53 in 2005 in Kingston, New York

• • •

A CANCER DIAGNOSIS is not a death sentence. It disturbs me that so many people in our small Italian town hate to mention the word cancer, and when they do, it is under their breath. Or they prefer to use phrases to describe cancer such as "an incurable illness" or "one of those modern illnesses that so many people die of." Yet, in this same small town, there are many people, like me, who have some form of cancer and are living with it—certainly struggling in many cases, even for many years, but still enjoying life. Everyone should know about those people, for they are living witnesses that cancer is not the invariable killer that so many people believe it to be. So we should talk openly about our cancer. I admit that when I was first diagnosed, I only told family and the closest of friends. Later, I began talking about it openly. I hope, by doing so, I have dispelled some of the worries that others may have about contracting a blood cancer like mine.

Colin, writer and author
Diagnosis of chronic lymphocytic leukemia at age 62 in 1998 in Roma (Italy)

TODAY, I DO NOT have cancer.

Mary, business assistant
Diagnosis of synovial sarcoma of the right forearm at age 44 in 2006 in McPherson, Kansas

· · ·

A CANCER SURVIVOR is someone who has faced a cancer diagnosis and did what they needed to do to be healed. I say "healed" because some people are never cured or never reach a point where they have no evidence of disease. Yet they live, enjoy life, and treat each day as being special.

Dorinda, retired teacher
Diagnosis of ovarian cancer at age 50 in 2005 in Edison, New Jersey

· · ·

I DO NOT CONSIDER myself lucky or, indeed, a "survivor." I am just someone who managed to get through treatment and maybe, just maybe, I will live for more years than I dare to wish for.

Pearl, nurse
Diagnosed at age 32 with breast cancer in 2004 in Glasgow (Scotland)

· · ·

> "Throughout life I have accepted what it brings: polio, cardiac bypass surgery, and cancer. I tell people I am a Triple Crown winner!"

SURVIVING MEANS THAT I'M so lucky and so blessed, that I'm stronger than I ever knew. I know that I can do things I'm afraid of because, if I can survive cancer, I can do just about anything. It also means I carry a certain fear with me that never goes away. When I carry them both—the strength and the fear—it makes me aware of how I cherish my life and how uncertain everything is. It's an interesting journey.

Cathi, clinical social worker
Diagnosis of breast cancer at age 52 in 2003 in Waban, Massachusetts

IT MEANS THAT I am strong. Stronger than I ever thought I was. It means I can really accomplish anything because I've accomplished this. It means that cancer was, is, and will be forever a part of my life and who I am. It also means that I have a duty to use my experience to help others with theirs. It means that I have to tell my story so that it helps others and also motivates others to make cancer programs a national priority. I don't want others to feel sorry for me because I am "so young" and have fought off two different cancers. I want people to see my strength and to see how cancer has positively influenced my life. It could have been a death sentence for me, but it was really a life sentence. It was a prescription to go out and live my life and touch others while doing so.

Todd, oncology social worker
Diagnosis of chronic myelogenous leukemia at age 25 in 1997 and kidney cancer in 2005 at age 33 in Warwick, Rhode Island

• • •

I AM IN ONE hell of a club.

Matt, carpenter
Diagnosis of chronic lymphocytic leukemia at age 51 in 2003 in Bath, New York

• • •

> "I feel weird saying I am a cancer survivor. Asking what that is like is like asking what it means to be me."

I AM A FOURTH-GENERATION breast cancer survivor. I always knew I would have breast cancer; I was just a little surprised to have it at age thirty-two. I knew right away I was going to survive. I just needed to get the facts and develop a plan of action. In doing that, I survived. I hope that doing what I did will leave a mark on the future. I believe I am a part of history in the fight against cancer.

Shelly, program coordinator for adults with disabilities
Diagnosis of breast cancer at age 32 in 2004 in Concord, New Hampshire

I HAVE BECOME A MEMBER of a "reluctant brotherhood." I mean, that I would still give anything not to have undergone what I've just been through, yet here I am, a survivor...and a member of a group no one wants to belong to. I do feel lucky that my cancer was detected early, and I am apparently "cured." Being a survivor also means having insights to an experience that non-cancer people do not, and perhaps cannot, have. This implies no special privilege...it just means that living through cancer changes the way I look at, and think about, the world and my life.

Bill, administrator
Diagnosis of prostate cancer at age 62 in 2007 in Jefferson, Wisconsin

• • •

BEING A CANCER SURVIVOR means living my life. I have chosen not to let the fact that I survived cancer define me as a person. Rather, I draw from the strength I found while I was recovering.

Sarah, paralegal
Diagnosis of breast cancer at age 28 in 2000 in Miami, Florida

• • •

ALTHOUGH MY OUTCOME was positive, I had an overlooked lung cancer and debated with several doctors on what to do about it. For whatever reason, I survived a bout with colon cancer and the removal of my left lung in the summer of 2004. I had enough radiation treatments to light up the entire East Coast, and I consumed enough chemo-juice to float a battleship. Logic and the odds said I would not make it, but I have! I lie awake at night, wondering why I survived. I have no answer. People have asked me how I was able to handle this or that treatment/process. My response was and still is, "What choice did I have?" You find doctors you trust, and then you do what they say. What happens, happens!

Bill, retired
Diagnosis of colon and lung cancer at age 63 in 2004 in Niceville, Florida

• • •

HONESTLY, IT MEANS I am not dead yet!

Evelyn, executive assistant
Diagnosis of colon cancer at age 33 in 2004 in Boston, Massachusetts

I'VE COPED with the "mack truck" collision that occurs when news of a cancer diagnosis brings your life and your plans to a screeching halt. I've known what it's like to be sicker than I ever thought possible...and to get better; to be so fatigued that I couldn't sit up; to know the kindness of hospital workers and friends; to feel so very alone...and at the same time part of a huge community of people out there who also proudly call themselves cancer survivors. To me, cancer survivorship is not about getting through cancer without dying. To me, it is about living through cancer treatment and then finding a way to integrate the impact of that news and that treatment back into your life.

Andrea, hospital administrator
Diagnosis of Ewing's sarcoma (a form of bone cancer) at age 15 in 1992 in Norfolk, Massachusetts

• • •

THIS MEANS that I am one of the fortunate ones who were able to get treatment and to keep cancer at bay. I feel so blessed!

Laura, housecleaner
Diagnosis of esophageal cancer at age 45 in 2002 in Schenectady, New York

• • •

I THINK that a "survivor" is someone who has really bad cancer and amazingly pulls through. I minimize my cancer because it was diagnosed early and was not life-threatening.

Sally, research laboratory administrator
Diagnosis of breast cancer at age 40 in 1990 in Salem, Massachusetts

• • •

I AM A SURVIVOR because I am here to talk about my cancer. The cancer was removed from my body in January 2007, and since that moment I have been a survivor. I survived my chemo treatments; now I will survive the rest of my life. I want to live a long life.

Debra, administrative assistant
Diagnosis of ovarian cancer at age 51 in 2007 in Chicago, Illinois

I'VE BEEN A CANCER survivor so long I don't know anything else. It means my life is different from that of most people at my age, and it takes a lot of strength to keep going.

Pamela, bookkeeper
Diagnosis of Hodgkin disease at age 23 in 1983, basal cell carcinoma (skin cancer) at age 41 in 2001, and breast cancer at age 46 in 2006 in Gardiner, Maine

Being a cancer survivor to me means that I'm still here. It's that simple. You can get very philosophical, pretentious, and even smug when referring to yourself as a cancer survivor. You can boast about how you overcame so much pain and fear and adversity, about how you are a fighter, and about how you are strong. But what's the bottom line? Being a cancer survivor simply means I am still alive. I am still here, and that is a very, very good thing. 'Nuff said.

JAMIE RENO is a *Newsweek* correspondent who received a diagnosis of stage IV, low-grade, follicular non-Hodgkin lymphoma at age 35. In his "other life," Jamie is an acclaimed singer-songwriter and guitarist whose CD, *Survivors' Songs*, is for lymphoma cancer awareness. This all-star album features a dozen music legends, including Peter Frampton, Charlie Daniels, and members of The Beach Boys family.

IT MEANS that my cancer was not my mother's cancer, and if my daughter has to go through this experience, hers will be easier. If there is any justice in the world, it means my granddaughter will not have to worry about it at all.

Pat, office manager
Diagnosis of breast cancer at age 53 in 2001 in Canton, Michigan

I FEEL EXTREMELY FORTUNATE. My cancer survivorship has become the latest phase of my life. I am fully engaged and seek to perpetuate it. I am enjoying it immensely. I wouldn't say that cancer has changed my life for the better—I wouldn't go that far. But it is certainly a very important phase in my life, along with the many others I've experienced. I've developed strengths, skills, and attitudes I never had or needed before, and they are all benefiting me now.

Mike, retired real estate developer and cattle rancher
Diagnosis of colon cancer at age 66 in 2006 in Red Lodge, Montana

• • •

WHILE I WAS GOING through treatment, all I wanted was to be a survivor. Now it represents a battle won. It represents strength, faith, perseverance—it's hard to fully articulate, because it is very emotional.

Eileen, teacher
Diagnosis of breast cancer at age 43 in 2006 in Hilton, New York

• • •

AT FIRST DIAGNOSIS, you might think it is the worst thing that could happen. But in reality, it has been the best thing for me. My priorities are in order, I have met so many wonderful people and have had so many opportunities to share, cry, and comfort others. Try to keep a positive attitude. Schedule your "pity party" day, and then live your life.

Beth, health educator
Diagnosis of liver cancer at age 32 in 1990 in Fort Hood, Texas

• • •

EVEN THOUGH I HAD an "easy" type of cancer, this is something that I will fight for the rest of my life. I hope that I can help educate people about the thyroid and the many functions it controls in your body. Although many people think that it's no big deal, to me and my family, it is a very big deal. We are proud to have gotten through it together, especially with two little children.

Nicki, homemaker
Diagnosis of thyroid cancer at age 20 in 2005 in Union, Missouri

I DON'T LIKE to call myself a cancer survivor. I'm not really sure why.

Kelley, massage therapist
Diagnosis of breast cancer at age 36 in 2006 in Rochdale, Massachusetts

• • •

BEING A CANCER SURVIVOR isn't easy. On the one hand, I am thrilled that the cancer has not come back. On the other hand, I am dealing with so many related issues that some days I find myself totally overwhelmed. People see me dressed well, with my makeup firmly in place, and they tell me how great I look. Some people tell me what a hero I am. I am not a hero—I fought a battle (and am still fighting). The alternative was not one I would even consider.

Eileen, technology specialist
Diagnosis of breast cancer at age 34 in 1984, acute myelogenous leukemia at age 49 in 1999, and basal cell carcinoma (skin cancer) at age 55 in 2005 in Framingham, Massachusetts

• • •

I DESERVE TO LIVE a good and happy life—to have another day to hug my kids, kiss my husband and hold hands, and tell them all how much I love them and how much they mean to me!

Rochelle, manicurist
Diagnosis of melanoma (skin cancer) at age 34 in 2007 in Las Vegas, Nevada

• • •

> "The mental fight is one that can wear people down. Having the right attitude, coupled with knowledge and its acquisition, helps..."

I FEEL PROUD. I feel strong. When faced with a challenge, I think back...if I could handle cancer, I can handle this.

Sheri, actress
Diagnosis of Hodgkin disease at age 29 in 1993 in Columbia, Maryland

I WILL NEVER SAY I am cured of cancer, and I don't think of myself as a survivor, even though I am considered one.

Joyce, educational assistant at an elementary school
Diagnosis of breast cancer at 41 in 1995 in Knoxville, Tennessee

• • •

TO BE A CANCER survivor means that you just went through hell. Your whole body and being are affected. Your whole life is affected. Your family's lives are affected. No one will know that feeling until you've personally experienced it. It's being able to get past the surgery, the treatments, the nausea, the possible hair loss, and then heal physically, emotionally, and spiritually. If you are waiting for the magic five years to pass, emotionally, it is very draining. Numerous testing...and the list goes on. This is a lot for a person to go through. Thank God when a person survives this ordeal. This is a cancer survivor: the one who does not give up hope, the one who gets another chance at life. This person deserves a medal.

Vera, personal assistant
Diagnosis of thyroid cancer at age 51 in 2002 in Milwaukee, Wisconsin

• • •

SINCE MY CANCER has recurred twice, being a survivor right now means that I have fought a good fight and that God has been very gracious to me. It also means that I am determined to keep fighting, so that I can be a five-year-plus survivor of ovarian cancer. I know that my cancer can return, and I do not take any day for granted.

Patti, financial administrator
Diagnosis of ovarian cancer at age 51 in 2005 in Colorado Springs, Colorado

Survivorship is a rocky road, but at least I'm still on it!

ELLEN STOVALL, president and CEO of the National Coalition for Cancer Survivorship, received three cancer diagnoses, including Hodgkin disease at age 24 in 1971, recurrent Hodgkin disease at age 36 in 1983, and breast cancer at age 61 in 2007.

USING THE TERM SURVIVOR to describe myself was one of the hardest things I had to overcome. I was superstitious about it and afraid to use it. It took me years to feel comfortable with it and to be able to say (in the past tense), "I had cancer."

Janet, elementary school teacher
Diagnosis of colon cancer at age 42 in 1993 in Philadelphia, Pennsylvania

• • •

I FEEL LIKE IT should be termed "cancer warrior" instead of "survivor."

Laurie, medical assistant
Diagnosis of breast cancer at age 43 in 2006 in Sacramento, California

• • •

I DON'T LIKE IT, but God has given me this gift and this voice, and He has allowed me to be a survivor. So, I receive every day as a gift and a blessing, and I take every opportunity to share my experience with someone else.

Julie, real estate agent
Diagnosis of thyroid cancer at age 34 in 1996 and breast cancer at age 43 in 2005 in Torrance, California

• • •

IS IT FUN? Hell, no. But after fifteen months, one mammogram, two ultrasounds, one MRI, one biopsy, two surgical procedures, six months of chemo, thirty-three radiation treatments, with the fun of third-degree radiation burns on my neck, I can gladly say, "I am a survivor."

Jerri, state employee
Diagnosis of breast cancer at age 48 in 2006 and endometrial (uterine) cancer at age 50 in 2008 in Standish, Michigan

• • •

I AM A MIRACLE and, according to all the statistics, I should not be here.

Susan, homemaker
Diagnosis of acute myelogenous leukemia at age 50 in 2003 in Medina, Ohio

> # "I can really accomplish anything because I've accomplished this."

IT MEANS A GREAT deal to me! I feel like I've accomplished something, that I beat it, and I'm proud of that.

Marla, executive assistant
Diagnosis of breast cancer at age 35 in 1994 in Jasper, Indiana

• • •

AFTER MANY DAYS and nights of denial and crying, I decided to live for today. To do what I wanted to do. To take one day at a time.

Audrey, disabled
Diagnosis of lung cancer at age 51 in 2007 in Baltimore, Maryland

• • •

IT MEANS THAT YOU can help other people get through it. I am proud every day, and I am thankful that I am okay. I feel that I am a special person for having survived. People make you feel special, especially at the Relay for Life®.

Lovey, homemaker
Diagnosis of uterine cancer at age 52 in 2000 in Cadiz, Kentucky

• • •

I HAVE A STRONG will to live. So, to be cancer free, to be a survivor, means that I have survived four bouts. I have won the battle! I want to help others win their battles!

Bryna, management development consultant
Diagnosis of tongue cancer at age 35 in 1985 in Brockton, Massachusetts

• • •

IT MEANS I'M a strong person. Being a cancer survivor means I'm lucky to be alive. Having survived the Big C, I know I can handle anything that life throws at me now.

Danielle, financial service specialist
Diagnosis of melanoma (skin cancer) at age 30 in 2000 in Ramstein (Germany)

IT MEANS I AM winning at life and here to prove it!
I have survived the diagnosis.
I have survived the physical and emotional part of cancer.
I have survived the financial part of cancer.
I will continue to survive the rest of the cancer baggage.

Kathryn, homemaker
Diagnosis of multiple myeloma at age 39 in 2001 and basal cell carcinoma
(skin cancer) at age 45 in 2007 in St. Charles, Missouri

• • •

WHEN FACED with my own mortality, I was able to take charge and become a better person. It means I'm someone people can come to when they need help dealing with adversity.

Maureen, manager
Diagnosis of breast cancer at age 40 in 2004 in Camarillo, California

> I absorb and fully experience more each day than I thought possible. You can never get a "non-cancer" survivor to understand those words. It is truly being handed a second chance. Forgive the Jersey vernacular, but, "You don't wanna screw it up!"
>
> **JOE PISCOPO**, actor and comedian, received a diagnosis of thyroid cancer at age 30 in 1981.

BEING A SURVIVOR MEANS I am thankful to everyone on my medical team and grateful for every day and every person in my life. It means that I enjoy living, loving, and working, and I do not take that for granted.

Barbara, nurse
Diagnosis of breast cancer at age 58 in 1995 in Stoneham, Massachusetts

There have been remarkable strides in cancer research over the past decade. Our understanding of the underlying biology of cancer is advancing more rapidly than ever before. More important, this understanding has led to a whole new generation of targeted cancer treatments that are making a major impact on the lives of many individuals with cancer. Hard work, dedication, and funding for cancer research will be indispensable, but I view the next decade of cancer research and cancer treatment with great optimism.

ERIC WINER, MD, is chief of the Division of Women's Cancers at the Dana-Farber Cancer Institute in Boston, Massachusetts. He is also the chief scientific advisor for Susan G. Komen for the Cure.

THAT I AM SPECIAL, a hero and, I hope, a good example to others faced with this.

Allie, Director, Distinguished Events; American Cancer Society
Diagnosis of thyroid cancer at age 46 in 2003 in Fair Haven, New Jersey

• • •

IT MEANS A LOT to me to be a cancer survivor. I did my first Relay for Life® with my company the year after my diagnosis, and I bawled like a baby during the survivors' lap.

Michele, facilities manager
Diagnosis of colon cancer at age 42 in 2006 in Charles Town, West Virginia

• • •

LIFE IS A JOURNEY, and just because the word cancer is spoken does not mean your life is over. I did not realize all the obstacles I could overcome.

Mariann, receptionist
Diagnosis of bladder cancer at age 50 in 2002 and endometrial (uterine) cancer at age 50 in 2003 in West Haven, Connecticut

I AM PROUD. I am strong.

Jocelyn, social worker
Diagnosis of breast cancer at age 43 in 2006 in Macedon, New York

• • •

AT THE TIME of my first cancer diagnosis in 1989, I had a vaginal hysterectomy, and no other treatment was necessary. It was almost as if I never had cancer. I did not include myself with other cancer patients; I had not suffered enough in my mind's eye. I actually really did not consider myself a survivor until after my 2005 diagnosis of stage IV colorectal cancer.

Cindy, staffing specialist
Diagnosis of cervical cancer at age 32 in 1989 and colorectal cancer at age 48 in 2005 in Maryville, North Dakota

• • •

IT'S A PRIVILEGE. I feel like I belong to a little secret society. We all understand. Most of us "get it" now—what's important.

Karen, real estate broker
Diagnosis of breast cancer at age 38 in 2001 in Loganville, Georgia

• • •

> "Logic and the odds said I would not make it, but I have! I lie awake at night, wondering why I survived. I have no answer."

EVERY DAY, THERE ARE more and more cancer survivors out here, running around, living their lives. Medical science hasn't yet found out how to eliminate it, but one day it will. Until then, they have some darn good ways of taking care of us, and as a survivor, I'm more grateful than I could ever say.

Judy, retired accounting clerk
Diagnosis of lung cancer at age 64 in 2004 in Norwalk, California

I WEAR IT LIKE a badge of courage, and I try to impart to others that they need not toss their hands up in defeat because there are exciting and promising new approaches being used right now. To be able to say that I stared cancer down gives me an enormous feeling of satisfaction.

Jerry, computer software instructor
Diagnosis of acute myelogenous leukemia at age 43 in 2003 in Anoka, Minnesota

I believe that having cancer didn't define my life; it simply added texture to it. I would not wish for this to happen to me again or to anyone, but I can say that it has enriched me in some way. I am more compassionate than before. I listen more closely than before. I walk more slowly than before.

TERRY MUSIC was 46 years old when her breast cancer was diagnosed. She is the chief mission delivery officer of the American Cancer Society.

SURVIVING CANCER MEANS that I'm going to be around to see my son grow up, get married, and have his own family. I'll be a grandmother and spoil my grandchildren like my mother spoils my son. I'll enjoy retirement with my husband. I won't be deprived of all of the things that I'm looking forward to as part of growing old.

Laura, unemployed psychiatric social worker
Diagnosis of breast cancer at age 43 in 2006 in Avon, Connecticut

• • •

TO HAVE A SECOND chance to be the kind of mom, grandma, wife, sister, daughter, friend, and aunt that I'm supposed to be.

Linda, purchasing agent
Diagnosis of breast cancer at age 47 in 2007 in Antioch, California

IT'S LIKE BACKGROUND MUSIC that only other survivors can hear. I will never be over cancer; it just will become a part of who I am.

Deborah, physician
Diagnosis of breast cancer at age 47 in 2007 in Overland Park, Kansas

• • •

EVERYTHING IN THE WORLD! I get to tell the young ladies how important it is to get a mammogram and do monthly breast exams. I beat that evil thing. I won the battle!

Jo Anne, nurse's aide
Diagnosis of breast cancer at age 51 in 2003 in Brownstown, Michigan

• • •

I'M HOPE, GRACE, AND MERCY walking. I'm literally flying without wings, one day at a time.

Tracey, radiation oncology information analyst
Diagnosis of breast cancer at age 37 in 2002 in Villa Park, Illinois

"To be able to say that I stared cancer down gives me an enormous feeling of satisfaction."

RESOURCES

• • •

American Cancer Society Programs

The following list includes American Cancer Society (ACS) programs mentioned by contributors to this book. For more information on these and other ACS programs, go to our Web site: **http://www.cancer.org**, or call our toll-free number at any time, 24 hours a day: **800-ACS-2345**.

Cancer Action Network™ (ACS CAN) is all about ensuring that fighting cancer is a top priority for our lawmakers. When constituents demand that legislators make fighting cancer a priority, they make a difference. All ACS CAN members are notified of cancer-related issues pending in government agencies. They are also notified when critical cancer issues are heading for a vote or are in danger of being ignored by our lawmakers.

Internet address: http://www.acscan.org/

The Cancer Survivors Network® comprises a community of cancer survivors, families, and friends! All have been touched by cancer and want to share their experiences, strength, and hope. Only those who have been there can truly understand. The Web site is completely non-commercial and provides a private, secure way to find and communicate with others to share similar interests and experiences. Members control access to personal information.

Internet address: http://www.acscsn.org/

Celebration on the Hill™, Washington, D.C., (last held, 2006) is an American Cancer Society Cancer Action Network event celebrating cancer survivorship and empowering survivors and others to advocate for laws that will help fight the disease.

Internet address: http://www.celebrationonthehill.org/

Look Good…Feel Better® is a free, community-based program that teaches beauty techniques to female cancer patients who are currently undergoing chemotherapy or radiation treatment, to help restore their appearance and self-image. The program is a partnership between the American Cancer Society; the Cosmetic, Toiletry, and Fragrance Association Foundation; and the National Cosmetology Association.

Internet address: http://www.lookgoodfeelbetter.org/

The *Patient Navigator* program is a service of the American Cancer Society (ACS), in which ACS staff members are made available to cancer patients in community hospitals, just after diagnosis. The "navigator" is a friendly, experienced, and approachable ACS staff person who helps patients have a better experience while they are receiving care.

Reach to Recovery® has helped people (female and male) cope with their breast cancer experience. This experience begins when someone is faced with the possibility of a breast cancer diagnosis and continues throughout the entire period that breast cancer remains a personal concern. Reach to Recovery volunteers offer understanding, support, and hope because they themselves have survived breast cancer and have gone on to live normal, productive lives.

Internet address: http://www.cancer.org

Relay For Life®, the American Cancer Society's signature event, is an overnight experience designed to bring together those who have been touched by cancer. At Relay, people from within the community gather to celebrate survivors, remember those lost to cancer, and to fight back against this disease. Relay participants help raise money and awareness to support the American Cancer Society in its life-saving mission to eliminate cancer as a major health issue.

Internet address: http://www.relayforlife.org/relay/

Other Resources

The following list comprises organizations and Web sites focused on cancer research, support services, and education. Many of these organizations were mentioned by contributors to this book. The list is not comprehensive, and inclusion here does not imply endorsement by the American Cancer Society.

American Academy of Physical Medicine and Rehabilitation (for locating physiatrists)
330 North Wabash Avenue
Suite 2500
Chicago, IL 60611-7617
Phone: 312-464-9700
Fax: 312-464-0227
E-mail: info@aapmr.org
Internet address: http://www.aapmr.org/

The American Academy of Physical Medicine and Rehabilitation is the national medical society representing more than 7,500 physicians who are specialists in the field of physical medicine and rehabilitation.

American Breast Cancer Foundation
1220 B East Joppa Road, Suite 332
Baltimore, MD 21286
Phone: 877-539-2543 (877-Key-2-Life)
Fax: 410-825-4395
Internet address: www.abcf.org

The American Breast Cancer Foundation is a nonprofit organization dedicated to providing a fighting chance to every individual threatened by breast cancer—regardless of age, race, or financial challenge—through screening assistance programs, research, and support.

American Occupational Therapy Association, Inc.
4720 Montgomery Lane
P. O. Box 31220
Bethesda, MD 20824-1220
Phone: 301-652-2682
Fax: 301-652-7711
Toll Free: 800-377-8555
Internet address: http://www.aota.org/

The American Occupational Therapy Association (AOTA) is the national professional association established in 1917 to represent the interests and concerns of occupational therapy practitioners and students of occupational therapy and to improve the quality of occupational therapy services.

American Physical Therapy Association
1111 North Fairfax Street
Alexandria, VA 22314-1488
Toll Free: 800-999-APTA (2782)
Fax: 703-684-7343
Internet address: http://www.apta.org/

The American Physical Therapy Association (APTA) is a national professional organization representing more than 72,000 members. Its goal is to foster advancements in physical therapy practice, research, and education.

American Speech-Language-Hearing Association
2200 Research Boulevard
Rockville, MD 20850-3289
Phone: 301-296-5700
Fax: 301-296-8580
E-mail: actioncenter@asha.org
Internet address: http://www.asha.org/

The American Speech-Language-Hearing Association (ASHA) is the professional, scientific, and credentialing association for more than 130,000 members and affiliates who are audiologists, speech-language pathologists, and speech, language, and hearing scientists.

(R.A.) Bloch Cancer Foundation, Inc.
Bloch Cancer Hotline
One H&R Block Way
Kansas City, MO 64105
Phone: 816-854-5050
Fax: 816-854-8024
Toll Free: 800-433-0464
Internet address: http://www.blochcancer.org/

The focus of the R. A. Bloch Cancer Foundation is to help all cancer patients in the process to successfully conquer their disease.

Bosom Buddies
11024 N. 28th Drive
Suite 200
Phoenix, AZ 85029
Phone: 602-265-2776
Fax: 602-279-5857
E-mail: info@bosombuddies-az.org
Internet address:
http://www.bosombuddies-az.org/

Bosom Buddies is a nonprofit organization of caring volunteers who have personal experience dealing with the trauma and challenges of breast cancer. The mission is to provide support through sharing of common experiences and knowledge.

Breast Cancer Network of Strength (formerly Y-Me National Breast Cancer Organization)
Toll Free: 800-221-2141 (National Hotline)
Toll Free: 800-986-9505 (Spanish Hotline)
Internet address: www.networkofstrength.org

CancerCare
275 Seventh Avenue
Floor 22
New York, NY 10001
Toll Free: 800-813-HOPE (4673)
Administrative: 212-712-8400
Fax: 212-712-8495
E-mail: info@cancercare.org
Internet address: http://www.cancercare.org/

CancerCare is a national nonprofit organization that provides free, professional support services for anyone affected by cancer.

CancerConnection
P. O. Box 60452
Florence, MA 01062
Phone: 413-586-1642
Internet address:
http://www.cancer-connection.org/

CancerConnection is a community-based,

nonprofit organization. Founded in 2000, it offers a haven where people living with cancer, their families, and their caregivers can learn how to cope with their changed lives and bodies and emotional turmoil by sharing strategies and resources. All offerings are free.

Cancer Hope Network
Two North Road, Suite A
Chester, NJ 07930
Phone: 877-467-3638
Fax: 908-879-6518
Internet address:
http://www.cancerhopenetwork.org

The Cancer Hope Network is a nonprofit organization that matches adult cancer patients with trained volunteers who have undergone and recovered from a similar cancer experience. Volunteers provide free and confidential one-on-one telephone support. Support for family members is also available.

Casting for Recovery®
P. O. Box 1123
3738 Main Street
Manchester, VT 05254
Phone: 802-362-9181
Fax: 802-362-9182
Toll Free: 888-553-3500
E-mail: info@castingforrecovery.org
Internet address:
http://www.castingforrecovery.org/

Casting for Recovery is a national nonprofit, support and educational program for women who have or have had breast cancer.

Colon Cancer Alliance
1200 G Street NW
Suite 800
Washington, DC 20005
Phone: 202-434-8980
Fax: 202-434-8980

Toll Free: 877-422-2030
Internet address: http://www.ccalliance.org/

The Colon Cancer Alliance is committed to ending the suffering and death caused by colorectal cancer.

FORCE: Facing Our Risk of Cancer Empowered
16057 Tampa Palms Blvd West, PMB 373
Tampa, FL 33647
Phone: 954-255-8732
Fax: 954-827-2200
Toll Free: 866-824-7475
Internet address: www.facingourrisk.org

Facing Our Risk of Cancer Empowered is a nonprofit organization for individuals and families affected by hereditary breast cancer and ovarian cancer, due to the BRCA mutation or a family history of these cancers.

Gilda's Club
322 Eighth Avenue
Suite 1402
New York, NY 10001
Phone: 888-GILDA-4-U
Fax: 917-305-0549
E-mail: info@gildasclub.org
Internet address: http://www.gildasclub.org/

Gilda's Club provides welcoming communities for everyone living with cancer—men, women, teens, and children. It is distinguished by its unique philosophy and program. Completely free of charge, Gilda's Club encourages a sense of "expertise" among members and emphasizes community-building, collective wisdom, and shared experience.

Inflammatory Breast Cancer Help
Internet address: www.ibchelp.org

Inflammatory Breast Cancer Help is a Web-based organization that provides information specific to inflammatory breast cancer.

Inflammatory Breast Cancer Research Foundation

321 High School Road NE, Suite 149
Bainbridge Island, WA 98110
Phone: 877-786-7422
Internet address: www.ibcresearch.org

The Inflammatory Breast Cancer Research Foundation is dedicated to the advancement of research in inflammatory breast cancer, in order to find its causes and to improve treatment. The organization also seeks to increase awareness of symptoms of inflammatory breast cancer, leading to better clinical methods of detection and diagnosis.

International Myeloma Foundation

IMF International Headquarters
12650 Riverside Drive, Suite 206
North Hollywood, CA 91607
Phone: 818-487-7455
Fax: 818-487-7454
Internet address: http://myeloma.org/

The International Myeloma Foundation is dedicated to improving the quality of life of myeloma patients while working toward prevention and a cure.

The Lance Armstrong Foundation

P. O. Box 161150
Austin, TX 78716-1150
Phone: 512-236-8820
Internet address: http://www.livestrong.org/

The Lance Armstrong Foundation was established to inspire and empower people affected by cancer. It provides practical information and tools people with cancer need to live life on their own terms. It takes aim at the gaps between what is known and what is done to prevent suffering and death due to cancer.

Leukemia & Lymphoma Society (LLS)

1311 Mamaroneck Avenue
White Plains, NY 10605
Phone: 914-949-5213
Fax: 914-949-6691
Toll Free: 800-955-4572
Internet address:
http://www.leukemia-lymphoma.org/hm_lls

The mission of the Leukemia & Lymphoma Society (LLS) is to cure leukemia, lymphoma, Hodgkin disease, and myeloma, and improve the quality of life of patients and their families.

Living Beyond Breast Cancer

10 East Athens Avenue, Suite 204
Ardmore, PA 19003
Toll Free: 888-753-5222
Internet address: www.lbbc.org

Living Beyond Breast Cancer is a national nonprofit education and support organization dedicated to empowering all women affected by breast cancer to live as long as possible with the best quality of life.

Make-A-Wish Foundation®

4041 North Central Avenue
Suite 555
Phoenix, AZ 85012
Phone: 602-230-9900
Fax: 602-230-9627
Internet address: http://www.wish.org/

The mission of the Make-A-Wish Foundation is to grant the wishes of children with life-threatening medical conditions to enrich the human experience with hope, strength, and joy.

Making Memories Breast Cancer Foundation, Inc.

270 Probe Street
Molalla, OR 97038
Phone: 503-829-4486
Fax: 503-829-3871
Business Hours: M-F 9 AM–5 PM PT
(If voicemail answers, leave a message for return call.)

Internet address:
http://www.makingmemories.org

Making Memories is a national nonprofit organization that uses donated items (such as wedding gowns and diamonds) to fulfill wishes of adult patients coping with stage IV terminal breast cancer. Cash and in-kind donations, airline vouchers, and time-share or vacation stays are some forms of donation.

Men Against Breast Cancer
P. O. Box 150
Adamstown, MD 21710-0150
Toll Free: 866-547-6222 (Leave a message for return call if answered by voice mail.)
Fax: 301-874-8657
Internet address:
www.menagainstbreastcancer.org

Men Against Breast Cancer is a nonprofit organization designed to educate and empower men to be effective caregivers when breast cancer strikes a loved one, and to mobilize men in the fight to eradicate breast cancer.

Mothers Supporting Daughters with Breast Cancer
21710 Bayshore Road
Chestertown, MD 21620-4401
Phone: 410-778-1982
Internet address: www.mothersdaughters.org

MSDBC encourages those with Internet access to use the Web site rather than the phone number.

Mothers Supporting Daughters with Breast Cancer is a nonprofit Web-based organization providing support services specifically to help mothers with daughters battling breast cancer.

Multiple Myeloma Research Foundation
383 Main Avenue
5th floor
Norwalk, CT 06851
Phone: 203-229-0464

E-mail: info@themmrf.org
Internet address:
http://www.multiplemyeloma.org/

The mission of the MMRF is to urgently and aggressively fund research that will lead to the development of new treatments for multiple myeloma.

National Asian Women's Health Organization
1 Embarcadero Center, Suite 500
San Francisco, CA 94111
Phone: 415-773-2838
Fax: 415-773-2872
Internet address: www.nawho.org

National Asian Women's Health Organization is a national nonprofit health organization whose mission is to achieve health equity for Asian women and their families.

National Breast and Cervical Cancer Early Detection Program
Centers for Disease Control and Prevention
Division of Cancer Prevention and Control
4770 Buford Hwy NE, MS K-64
Atlanta, GA 30341-3717
Toll Free: 800-232-4636; Select Option 1, "General Health Information"
Fax: 770-488-4760
Internet address: www.cdc.gov/cancer

The National Breast and Cervical Cancer Early Detection Program (NBCCEDP) provides screening services, including clinical breast examination, mammograms, pelvic examination, and Pap tests to women underserved in the health care community. The NBCCEDP also funds post-screening diagnostic services, such as surgical consultation and biopsy, to ensure that all women with abnormal results receive timely and adequate referrals.

National Breast Cancer Coalition
1101 17th Street NW, Suite 1300

Washington, DC 20036
Toll Free: 800-622-2838
Fax: 202-265-6854
Internet address: www.stopbreastcancer.org

The National Breast Cancer Coalition is a grassroots membership organization whose mission is to eradicate breast cancer through action and advocacy.

National Cancer Institute
NCI Public Inquiries Office
6116 Executive Boulevard
Room 3036A
Bethesda, MD 20892-8322
Toll Free: 800-4-CANCER (1-800-422-6237)
Internet address: www.cancer.gov

The National Cancer Institute, a component of the National Institutes of Health, supports and conducts groundbreaking research in cancer biology, causation, prevention, detection, treatment, and survivorship.

National Marrow Donor Program (NMDP)
National Marrow Donor Program
3001 Broadway Street NE
Suite 100
Minneapolis, MN 55413-1753
Phone: 612-627-5800
Toll Free: 800-627-7692
E-mail: patientinfo@nmdp.org
Internet address: http://www.marrow.org/

Support for the National Marrow Donor Program adds donors to the Registry, helps patients with transplant costs, and funds research to improve transplant outcomes.

National Women's Health Information Center
8270 Willow Oaks Corporate Drive
Fairfax, VA 22031
Phone: 800-994-9662
Internet address: www.womenshealth.gov

The National Women's Health Information

Center is a service of the Office on Women's Health in the Department of Health and Human Services. NWHIC provides a gateway to the vast array of federal and other women's health information resources.

Patient Access Network Foundation
PO Box 221858
Charlotte, NC 28222-1858
Phone: 866-316-7263
Internet address: www.patientaccessnetwork.org

Patient Access Network Foundation encourages those with Internet access to use the Web site rather than the toll free number.

Patient Access Network Foundation is an independent, nonprofit organization dedicated to assisting underinsured patients who cannot afford the out-of-pocket medication costs associated with their treatment. Patients must be U.S. residents and meet certain financial, insurance, and medical criteria. In addition, the drugs must be covered by the patient's insurance.

Planet Cancer
314 E. Highland Mall Blvd., Suite 306
Austin, TX 78752
Phone: 512-452-9010
Fax: 512-857-1058
Internet address: http://www.planetcancer.org/

Planet Cancer is an international network—a community of support and advocacy for young adults with cancer in their 20s and 30s, ready and willing to help each other through what may well be the most difficult experience of their lives. "We know it's a big dream, but we figure that once you face cancer, there's little you can't do."

SHARE: Self Help for Women with Breast or Ovarian Cancer
1501 Broadway, Suite 704A
New York, NY 10036

Phone: 212-719-0364
Fax: 212-869-3431
Toll Free: 866-891-2392; Breast Cancer
Hotline & Spanish-speaking Hotline
Internet address: http://sharecancersupport.org

SHARE: Self Help for Women with Breast or
Ovarian Cancer serves women, men, and
children who have been affected by breast
cancer or ovarian cancer. Services include
hotlines, survivor support groups, public
education, advocacy, and wellness programs.

Sharsheret
1086 Teaneck Road, Suite 3A
Teaneck, NJ 07666
Phone: 866-474-2774
Internet address: www.sharsheret.org

Sharsheret is a nonprofit organization of
cancer survivors dedicated to addressing the
challenges facing young Jewish women living
with breast cancer.

Shop Well with You
PO Box 1270
New York, NY 10009
Phone: 800-799-6790
Internet address: www.shopwellwithyou.org

*Shop Well with You encourages those with
Internet access to use the Web site rather than
the toll free number.*

Shop Well with You is national nonprofit
body-image resource for women surviving
cancer. The organization also provides support for caregivers and health care providers.

Sisters Network™ Inc.
8787 Woodway Drive, Suite 4206
Houston, TX 77063
Phone: 713- 781-0255
Toll Free: 866-781-1808
Fax: 713-780-8998
Internet address: www.sistersnetworkinc.org

Sisters Network Inc. is a national African-
American breast cancer survivorship
organization. This nonprofit organization is
committed to increasing local and national
attention on the devastating impact that breast
cancer has in the African-American Community.

Susan G. Komen for the Cure
5005 LBJ Freeway, Suite 250
Dallas, TX 75244
Toll Free: 1-877-465-6636
Internet address: www.komen.org

Susan G. Komen for the Cure is an international
nonprofit organization of breast cancer survivors
and activists dedicated to eradicating breast
cancer as a life-threatening disease by advancing
research, education, screening, and treatment.

Wellness Community
919 18th Street NW
Suite 54
Washington, DC 20006
Phone: 202-659-9709
Fax: 202-659-9301
Toll Free: 888-793-WELL
Web site:
http://www.thewellnesscommunity.org/

The Wellness Community is an international
nonprofit organization dedicated to providing
free support, education, and hope to people
with cancer and their loved ones at over 100
locations worldwide, including 24 U.S. based
and 2 international centers with 73 satellite
and offsite programs, and online at The Virtual
Wellness Community.

WomenStories
1807 Elmwood Avenue
Buffalo, NY 14207
Phone: 716-873-3689
Fax: 716-873-5361
Toll Free: 800-775-5790

Internet address: www.womenstories.org

WomenStories, a nonprofit organization, benefits those who have been diagnosed with breast cancer and need the information and comfort that only other breast cancer survivors can provide. WomenStories is a series of videos in which breast cancer survivors offer emotional support.

Young Survival Coalition

61 Broadway, Suite 2235
New York, NY 10006
Phone: 646-257-3000
Fax: 646-257-3030
Toll Free: 877-972-1011
Internet address: www.youngsurvival.org

The Young Survival Coalition is dedicated to the concerns and issues that are unique to women aged 40 and younger with breast cancer.

Other Useful Web Sites*

*Some are mentioned in this text.

American Pain Foundation

Toll Free: 888-615-7246 (888-615-PAIN)
Internet address: www.painfoundation.org

Centers for Medicare and Medicaid Services (CMS)

Toll Free: 877-267-2323
Internet address: www.cms.hhs.gov

Family and Medical Leave Act

Toll Free: 866-487-9243 (866-4USWAGE)
Internet address: www.dol.gov/esa/whd/fmla

Family Caregiver Alliance

Toll Free: 800-445-8106
Internet address: www.caregiver.org

National Alliance for Caregiving (NAC)

Internet address: www.caregiving.org

Substance Abuse and Mental Health Services Administration (SAMHSA)
Mental Health Information Center

Toll Free: 800-789-2647

CONTRIBUTORS INDEX

• • •

Alejandra, Torrance, California 20, 60, 89, 110, 148, 173, 200, 241

Allie, Fair Haven, New Jersey 128, 169, 223, 330

Alycia, East Berlin, Connecticut 305

Amelia, Long Beach, California 197

Andrea, Norfolk, Massachusetts 9, 26, 49, 75, 217, 228, 254, 301, 322

Andrew, Greater Manchester (England) 54, 192

Angela, Fulton, Mississippi 202, 239

Angie, Anderson, South Carolina 181, 209, 245, 317

Ann, Mechanicsburg, Pennsylvania 98, 118, 210, 246, 295

Ann, Random Lake, Wisconsin 226

Anne, Boston, Massachusetts 90, 120, 226

April, Wichita, Kansas 15, 33, 55, 155, 195, 234

Audrey, Baltimore, Maryland 32, 80, 328

Barbara, Conway, Arkansas 14, 54, 83, 105, 195, 307

Barbara, Golden, Colorado 85, 199

Barbara, Stoneham, Massachusetts 32, 56, 107, 169, 195, 235, 259, 286, 329

Bernadette, Oxnard, California 95, 252

Beth, Fort Hood, Texas 4, 75, 97, 124, 162, 206, 228, 253, 273, 310, 324

Beth, Tempe, Arizona 133, 161, 181, 246, 295

Bill, Jefferson, Wisconsin 7, 48, 72, 117, 136, 150, 165, 185, 215, 227, 277, 299, 321

Bill, Niceville, Florida 48, 150, 321

Brenda, Madison, Tennessee 18, 155, 171, 288, 309

Bryna, Brockton, Massachusetts 14, 54, 127, 154, 194, 259, 285, 306, 328

Buffy, Bobcaygeon, Ontario (Canada) 86, 108, 172

Candy, El Paso, Texas 60, 87, 142, 201, 264, 314

Carlyn, Willow Spring, North Carolina 21, 88, 109, 148, 174, 200, 235, 263, 315

Carmela, Clinton Township, Michigan 13, 54, 127, 169, 234

Carrie, New York City, New York 147, 181, 209, 237, 294

Cathi, Waban, Massachusetts 6, 47, 73, 136, 150, 165, 185, 214, 240, 251, 275, 299, 319

Cathy, Columbus, Ohio 3, 44, 163, 210, 245, 294

Celestine, Rosedale, Maryland 73, 152, 180, 314

Charles, Colorado Springs, Colorado 314

Charose, Omaha, Nebraska 11, 29, 50, 139, 151, 189, 219, 257, 282

Cheryl, Garland, Texas 57, 84, 107, 141, 155, 225, 236, 287

Cheryl, Malden, Massachusetts 79, 194, 257, 285

Chris, Yardley, Pennsylvania 170

Cindy, Maryville, North Dakota 57, 197, 224, 331

Colin, Roma (Italy) 72, 161, 250, 318

Cynthia, Highland Lakes, New Jersey 53, 80, 138, 191, 284

Danielle, Ramstein (Germany) 31, 105, 154, 167, 193, 222, 234, 259, 328

David, Missoula, Montana 4, 75, 124, 189, 206, 310

Deb, Evansville, Indiana 27, 43, 216

Debbie, New York City, New York 32

Debbie, Phoenix, Arizona 84,196, 236, 259, 307

Deborah, Overland Park, Kansas 18, 36, 130, 140, 157, 172, 225, 262, 311, 333

Debra, Chicago, Illinois 49, 101, 179, 217, 255, 322

Dee, Wood Dale, Illinois 45, 316

Don, Ocean Pines, Maryland 208, 294, 315

Dorinda, Edison, New Jersey 26, 47, 149, 184, 319

Doris, Carmichael, California 305

Dorothy, Chesapeake, Virginia 14, 25, 55, 223

Edward, Chapel Hill, North Carolina 276

Eileen, Charlotte, North Carolina 73, 282

Eileen, Framingham, Massachusetts 28, 50, 77, 123, 137, 151, 187, 218, 256, 280, 302, 325

Eileen, Hilton, New York 30, 76, 133, 153, 188, 206, 254, 324

Eileen, Maple Glen, Pennsylvania 298

Elena, Silver Spring, Maryland 95, 180, 208, 237, 308

Elizabeth, Des Moines, Iowa 121, 275
Elizabeth, Plymouth, Devon (England) 27, 217, 254, 279
Elizabeth, Sanford, Florida 272
Evelyn, Boston, Massachusetts 9, 27, 48, 137, 150, 166, 217, 253, 300, 321

Federico, Brookline, Massachusetts 98, 147, 182, 210, 245, 274, 295, 317
Fran, LaVergne, Tennessee 16, 34, 156, 196, 236, 287

Glenda, Chanute, Kansas 55, 232
Greg, Orland Park, Illinois 46, 126, 162, 189, 206

Iris, Santa Fe, New Mexico 18, 50, 182

James, Sheridan, Wyoming 3, 31, 46, 134, 153, 162, 188, 308
Jamie, Blackwood, New Jersey 211, 247, 296
Jan, Wichita, Kansas 13, 80, 139, 191, 221, 231, 285
Janet, Philadelphia, Pennsylvania 52, 103, 167, 221, 231, 258, 284, 306, 327
Jennifer, Craig, Colorado 17, 129, 174, 225
Jennifer, Montreal, Quebec (Canada) 38, 60, 86, 130, 142, 147, 173, 200, 207, 263, 317
Jennifer, Pennington, New Jersey 4, 99, 213, 248
Jennifer, San Diego, California 19, 58, 141, 171, 262, 310
Jerri, Standish, Michigan 13, 81, 167, 286, 327
Jerry, Anoka, Minnesota 15, 33, 56, 84, 107, 154, 169, 194, 223, 234, 286, 332
Jitendra, Cleveland, Ohio 134, 164, 179
Jo Ann, Lanoka Harbor, New Jersey 19, 34, 95
Jo Anne, Brownstown, Michigan 19, 240, 333
Jocelyn, Macedon, New York 17, 170, 224, 331
John, Jacksonville, Florida 85, 129, 199
John, Jamestown, North Carolina 61, 108, 142, 201, 206, 241, 292, 314
Joyce, Knoxville, Tennessee 11, 51, 77, 102, 190, 220, 230, 283, 303, 326
Joyce, South Amboy, New Jersey 98, 134, 162, 211, 238, 246
Judi, Pen Argl, Pennsylvania 37, 60, 88, 143, 172, 200, 240, 272, 287, 293, 315
Judy, Cudahy, Wisconsin 16, 35, 58, 171, 197, 287, 309
Judy, Norwalk, California 35, 57, 84, 155, 170, 198, 236, 261, 312, 331
Julie, New York City, New York 31, 76, 135, 253

Julie, Torrance, California 30, 52, 79, 104, 126, 230, 327

Karen, Cincinnati, Ohio 18, 108, 199, 289
Karen, Loganville, Georgia 18, 58, 107, 129, 141, 171, 197, 205, 261, 287, 307, 331
Kathi, Wrightstown, Wisconsin 10, 49, 166, 187, 229, 255
Kathie, Kingston, New York 3, 96, 121, 212, 239, 297, 318
Kathleen, Lisbon, Connecticut 30, 102, 231
Kathleen, Washington Township, New Jersey 17, 82, 140, 196, 286
Kathryn, St. Charles, Missouri 32, 82, 105, 194, 222, 233, 329
Kathy, Niles, Illinois 143, 263, 311
Kelley, Rochdale, Massachusetts 28, 101, 150, 187, 218, 229, 280, 303, 325
Kelly, Arlington, Virginia 26, 127, 183, 298
Kelly, Holland, New York 316
Kenneth, San Diego, California 183, 248
Kimatha, Edinburgh, Indiana 133, 163, 182, 247, 313
Kirsten, Buford, Georgia 9, 186, 215, 228, 278, 300
Kyle, Johnstown, Pennsylvania 38, 46, 121, 148, 163, 183, 248, 318

LaDonne, Mundelein, Illinois 30, 124, 220, 304
Laura, Avon, Connecticut 17, 34, 58, 85, 106, 129, 141, 156, 198, 224, 259, 289, 332
Laura, Hope Mills, North Carolina 59, 109, 241, 263
Laurie, Sacramento, California 13, 136, 220, 230, 283, 327
Laura, Schenectady, New York 10, 75, 122, 137, 179, 254, 278, 322
Leslie, Prescott, Arizona 118, 161
Linda, Antioch, California 36, 130, 142, 199, 226, 261, 289, 332
Linda, Placentia, California 8, 74, 165, 186, 252
Linda, Selden, New York 247, 318
Linda, Sulphur, Louisiana 45, 119, 219
Linda, Superior, Colorado 45, 121, 316
Lindy, Lexington, Massachusetts 185, 215, 251, 300
Lisa, Colebrook, New Hampshire 85, 109, 201, 235
Lisa, Owings Mills, Maryland 37, 87, 142, 173, 293
Lorraine, Skaneateles, New York 85, 109
Lovey, Cadiz, Kentucky 81, 192, 328

Luann, Charleston, West Virginia 35, 141, 155
Luanne, Morris, Illinois 83, 161, 229
Lynne, Rome, New York 182, 274

Marguerite, Cheltenham, Maryland 172, 198
Mariann, West Haven, Connecticut 83, 197, 236, 330
Marie, Lebanon, Ohio 15, 82, 168, 193, 235
Mark, Bay Shore, New York 5, 214, 239, 296
Marla, Jasper, Indiana 31, 79, 103, 191, 222, 233, 284, 328
Mary, Brookline, Massachusetts 205, 293
Mary, McPherson, Kansas 70, 277, 319
Mary, Simi Valley, California 78, 103, 151, 191, 221, 231, 284
Mary Anne, Dixon, California 35, 171, 262, 288, 310
Matt, Bath, New York 100, 122, 149, 165, 185, 214, 216, 251, 277, 298, 320
Maureen, Camarillo, California 56, 329
Megan, Milford, Connecticut 25
Melody, Jessup, Maryland 154, 192
Michele, Charles Town, West Virginia 196, 330
Michele, Detroit, Michigan 209, 239, 273
Midge, Westford, Massachusetts 99, 120, 212, 238, 248
Mike, Red Lodge, Montana 5, 44, 135, 153, 160, 188, 253, 274, 309, 324
Mike, Rochester, New York 26, 43, 119, 229, 283, 298, 314
Mollie, Seward, Alaska 45, 51
Myra, Sharon, Massachusetts 44, 247

Nancy, Fowlerville, Michigan 53, 79, 126, 140, 153, 222, 258
Nancy, Levittown, New York 70, 276
Nicki, Union, Missouri 10, 100, 187, 218, 230, 255, 279, 302, 324

Pam, Lakeland, Florida 22, 89, 110, 202, 207, 271, 313
Pamala, Gardiner, Maine 229, 255, 323
Pat, Canton, Michigan 9, 100, 123, 186, 217, 279, 302, 323
Pat, Como (Western Australia) 78, 103, 139, 152, 190, 258, 306
Patti, Colorado Springs, Colorado 78, 126, 152, 166, 191, 283, 326
Pearl, Glasgow (Scotland) 5, 47, 88, 122, 149, 163, 184, 213, 240, 249, 319
Peggy, St. Augustine, Florida 27, 74, 101, 136, 151, 250

Phil, Pawcatuck, Connecticut 316
Polly, Port Gibson, Mississippi 59, 172, 226

Randy, Ewa Beach, Hawaii 29, 123, 157, 219, 256, 280, 303
Ric, Londonderry, New Hampshire 71, 164, 211, 297
Robert, La Habra, California 4, 273
Robin, Costa Mesa, California 16, 57, 170, 225, 288
Rochelle, Las Vegas, Nevada 10, 29, 97, 123, 137, 188, 230, 256, 276, 304, 325
Ronald, Dover, New Hampshire 122, 209, 271, 316
Rose, Centreville, Virginia 104, 127, 295
Rosi, Austin, Texas 44, 76, 161, 205, 273
Roxanne, Palm Beach Gardens, Florida 190, 258
Ruthanne, Thorne Bay, Alaska 12, 52, 77, 102, 190, 257, 281

Sally, Salem, Massachusetts 228, 278, 322
Sandra, Atlanta, Georgia 71, 97, 181, 208, 237, 245
Sarah, Miami, Florida 7, 24, 48, 74, 136, 227, 252, 300, 321
Sheila, Walnut Creek, California 21, 36, 88, 241, 292
Shelly, Concord, New Hampshire 7, 47, 110, 186, 215, 240, 278, 320
Sheri, Columbia, Maryland 11, 29, 50, 76, 124, 139, 189, 220, 258, 282, 325
Sherri, Bruceville, Indiana 43, 96, 184, 212, 248
Susan, Graham, Washington 179
Susan, Medina, Ohio 80, 104, 168, 192, 221, 284, 327
Susan, Mobile, Alabama 180, 293
Sigrid, Oceanside, California 108, 156, 264
Suza, Johannesburg, Gauteng (South Africa) 119, 148, 163, 182, 274
Suzanne, Canton, Texas 70, 276, 297

Teri, Fort Langley, British Columbia (Canada) 14, 81, 128, 140
Tim, Memphis, Tennessee 305
Todd, Warwick, Rhode Island 6, 59, 73, 134, 143, 165, 184, 214, 239, 250, 320
Tracey, Villa Park, Illinois 20, 141, 208, 333

Vera, Milwaukee, Wisconsin 52, 220, 231, 326

Yvonne, San Antonio, Texas 17, 34, 83, 106, 140, 195, 235, 285, 307

ADDITIONAL CONTRIBUTORS INDEX

• • •

Adams, Heidi 125
Armstrong, Lance 55, 77, 213

Blum, Diane 242
Brinker, Nancy 89, 157, 279
Brooke, Edward W. 81

Caban, Mabel 289
Caplan, Elyse 20, 106, 156, 288

Eib, Lynn 193

Gafni, Ramy 257
Ganz, Patricia 304
Grose, Amy 232–233

Hahn, Karin 86
Hamilton, Scott 272
Harpham, Wendy S. 99
Hilliard, Anita Joy 135, 149
Hobson, Alan 260–261, 311
Hutchison, Nancy A. 290

Johnson, David 33

LaTour, Kathy 296
Lockaby, Jay 174

Mardigan, Tara 143
Mazan, Steve 167
Miller, Ken 218
Moddelmog, Hala 38, 111, 264
Music, Terry 21, 290, 312, 332

Nathanson, David 89

O'Reilly, Mary Beth 238
Osbourne, Sharon 7, 58, 82, 285, 308

Paul, Kelly 207
Perlis, Cynthia 168
Piscopo, Joe 329
Planchon, Claude-Alain 216
Pories, Susan 19, 51, 223

Rauch, Paula 112
Reno, Jamie 16, 37, 224, 323
Richer, Alice 138
Runowicz, Carolyn 210, 317

Schimmel, Selma 315
Schnipper, Hester Hill 249
Schoenthaler, Robin 8
Shilling, Shonda 275
Shin, Ki Y. 152
Shipp, Laura 61
Siegel, Bernie 34
Simon, Carly 15, 46
Sommer, Karen 164
Stovall, Ellen 28, 281, 326

Tuthill, Kelley 53

Verbeek, Jos 120
Vreeland, Susan 12, 72, 198

Warrick, Heather 173, 278
Willis, Jack 128, 186
Winer, Eric 330
Woods, Marc 301
Wright, Alan 183

INDEX

· · ·

A

The ACS Complete Guide to Complementary and Alternative Cancer Therapies, 160
Activities of daily living, 120
Adolescent peer counseling, informal, 75
Adults, single, with cancer, 116–117
American Academy of Physical Medicine and Rehabilitation, 336
American Breast Cancer Foundation, 336
American Cancer Society
    Cancer Action Network™, 306, 335
    Cancer Survivors Network®, 82, 307, 335
    Celebration on the Hill®, 306, 335
    as connection to other patients, 79, 121
    as connection to other resources, 82
    as employer, 121, 128
    Look Good…Feel Better®, 16, 19, 78, 206, 335
    Patient Navigator Program, 206, 335
    Reach to Recovery®, 10, 87, 103, 256, 293, 336
    reassurance from, 82
    Relay for Life®, 102, 105, 292, 306, 328, 330, 336
    telephone number, 335
    Web site, 31, 79, 335
American Occupational Therapy Association, 336
American Pain Foundation, 343
American Physical Therapy Association, 337
American Speech-Language-Hearing Association, 337
Art for Recovery, 168

B

Belief in humanity, 15
Bible, reading, 12, 178, 182, 191, 195
Bloch Cancer Foundation, 337
Body image. *See also* Hair, losing; Intimacy, emotional; Intimacy, sexual
    acceptance by partner, 251, 255, 261, 262, 263, 265
    beauty of, no matter what, 265
    betrayal by body and, 247
    breast prosthesis and, 247
    breast reconstruction and, 252, 282
    counteracting negative, 257
    hair recovery and, 252
    more precious after therapy, 251
    negative, 248, 262, 263
    partner's messages about, 251, 252, 261, 262, 263, 265
    positive, 256
    public dressing room and, 246, 262
    reconstructed breast and, 249, 250, 252, 257
    recovering, 247, 262, 264
    scars and identity, 253, 254, 255, 263
    sexy to husband, 259
    struggle with, 244, 257, 259
    time's effect on, 245, 259
Bosom Buddies, 219, 337
Boss, as source of support, 57, 124
Breast Cancer Network of Strength, 161, 337
Breastcancer.org, 79

C

Cancer. *See also* Cancer experience; Life changes caused by cancer
    as change agent, 129, 260-261, 291–312
    as chronic illness, 115-116
    as enemy, 286
    avoiding panic about, 286
    and increasing dependence on others, 197
    as monster, 121
    as something to manage, 120, 129
    not synonymous with death, 217, 318, 330
CancerCare, 242, 337
CancerConnection, 161, 337
Cancer experience
    bringing family closer, 104
    dichotomy of life, 115-116, 130, 296
    as emotional, 191
    expanded community, 309
    flashback to, 287
    gift of time from, 297
    impact on day-to-day life, 106, 291–312

as inspiration for child's future career, 103
as inspiration for regular screening, 108
as journey, 279
life changing, 4, 291-312
motivating work, 295
prompting appreciation, 281
prompting empathy, 295, 297
as teacher, 203
as test of strength, 294
Cancer Hope Network, 338
Captain of Kindness, 94
Caregiver, role of, 126
Casting for Recovery, 338
Celebrating milestones, 3
Centers for Medicare and Medicaid Services, 343
Chalke, Sarah, 243
Changes caused by cancer. *See* Life changes caused by cancer
Chat rooms, Internet, 17, 69, 82, 206
Children
    adjustment to parent's diagnosis, 109
    adult, of parents who are ill, 100, 108, 110
    being truthful with, 95, 97, 99, 106, 107, 109
    communicating to, about cancer, 106, 113
    as communicators to health care team, 103
    coping with books, 103
    diet of, improving, 132-133
    difficulty of separation from, 100
    easing cancer journey, 94, 97, 107, 108, 304
    fear of parent's death, 99, 106, 110
    focus for survival, 75, 109, 194
    friends' and family's help with, 42, 105, 112
    helping, cope, 93-113
    as motivators, 137
    responsibility for cancer, relieving them of, 106, 113
    relationship ups and downs, 97, 98
    sheltering, 98
    support from, 96, 100, 108, 110, 294
    teachers of, as source of support, 47
    tips to help, and families, 112
Clinical trials, 91
Colon Cancer Alliance, 338
Cooking, 25
Coping strategies. *See* Self-nurturing; Stress, relieving
Courage, 286
Coworkers, 45, 121, 123, 127
Cure for cancer, 69-70, 287, 331

D

Depression, 71, 149, 280, 284, 304
Diagnosis of cancer. *See also* Diagnosis of cancer, what patients wish they had known at
    announcing, to friends, 45
    becoming survivor with, 317
    as catalyst for diet change, 133
    difficulty of absorbing, 86, 87
    difficulty of delivering, 89
    deepening faith, 193
    life-changing effect of, 161, 291-312
    not disclosing, 120, 211
    partner's response to, 265
    physician's poor delivery of, 79
    second, in family, 199
    spirituality result of, 187
    stress related to, 159
    what to know at, 203-226
Diagnosis of cancer, what patients wish they had known at, 203-226
    adaptability to crisis, 208, 216, 225
    about advocacy for self, 212, 213, 214, 221, 225
    about avoiding negative reports, 221
    about breast cancer, 210, 211, 214, 221, 225, 226
    cancer as process, 206, 207, 212
    about death, 213, 219, 222
    emotional aspects of cancer journey, 210, 215
    fear normal and controllable, 223, 224
    genetic susceptibility to illness, 215
    importance of communicating, 208, 211, 215, 220, 22
    importance of family, 220
    importance of focusing outside self, 209
    importance of health care team, 208, 220
    importance of screening, 216
    importance of second opinions, 209, 213, 218
    about keeping records, 214, 219, 223
    knowledge of disease, 218, 222
    about loss of friends, 222
    lymphedema's effect, 208
    possibility of earlier diagnosis, 207
    possibility of feeling well, 205
    possibility of fertility options, 209, 214
    possibility of survival, 214, 216, 217, 218, 222, 223, 226
    quality life after treatment, 205, 210, 213, 214, 225

about risk factors, 220
about side effects, 206, 207, 208, 217
about support and support groups, 206,
    210, 211, 212, 219, 222
transformative nature of cancer, 214
about treatment choices, 209, 210, 211,
    213, 218, 225
Diet. *See also* Nutrition, improving
    advice about, 135, 138, 143
    antioxidants in, 140
    avoiding processed foods, 135, 139
    changes after diagnosis, 131–144
    to combat nausea, 138
    eliminating alcohol, 140
    eliminating chocolate, 140
    eliminating red meat, 136, 140, 141, 142
    fruits and vegetables in, 131, 132–133, 138,
        140, 141, 142, 144
    guidelines for, 131–133
    and supplements, 138, 141, 144
    tips for improving, 144
    vegetables and fruits in, 131, 132–133, 138,
        140, 141, 142, 144
    and water, 141
    ways to improve, 138, 139, 144
Divine intervention, 177
Divorcing and healing, 247

E

E-mailing status report, 5
Emotional intimacy. *See* Intimacy, emotional
Employer, 126, 127
Estrogen, 149
Exercise. *See also specific types of exercise*
    benefits of, 145–147, 149, 152, 154
    and side effects, 148
    easing depression with, 149
    importance of, 134, 138
    psychological benefits of, 147, 149, 154

F

Faith, 180, 189, 190, 192, 193, 198, 201.
    See also Faith, family of; God; Religion;
    Spirituality
Faith, family of, 55, 181
    and humor, 180
    organizing support in, 200
    as prayer warriors, 192
Family and Medical Leave Act, 343

Family Caregiver Alliance, 343
Family members, support from, 23–38. *See
    also* Children; Spousal or partner support
    accepting, 24, 123, 124
    from aunt, 195
    from brother, 30, 31
    from brothers-in-law, 196
    child care management, 26, 29, 105
    despite dislike of hospitals, 27
    from fiancé, 36
    financial, 34, 105
    from grandmother, 35, 37
    and hope, 33
    husband's assumption of household duties,
        27, 28
    importance of, 38
    from mother, 26, 27, 29, 30
    as motivator, 33, 137
    from parents, 29, 184
    as purpose for survival, 31
    rejection of, 31
    request for, 32
    from sister, 27, 28, 30, 34
    from son, 25, 35, 108
    threat of loss, 25
Family-work balance, 115–130
Fatigue, 1
Fear, 287
Fertility, 255, 266
Financial security, 127
Flying Crooked, 177
FORCE: Facing Our Risk of Cancer
    Empowered, 338
Friends
    absent, 48, 58
    as advisors, 46
    as blessing from God, 53
    at appointments, 39
    business, 58, 60
    cards and letters from, 44, 48, 51, 56, 58, 126
    as child care support, 59
    difficulty in asking for help, 40, 51
    expressing need to, 43, 55
    financial support from, 56
    frustration of, 46
    humor, 51, 52, 53, 54, 56
    involving friends in experience, 42, 51
    listening, 42, 52, 55, 60
    long-distance, 41
    prayers from, 50, 55, 60, 179
    support from, 39–63

true, revealed during illness, 48, 49, 50, 56
visitation, 48, 49, 54, 58, 59, 61, 62
on Web, 41–42
Fruits, 131, 132–133, 138, 140, 141, 142.
  See also Diet

G

Gafni, Ramy, 257
Gawande, Atul, 65
Gifts
  affordable luxuries, 62
  at each chemotherapy round, 108
  cancer experience as, 299
  financial, 60
  gift certificates, 55
  haircut, 57
  laughing stick, 53
  from long distance, 63
  manicure, 57
  pedicure or foot massage, 57, 62
  with scripture verses, 54
  time, 60
Gilda's Club, 16, 171, 338
Goals, setting, 156
God
  blaming, 193, 199
  faith in, and surviving, 76, 81, 178, 192,
    193, 198, 201
  feeling presence of, through nurse, 73
  grace of, 194
  and hope, 186, 191, 198
  plan of, and cancer diagnosis, 186
  presence of, 194
  and purpose for life, 179, 182, 189
  rediscovery of, 188, 191
  rejection of, 178
  speaking through pastor, 196
  support from, 35, 182
  trust in, 83, 180, 192, 193
Greater good, belief in, 182

H

Hair, losing. *See also* Body image; Intimacy,
    emotional; Intimacy, sexual
  and children's response to, 95, 98, 103
  effect over time, 247
  family support during, 24, 25, 245
  friends' support during, 39–40, 58
  freedom of, 20
  hat party, 181

insignificance of, 4
  no bad hair day, 20, 258
  sexual intimacy and, 245, 246, 263
Hat party, 181
Healer, hands-on, 180
Healing, 269-290. *See also* Body image
  by admitting to having cancer, 271
  amazing, 308
  attitude, positive, and, 278, 284, 285
  combination of factors in, 272, 281, 287
  with complementary therapies, 279
  through counseling, 283, 285, 287
  by doing what you love, 289
  emotional, 274, 283, 284
  faith and, 273
  friends' role in, 277, 283
  guide to, 270
  impossible to rush, 269, 270, 271, 274
  motivation for, 272
  through nature, 273, 276, 281
  through new hobby, 288
  through not feeling alone, 274
  optimal, 66–67
  pet's help in, 273, 281
  physical therapy's role in, 67, 273, 282, 284
  as process, 274
  sleep and, 278, 285
  over time, 275, 276
  trust in survival, 290
Health care, traveling to get best, 71
Health care team. *See also* Nurse; Physician
  embarassing with humor, 86
  errors in predictions, 68, 85, 86
  finding time for questions, 80
  finding aggressive, 75
  outlook of, 80, 84
  questions to ask, about sex, 266
  source for advice, 19, 67, 80
  source of hope, 87
  thankful for, 329
  trust in, 80, 81
  valuing patient's wishes, 86
Health insurance, 75
Honesty, 278
Hope, 33, 70, 76
Housekeeping, forgoing, 9

I

Inflammatory Breast Cancer Help, 338
Inflammatory Breast Cancer Research
    Foundation, 339

Immune system, 1, 177
International Myeloma Foundation, 82, 339
Intimacy, emotional. *See also* Intimacy, sexual
    throughout cancer experience, 255
    during chemotherapy sessions, 264
    greater after therapy, 245, 261, 306
    improving, 267
    infidelity's effect on, 254
    messages from partner, 265
Intimacy, sexual, 243-267. *See also* Intimacy, emotional
    desire for in seventies, 258
    fear of loss of appeal to partner, 246
    intercourse, painful, 266
    loss of, 254
    loss of desire for, 246, 248, 249, 253
    male performance and, 245
    medications' effect on, 248
    return of, over time, 253, 258, 263
    testosterone's drop, 250

J

Jeffers, Susan, 159-160
Journal (Things I want you to know), 112

K

Kindness, ripple effect of, 117
Kliewer, Stephen, 177

L

Lance Armstrong Foundation, 339
Leukemia and Lymphoma Society, 6, 339
Life changes caused by cancer, 129, 197, 260–262, 291–312
    absence of road rage, 300
    advocacy for others with cancer prompted, 292, 294, 295, 299, 307, 310
    closeness with family improved, 298, 300, 311
    closeness with God increased, 311
    compassion increased, 307, 311
    determination to live strengthened, 302
    empathy for others prompted, 295, 297
    family and friends embraced, 293, 298
    insecurity prompted, 303
    kindnesses prompted, 306
    life became better, 294, 295, 303, 308, 309
    life became precious, 292, 295, 299, 303, 312
    love of life underscored, 303
    perspective changed, 298
    push for perfection relinquished, 307, 308
    worry increased, 311
Living Beyond Breast Cancer, 339
Long-distance support, 63
Lucas, Geralyn, 243
Lumpectomy, 211

M

Make-A-Wish Foundation, 339
Making Memories Breast Cancer Foundation, 339
Mantras
    Life's a trade, 251
    No heroics, 164
    for radiation therapy, 54
Marathon, cancer experience as, 226
Medical practice, 65. *See also* Health care team; Physician
Men Against Breast Cancer, 340
Menopause, 246, 251, 252, 266
Mental battle in head, 88
Merle Norman, 256
Michael, Jan, 177
Michaud, Ellen, 1
Mindfulness, 186
Mothers Supporting Daughters with Breast Cancer, 340
Multiple Myeloma Research Foundation, 82, 340

N

Napping, 8, 20, 39, 165
National Alliance for Caregiving, 343
National Asian Women's Health Organization, 340
National Breast and Cervical Cancer Early Detection Program, 340
National Breast Cancer Coalition, 340
National Cancer Institute, 341
National Marrow Donor Program, 6, 341
National Women's Health Information Center, 341
Nature as consoler, 7, 186
Nausea, 7, 25, 80, 138, 143, 326
Needles, coping with, 83
Normalcy
    exercising as, 153
    importance to healing, 282, 284, 285
    need for, 13, 20, 32, 54, 56, 124

new, 66
working as, 121, 129
Nurse
  as careful listener, 72
  compassion of, 88
  encouragement from, 80
  knowing what calms, 73
  knowing what is needed, 84
  as inspiration for foundation, 77
Nutrition, improving, 132-133, 136, 138, 139,
  140, 144

O

One-day-at-a-time philosophy, 3, 25, 186, 208,
  328, 333
One-step-at-a-time philosophy, 157, 173, 305
Our Dad Is Getting Better, 132
Our Mom Is Getting Better, 132

P

Patient Access Network Foundation, 341
Patient Navigator program, 206, 335
Pets, therapeutic effect of, 9, 46, 151, 155,
  281, 309
Phlebotomists, 76
Physical therapy, 284
Physician. *See also* Health care team; Nurse
  critical of patient, 78, 81
  difficulty understanding, 66
  education of, 203–204
  excellent, 77
  firing, 84
  five things, should tell patient, 91
  humor of, 85
  importance of listening, 83
  information giving as therapeutic, 5, 6
  need for encouragement from, 84
  negative effect of bluntness of, 83
  off-site consultation with, 77
  positive outlook of, 79
  preparing patients for future, 73
  preparing patients for treatment side effects,
    74
  questions to ask, about sex, 266
  reassurance of, 88
  sharing determination, 80
  staff of, effect on patients, 85
  who did not say "cancer," 88
Plan, survivorship, 67
Planet Cancer, 125, 341

Port, chemotherapy, 258
Positive frame of mind, keeping, 10
Praver, Frances Cohen, 1
Prayer
  belief and, 179, 188
  for cure, 187, 197, 284
  for help with illness, 182, 192, 194
  first step, 202
  from friends, 181, 189, 197
  greatest help, 201
  lessons in truthfulness, 190
  as self-help, 178, 181, 190
  from strangers, 191
  supportive nature of, 202
  as wonderful thing, 195
Preparation for future, 73
Present, living in, 71
Prevention, cancer, 145
Priapism and leukemia diagnosis, 250
Prognosis
  honesty in presentation, 72
  need for, 73
  understanding, 90
  unpredictability of, 72, 159
Psychologist, 74

R

*Ramy Gafni's Beauty Therapy: The Ultimate
  Guide to Looking and Feeling Great While
  Living with Cancer*, 257
Rauch, Paula, 94
Recurrence, preventing
  taking responsibility for, 136
Rehabilitation services, 289. *See also* Physical
  therapy
Relaxing, 160, 175
Religion, 177
  comfort from, 184, 195, 198
  effect of, 17, 187
  fostering health, 177
  healing service, 284
  rejection of, 182, 185
  support from church, 200
Research, new, on horizon, 91
Rest, as self-nurturing, 10. *See also* Sleep
Rich, Katherine Russell, 115–116
Rodgers, Joni, 39
Rollin, Betty, 93
Rosary, as comfort, 183, 184
Rotary Club, 58
Running, 150

S

Screening, importance of, after diagnosis, 91
Secure, feeling, 2
Self-esteem, 261. *See also* Body image
Self-image, changes in, 15. *See also* Body image
Self-nurturing, 1-22
    avoiding activity, 17
    baths, warm, as, 10, 15
    bed clothes as, 22
    bed purchase as, 21
    belief in life, 16
    biking as, 7
    book reading as, 8
    celebrating events, 16
    child care as, 7, 21
    doing things you love, 8
    eating out with friends, 10
    educating self as, 6, 10, 16
    exercising, 11
    favorite things as, 12, 18
    friends, 11, 12
    gifts for self, 13, 15, 18
    honoring others with cancer, 15
    hot tubbing as, 14
    housekeeping, forgoing, 9
    humor, 13
    journaling, 17, 20
    making time for self, 18
    movie watching as, 8, 20
    music as, 12
    need for, 1, 18
    nutrition as, 11, 14
    pet ownership as, 9, 17
    pool, playing, as, 15
    prayer and meditation as, 13, 14
    reading as, 20
    rewards as, 11
    scheduling special events as, 9, 11
    scrapbooking, 7
    shopping as, 9, 17
    sleep as part of, 1, 8, 11, 14, 20, 22
    slowing down, 18
    song writing as, 15
    support group participation as, 9, 10, 15, 19
    talking, 21
    travel, 4, 5, 11, 16, 19, 32, 50
    volunteering as, 6
    walking as, 5
    watching television, 18, 19
    Web forums and information as, 5, 10, 13, 17
    writing e-mail health report, 5
    writing poetry, 14
Sex. *See* Intimacy, sexual
SHARE: Self Help for Women with Breast or Ovarian Cancer, 341
Sharsheret, 342
Shop Well with You, 342
Side effects, warnings needed about, 66
Sisters Network™ Inc., 342
Sleep, 1, 8, 11, 14, 20, 22
Sleeping pills, 8
Social worker, 71
Soldiers, perspective from seeing, 280
Soy in diet, 131, 139
Spirituality, 177–202. *See also* Faith, family of;
    God; Prayer; Religion
    angels as protection, 199
    blessing from illness, 195
    Buddhist, 198
    comfort from, of other cultures, 185
    day-to-day, 187
    defining, 177
    dying not feared, 199
    gratitude as, 185, 198
    learning "to be," 190
    in nature, 196
    and positive mindset, 199
    and prayer, 177, 184, 187
    reflection and peace, 200
    result of cancer, 185
    science behind effects, 177
    as source of strength, 179
    and survival, 198
Spousal or partner support, 34, 37, 38
    through assurances, 30
    through deeds, 35
    at diagnosis, 24
    from divorced mate, 33
    faith in recovery, 35
    during hair loss, 24, 25
    through humor, 36
    improving emotional intimacy, 267, 306
    despite irrationality, 37
    messages to partner with cancer, 265
    retiring to help, 119
    in sharing burden, 38
    understanding of support role, 32
Sterility, as consequence of therapy, 256
Stress, as cause of cancer, 159. *See also* Self-
    nurturing; Stress, relieving
Stress, relieving. *See also* Self-nurturing
    with acupuncture, 170
    with art, 168, 175

with audio books, 168
by asserting self, 165
baths, hot, 162
to collect strength, 164
complementary therapies, 166
controlling stressful input, 170
crying, 166
deep breathing, 166, 172
by disengaging, 170
with exercise, 173, 175
guided imagery, 161
with hope, 167
with humor, 167
journaling, 162, 166
laughter, 173
massages, 161, 170
meditation, 161, 164, 165, 170, 171
with music, 162, 163, 168, 169, 170, 171,
    175
napping, 165
through nature, 175
needlework, 167, 172, 175
nutrition, improving, 172
with pet, 169, 171
with plants, 171
positive thinking, 162
prayer, 172, 173, 174
by reading, 168, 170, 173, 175
reflexology, 163, 166
Reiki, 163, 169, 174
relaxation tape, 163, 167
running, 165
self-hyponosis, 165
stretching, 171
visualization, 166, 167, 172
walking, 165
writing, 175
yoga, 161, 163, 164, 165, 171, 173
Substance Abuse and Mental Health Services
    Administration, Mental Health Information
    Center, 343
Support, identifying needs, 232–233. See also
    Support group; Support too difficult to
    request
Support group. See also Support, identifying
    needs; Support too difficult to request
    of cancer survivors, 47, 69
    inspiring courage, 288
    during therapy, 76, 78, 79
Support too difficult to request, 227–242
    any, 230, 234, 237
    child care, 240, 241

care for mother with Alzheimer's, 231
company during treatment, 238, 240
concrete plan for therapy, 239
counseling, 233
emotional support, 234, 240, 241, 242
empathetic acknowledgment of fear, 239
financial help, 235, 240, 242
family support, 229, 231, 232, 236, 241
housekeeping help, 228, 229, 230, 231,
    233, 234, 235, 238, 239, 241
intimacy with partner, 231, 236
permission to admit illness, 239
permission to fall apart, 236
physical contact or presence, 227, 228, 230,
    237
prognosis, 239
psychological help, 240, 242
reassurance, 231, 235
shoulder to cry on, 227, 234
someone to visit or talk to, 229, 236
support group, 228, 241
survivor to talk to, 229, 231, 241
time alone, 227, 237
transportation aid, 228, 236
Survival
    as battle, 324, 325, 326
    ability to pursue passion, 316
    as attitude, 315
    a badge of courage, 332
    being part of cancer history, 320
    having another day, 325
    as identity, 316
    as impetus to fight additional illness, 280
    being alive, 321, 323
    conquering sense of hopelessness, 315
    difficulty of, 325
    everything in the world, 333
    gift of God, 327
    looking forward to granddaughter's birth,
        107
    as meaning, 318
    means a different life, 323
    means being lucky, 328
    optimism about, 330
    as peace, 316
    possibilities of, 313, 315
    privilege of, 331
    reason to celebrate, 314, 316
    reason to smile, 313, 314
    "reluctant brotherhood," 321
    resilience from, 317
    setting goal to see son's graduation, 104

strength for other challenges, 325,328, 331
successfully confronting diagnosis, 319
to be with children, 315
uncertain journey of, 319
what it means, 313–333
Survivor (as term). See also Survival; Survivors,
   as source of support; Survivorship
   other word for miracle, 327
   rejection of term, 325, 326, 327
   cancer warrior, 327
Survivors, as source of support, 57, 82, 151,
   197, 288, 306. See also Survivor; Survivorship
Survivorship. See also Survivor; Survivors, as
   source of support
   length of recovery, 91
   optimal, 66–67
   plan, 67
   possibilities, 313
   a rocky road, 326
   what it means, 313–333
Susan G. Komen for the Cure, 87, 342

T

Talking, 3, 4, 21, 318
Tanning beds, 310
There's Always Help; There's Always Hope,
   204–205
Tips, 62, 63, 112, 144, 175, 267
Trials, clinical, 91
Treatment options, 91
Tuthill, Kelley, 23, 53
Twins, simultaneous cancer diagnosis in, 27

U

U.S. Navy, 123

V

Vacation, 4, 5, 8, 32, 112, 284
Vegetables, 132–133, 135, 136, 138, 139, 140,
   142, 143, 144
Vital Options International, 216

W

Walking
   as exercise, 119, 147, 148, 149, 151, 155,
      156
   during hospital stay, 154

motivated by dog, 149, 150, 151, 152, 155,
   157, 281
Web sites, 69, 335–343
Weight, gaining, 134, 140, 259
Weight, losing
   methods for, 136, 137
   during therapy, 108, 143
Weight Watchers, 137
Wellness Community, 174, 342
Why I Wore Lipstick to My Mastectomy, 243
Wig, 70, 100, 102, 109, 127, 181, 258
Will to survive, 58, 285
WomenStories, 342
Wood, Eve, 204–205
Work
   benefits of, 19
   cancer-related career change, 121
   employer support, 57, 117, 123, 124
   and family balance, 115–130
   forgoing during treatment, 122
   inability to cope with, 122, 129
   loss of, 118
   for normalcy, 121, 122, 129
   not disclosing diagnosis at, 120
   as passion, 121, 122, 128
   resuming, 120
   sustaining work through therapy, 124
Work-family balance, 115–130
Worry, 160, 166

Y

Y-me, 161. See also Breast Cancer Network of
   Strength
Young Survival Coalition, 343

BOOKS PUBLISHED BY
THE AMERICAN CANCER SOCIETY

• • •

Available everywhere books are sold and online at
http://www.cancer.org/bookstore

Information

American Cancer Society's Complete Guide to Colorectal Cancer

American Cancer Society's Complete Guide to Prostate Cancer

Breast Cancer Clear & Simple: All Your Questions Answered

The Cancer Atlas (available in English, Spanish, French, and Chinese)

Cancer: What Causes It, What Doesn't

QuickFACTS™ - Advanced Cancer

QuickFACTS™ - Bone Metastasis

QuickFACTS™ - Colorectal Cancer, Second Edition

QuickFACTS™ - Lung Cancer

QuickFACTS™ - Prostate Cancer

The Tobacco Atlas, Second Edition (available in English, Spanish and French)

Day-to-Day Help

American Cancer Society's Guide to Pain Control: Understanding and Managing Cancer Pain, Revised Edition

Cancer Caregiving A to Z: An At-Home Guide for Patients and Families

Caregiving: A Step-By-Step Resource for Caring for the Person with Cancer at Home, Revised Edition

Eating Well, Staying Well During and After Cancer

Get Better! Communication Cards for Kids & Adults

Lymphedema: Understanding and Managing Lymphedema After Cancer Treatment

Social Work in Oncology: Supporting Survivors, Families and Caregivers

When the Focus Is on Care: Palliative Care and Cancer

Emotional Support

Angels & Monsters: A child's eye view of cancer

Cancer in the Family: Helping Children Cope with a Parent's Illness

Couples Confronting Cancer: Keeping Your Relationship Strong

Crossing Divides: A Couple's Story of Cancer, Hope, and Hiking Montana's Continental Divide

I Can Survive

Just for Kids

Because...Someone I Love Has Cancer: Kids' Activity Book

Healthy Me: A Read-Along Coloring & Activity Book

Kids' First Cookbook: Delicious-Nutritious Treats To Make Yourself!

Mom and the Polka-Dot Boo-Boo

Our Dad Is Getting Better

Our Mom Has Cancer (hardcover)

Our Mom Has Cancer (paperback)

Our Mom Is Getting Better

Prevention

The American Cancer Society's Healthy Eating Cookbook: A celebration of food, friendship, and healthy living, Third Edition

Celebrate! Healthy Entertaining for Any Occasion

Good for You! Reducing Your Risk of Developing Cancer

The Great American Eat-Right Cookbook: 140 Great-Tasting, Good-for-You Recipes

Healthy Air: A Read-Along Coloring & Activity Book (25 per pack: Tobacco avoidance)

Healthy Bodies: A Read-Along Coloring & Activity Book (25 per pack: Physical activity)

Healthy Food: A Read-Along Coloring & Activity Book (25 per pack: Nutrition)

Kicking Butts: Quit Smoking and Take Charge of Your Health

National Health Education Standards: Achieving Excellence, Second Edition (available in paperback and on CD-ROM)